# *Progress in Lymphology*

# *Progress in Lymphology*

*Edited by*
*R. C. MAYALL*
The International Cardiovascular Society
Rio de Janeiro, Brazil

*and*

*MARLYS H. WITTE*
University of Arizona
Tucson, Arizona

*PLENUM PRESS · NEW YORK AND LONDON*

Library of Congress Cataloging in Publication Data

International Symposium on Lymphology, 4th, Tucson, Ariz., 1973; 5th, Rio de Janeiro, 1975.
Progress in Lymphology.

Includes index.
1. Lymphatics—Diseases—Congresses. 2. Lymphatics—Congresses. 3. Lymphangiography—Congresses. I. Mayall, R. C. II. Witte, Marlys H. III. Title. [DNLM: 1. Lymphatic system—Congresses. 2. Lymphoid tissue—Congresses. W3 PR947J]
RC646.I56 1975 616.4'2 76-46410
ISBN 978-1-4684-9032-9 ISBN 978-1-4684-9030-5 (eBook)
DOI 10.1007/978-1-4684-9030-5

Selected lectures from the Fourth and Fifth International Congresses
in Lymphology held in Tuscon, Arizona, March 6-10, 1973
and Rio de Janeiro, Brazil, March 27-29, 1975


Softcover reprint of the hardcover 1st edition 1977

A Division of Plenum Publishing Corporation
227 West 17th Street, New York, N.Y. 10011

# Acknowledgments

The Fourth International Congress of Lymphology
was supported by funds from:

National Cancer Institute (USPHS)

American Heart Association

Arizona Cancer Society

Arizona Regional Medical Program

Eli Lilly Company

Mead Johnson Company

Roche Laboratories

Claudia Gips Foundation

The Fifth International Congress of Lymphology
was supported by funds from:

Brazilian Federal Government

Brazilian Society of Angliology

World Health Organization

Government of the Republic of Argentine

# Preface

Publication of the Proceedings of the Fourth and Fifth International Congresses of Lymphology celebrates the 10th anniversary of the founding of the International Society of Lymphology, a 500-member scientific association representing the world's foremost authorities on lymph nodes, lymphatics, lymphocytes, and lymph in health and disease. Utilizing a multidisciplinary approach and a wide variety of techniques including visualization, interruption, ablation, diversion, sampling, and characterization of regional lymph and lymphatic pathways, Congress participants from more than 40 different nations delved into such varied topics as lymphatic spread of cancer, tumor immunology, propulsion of lymph, microcirculatory physiology, improved methods of tumor detection and diagnosis, electron microscopy of lymphatic capillaries, lymphoscopy, immunoprotein chemistry, relationship of viruses to neoplasia, radiotherapy of lymphomas, structure and function of normal and abnormal lymphocytes, transplantation biology, lymphvascular surgery, edema including lymphedema and effusion, portal hypertension, filariasis, congenital lymphatic malformations, and protein-losing enteropathy and nephropathy.

Only a few years after William Harvey discovered the circulation of blood, Gaspar Asellius "discovered" the lymphatic system. When asked in the twilight of his career to enter the raging controversy about this new circulation, Harvey responded, "It is useless for you to spur me to gird myself to any new investigations seeing now that I am not only ripe in years but also weary. It seems to me indeed that I am entitled to ask for my honorable discharge from duty." Only in the past few decades has there been a vigorous and concerted effort by clinicians and basic scientists alike to take on the challenge, which Harvey declined, to study the elusive tissue fluid circulation. The Fourth and Fifth International Congresses of Lymphology — twin Pan-American gala events — only "scratched the surface" on the vast amount of information that lies hidden within the lymphatic network. But the new frontier opened by lymphologists holds promise of bringing us just one step closer to the living process.

Marlys Hearst Witte, M.D.

Rubens Carlos Mayall, M.D.

## Contents

BASIC LYMPHOLOGY

## LYMPHOGRAPHY

LYMPHEDEMA

## MISCELLANEA

# Basic Lymphology

# LYMPHOLOGY AND THE MICROCIRCULATION--A SYNOPSIS OF FOURTH INTERNATIONAL CONGRESS OF LYMPHOLOGY SYMPOSIA

Marlys Hearst Witte, M.D.

Department of Surgery
University of Arizona College of Medicine
Tucson, Arizona 85724

Lymph is a mirror of tissue fluid (the "milieu interieur" of Claude Bernard) as well as a barometer of dynamic microcirculatory events. This important facet of lymphology pervaded the 4th International Congress and was explored in depth in several symposia. The symposium entitled "What and Where is Lymph?" (M. Witte, J.R. Casley-Smith, F.C. Courtice, M. Papp, G. Szabo, P.J. Johnson, S. Rodbard, and A.E. Taylor) delved into the nature and location of "lymph". The panel examined the relationships of lymph in lymphatic collecting channels to capillary filtrate and tissue fluid as well as the barriers that separate these fluids and the differences in their composition. Casley-Smith postulated a concentrating mechanism in initial lymphatic channels and proposed the existence of an "oncotic pump" to propel lymph onward (i.e., he maintained that lymph is higher than tissue fluid in protein content). Rodbard, on the other hand, introduced the concept of a "tissue module" constructed of a fibrous connective tissue capsule containing a cluster of parenchymal cells, blood capillaries, and ultrafiltrate permeating the intracapsular space. Lymphatic vessels are restricted to extracapsular clefts and intracapsular and extracapsular tissue fluid are discrete pools (i.e., Rodbard postulated that lymph is somewhat lower than tissue fluid in protein content). In contrast, Taylor's simple mathematical model predicted that protein concentration in an upstream lymphatic vessel is essentially the same as tissue protein concentration adjacent to the blood capillary wall. He reported that a subcutaneously implanted Guyton capsule contained fluid identical in protein content to draining regional lymph. After a lively discussion, there was general agreement on at least one point--that further investigation in this area was greatly needed and direct measurements had to be made.

The symposium on "Lymph Flow" (K. Arfors, Moderator; L. Beltz, S. Godart, M. Intaglietta, M. Papp and G. Szabo) examined the factors influencing lymph formation (net capillary filtration) and lymph absorption. Intaglietta postulated that lymph is continually forming from a slight imbalance in the Starling forces at the capillary level, in contrast to the classical teaching of to-and-fro motion of transcapillary fluid with filtration at the arterial end of the capillary exceeding reabsorption at the venous end. According to measurements in rabbit omentum, lymph formation approximated 0.1% of regional blood flow. Lob described the rapid opening of lymphatic-venous communications after thoracic duct ligation and visualized intrinsic contractility of the major collecting lymphatic ducts on cinelymphangiography. Using vital dye injections, Godart demonstrated lymphatic capillaries in the dermis and lymphatic collectors in the subcutaneous tissue. Dye entered the lymphatics slowly after subcutaneous injection but rapidly after intradermal injection. General discussion centered on microcirculatory physiochemical forces governing lymph formation and on techniques to quantitate lymph flow, including cannulated lymph flow rates and rates of disappearance of protein and colloidal particles injected into tissues. There was general agreement that lymph flow derived primarily from net capillary filtration but depended further upon intrinsic lymphatic contractility and external compressive forces. The participants disagreed, however, on the nature of the tissue "pump" (hydrostatic or oncotic) promoting the filling of lymphatic channels with surplus capillary filtrate.

The session on "Composition of Lymph" (F.C. Courtice, Moderator) began with opening comments by Hyman Mayerson on the origin of lymph. He reviewed experimental evidence for the derivation of lymph from leaky capillaries of differing permeability--observations on the entry into regional lymph of intravascularly administered dextrans of varying molecular weight and radioactively tagged albumin and the partition of immunoglobins of differing molecular weight between lymph and blood. The theory of two different sizes of capillary pores, small and large, was examined in the light of available physiological data and electron microscopic structure of the capillary. The function of the lymphatic circulation in returning plasma proteins and of the venous circulation in returning extravascular fluid to the vascular compartment was reviewed. It was acknowledged, however, that most studies have involved relatively impermeable capillary beds (e.g., the extremities) and that in more permeable beds (e.g., liver or intestine) the "division of labor" between lymphatics and veins in returning protein and fluid may differ strikingly. Courtice reported that during shock and limb ischemia lysosomal enzymes enter the bloodstream directly and then pass according to molecular size and regional capillary permeability into tissues and draining lymph. Ischemia enhanced capillary permeability to macromolecules but without any appreciable release of lysosomal enzymes from injured cells or invading phagocytic cells.

Szabo presented data supporting the thesis that protein molecules in tissues are returned to the bloodstream via venous as well as lymphatic channels. He noted direct entry into veins of colloidal particles injected under controlled pressure into various tissues as well as a significant arteriovenous concentration difference for endogenous proteins, specifically enzymes (lactic dehyrogenase, maleic dehyrodgenase, glutamic oxaloacetic transaminase) escaping from cells during ischemia or exercise. This finding, which was challenged by several discussants, suggested that venous channels reabsorb proteins under conditions of altered vascular permeability. Utilizing a variety of tissues and polyvinylpyrrolidone (PVP) of different molecule weights, Vogel described experiments to detect alterations in the blood-lymph barrier to macromolecules. He recommended the hind limb model and the use of horse chestnut seeds as a powerful "capillary active" agent. The blood-lymph barrier was also examined by other investigators looking into transcapillary exchange of protein-bound thyroxine between testicular blood and afferent testicular lymph, protein distribution in fetal sheep lymph, and blood coagulation factors in human thoracic duct lymph as compared to plasma levels. In each instance, lymph protein content was lower than that in plasma and reflected restrictive diffusion ("molecular sieving").

The critical role of the lymph circulation in edema formation (high and low output failure of the lymph circulation) was examined in the symposium on "Edema and Effusion: A Problem in Lymph Drainage?" (M. Witte, Moderator). Taylor analyzed the tissue safety factors in edematogenic states, including increased interstitial fluid pressure, decreased tissue oncotic pressure, and increased lymph flow. Experiments using either saline infusion or venous occlusion techniques in dogs yielded a "tissue protein washout factor" of 4 mmHg, increased tissue pressure of 6.5 mmHg, and increased lymph flow during edema formation of 7.4 mmHg (a total of 17.9 mmHg) as subcutaneous tissue safety factors guarding against edema formation. Each panel member pretended to be a drop of capillary filtrate destined to traverse the lymph circulation before returning to the bloodstream via the lymphatic-venous junction in the neck. During this "fantastic voyage", the panel examined and debated the numerous obstacles encountered along the way--i.e., resistance in prelymphatic tissue spaces, impaired uptake by lymphatic capillaries, defective lymphatic contractility, excessive lymphatic permeability, overdistention of lymph ducts with fluid ("Starling's Law of the Lymphatics"), funnel structure of lymphatic valves, gravitational forces, and finally central venous pressure and the local anatomy of the cervical lymphatic-venous junction. These obstacles have not been well studied and should provide fruitful areas for future basic and clinical research.

In summary, Congress participants agreed that the full study of the microcirculation must include further analysis of events on the "other side" of the capillary membrane. These tissue events should be examined directly, and the changing composition of tissue fluid or lymph analyzed as local conditions vary in normal and pathologic states. It was this very line of reasoning that led Starling to the experiments that uncovered the laws governing the net exchange of fluid between capillaries and tissues, a process for which he reserved the term "lymph formation". Furthermore, Starling acknowledged that the strongest argument favoring his "filtration hypothesis" was the predictable effect on regional lymph flow after altering the gradient of transcapillary hydrostatic or oncotic pressure. Since Starling, more precise and direct measurements of the capillary forces and fluxes governing lymph formation by highly sophisticated techniques have affirmed the validity of the filtration hypothesis and at the same time provided a potent stimulus to technical advances in the study of the blood circulation. This technology has already been extensively applied to physiologic measurements in the blood vascular system in patients. More recently similar techniques have been developed and applied to the study of the lymph circulation, although only to a limited extend in man. Thus, the tools are ready and the time is ripe for lymphologists to undertake a comprehensive examination of the lymph circulation as an integral component of the microcirculation in health and disease.

VARIATIONS OF LYMPHATIC ENDOTHELIAL CELL JUNCTIONS IN EXPERIMENTAL CONDITIONS

T.V. Kalima, Y. Collan and S.H. Kalima

Second Department of Surgery and
Second Department of Pathology,
University of Helsinki, Helsinki, Finland

## Introduction

In the lymphatic endothelium there are different kinds of contact areas of adjacent endothelial cells, and some of these appear to function as valves through which interstitial fluid can enter the initial lymphatics. We have presented a model describing interdigitation of the borders of lymphatic endothelial cells and thus explaining various kinds of contact areas seen in electron microscopial sections. This model (Fig. 1) shows that the walls of the initial lymphatics have areas potentially capable of functioning as inlet valves and indirect proof of such a function has been presented in many earlier experiments.

In this study we want to clarify further the role of contact areas in the filling of initial lymphatics. This is done by examining the quantitative amount of various types of contact areas under three experimental conditions: in normal animals, in venous stasis and in lymphostasis.

## Material and Methods

In three animals venous stasis was produced by ligating the veins at the base of the mesentery and carefully avoiding any damage of lymphatics or arteries. After five minutes (3% phosphate buffered 4°C) glutaraldehyde was injected into the lumen of the ileum.

In three rats lymphostasis was produced by carefully ligating the lymphatics at the base of the mesentery without causing damage to veins or arteries. After 30 minutes samples were

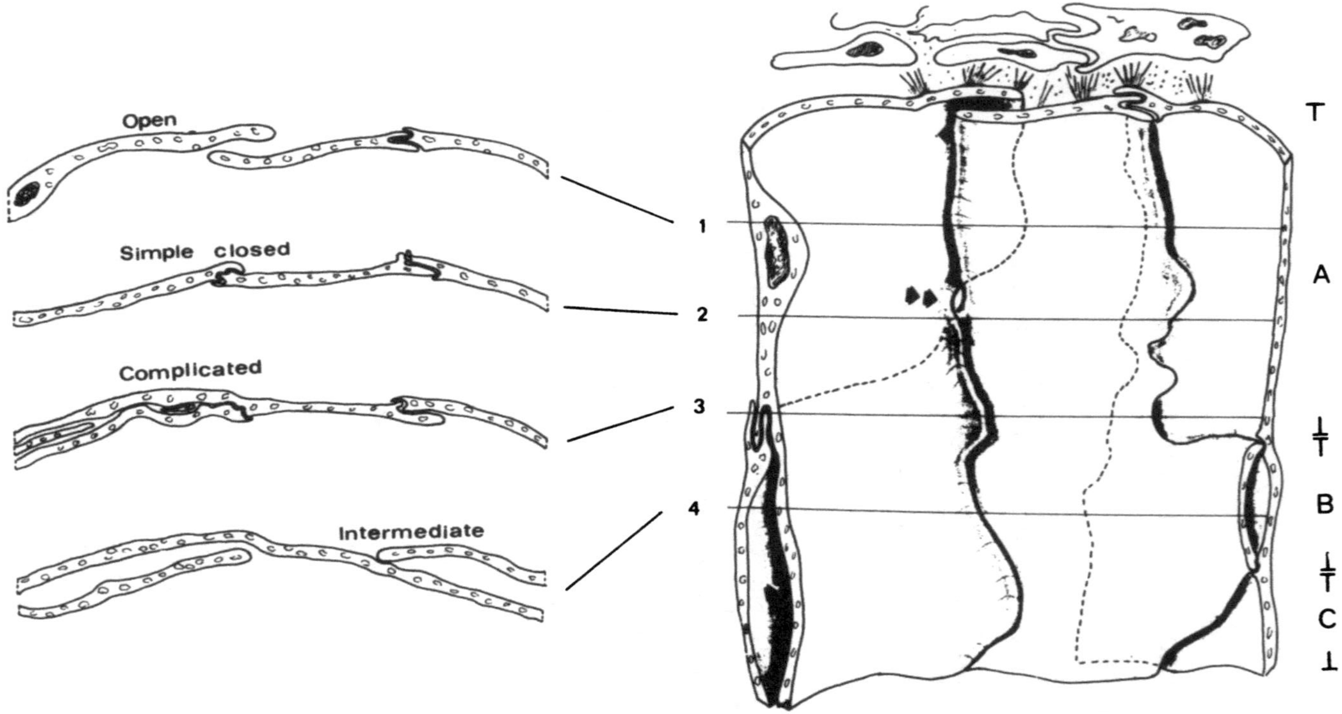


Fig. 1 -

In two dimensional sections the calculated number of closed cellular junctions divided with the number of open cellular junctions must be the same as $\frac{A\ um + C\ um}{B\ um}$ in the three dimensional model

collected as in the former group.

There were three controls. Sections were cut perpendicular to the long axis of the villi so that sections were got from the middle third of the villus. From each animal 5 blocks were cut and from each of them two thin sections about 20 um apart. Sections were stained with lead citrate and uranyl acetate in 50% ethanol. From these sections the number of various kinds of contact areas were calculated. All the visible parts of lymphatics were studied in every section. Calculating numerous cellular junctions we have tried to minimize the fact that endothelial cell junctions may appear in two dimensional sections in many forms depending on sectioning directions.

The contact areas were classified into 5 groups.

I Gaps - the cytoplasmic leaves of the adjacent endothelial cells were stretched apart creating a gap between them.

II Open valves - the cytoplasmic leaves of the adjacent endothelial cells were on each other but did no have contacts.

III Intermediate valves - the cytoplasmic leaves of the adjacent endothelial cells were in slight contact with one another but only at one point due to bulging of the luminal leaf into the lumen.

IV Closed, simple valves - the cytoplasmic leaves of the adjacent endothelial cells were in continuous touch with each another but formed only two layers.

V Complicated contact areas - the cytoplasmic leaves of the adjacent endothelial cells were in contact with each other and formed more than two layers at the contact area.

## Results

The number of lymphatics calculated and the distribution of various contact areas into these groups is shown in table 1. In this table it is shown that changes do appear in the lymphatic endothelium. In venous stasis the number of contact areas "capable for opening" (gap, open, intermediate and simple closed) increases and in lymphostasis complicated contact areas decreases in number at the same time the initial lymph vessels are dilated. The statistical analysis is not ready but in preliminary calculatives it seems that differences are significant.

Table 1

| Experimental situation | No. of lacteals calculated | No. of junctions calculated | Gap | Open | Inter-mediate | Simple closed | Complicated closed |
|---|---|---|---|---|---|---|---|
| normal | 110 | 911 | 2(0,2%) | 14(1,5%) | 102(11,2%) | 349(38,3%) | 444(48,7%) |
| venous stasis | 189 | 1077 | 3(0,3%) | 15(1,4%) | 241(22,4%) | 492(45,6%) | 326(30,3%) |
| lymphostasis | 103 | 724 | 1(0,1%) | 0(0 %9 | 54( 7,6%) | 432(59,5%) | 237(32,6%) |

Table 2

| | Open | Inter-mediate | Closed simple | Closed complicated |
|---|---|---|---|---|
| Normal lacteals | 2% | 11% | 38% | 49% |
| Very early venous stasis | 4% | 25% | 36% | 35% |
| Lymphostasis | 0% | 8% | 60% | 32% |

## Discussion

Increase in the number of simple contact areas in relation to complicated ones can most easily be explained on stertching of the lymphatic wall. In the complicated contact areas there are numerous tight junctions and more over the endothelial cytoplasms of cells are overcrossing in many of these complicated junction regions. During distension of the initial lymphatic these contact areas can hardly be changed in number but during distension unravelling can occur at marginal regions with more simple junctions. So, in two dimensional sections the frequency of complicated junctions is decreased when compared to more simple or even open endothelial valves. In our experiments both during venous stasis and lymphostasis the initial lymphatics dilated and so there was a decrease in complicated contact areas with a parallel increase in uncomplicated ones.

The number of open contact areas can be suggested to correspond to the flow of extracellular fluid into the lymphatic. Accordingly few really open contact areas are seen during lymphostasis whereas during venous stasis there are many open valves. Outside this material we have also investigated initial lymphatics in a very early phase of venous stasis and the number of open valves was about three times greater than in this material with a venous stasis of five minutes duration (Table 2). This observation can be interpretated as follows: During venous stasis the absorption into initial lymphatics is increased and so relatively numerous contact areas are open whereas in lymphostasis the intralymphatic pressure is increased and these valve-like formations are compressed and visualized in sections as simple, closed or at least intermediate contact areas.

## Conclusions

During increased lymph production the cellular contact areas of initial lymphatic endothelial cells are more often open than in normal conditions and during decreased lymph production they are more often closed. Moreover, these opening can be twice as wide as in normal conditions whereas tightly closed contact areas are correspondently narrower. When the endothelium of initial lymphatics is stretshed, complicated junctions seem to be unravelled to more simple ones thus increasing the endothelial surface without rupturing its continuity. As a physiological point of view this unrigid system can explain why lymphatics can increase their lymph producing capacity enormously when neede.

References

1. Casley-Smith, J.R.: The functioning of lymphatic system under normal and pathological conditions: Its dependence on the fine structures and permeabilities of the vessels. A. Rüttiman (ed), in: Progress in Lymphology. Thieme, Stuttgart (1967) 348-359.

2. Collan, Y. and Kalima, T.V.: Topographic relations of lymphatic endothelial cells in the initial lymphatic of the intestinal villus. Lymphology 7 (1974) 1975-184.

3. Leak, L.V. and Burke, J.F.: Ultrastructural studies on the lymphatic anchoring filaments. J. Cell Biol. 36 (1968) 129-149.

TISSUE AND CAPILLARY FORCE CHANGES DURING THE FORMATION OF INTRA-ALVEOLAR EDEMA

R. E. Drake and A. E. Taylor

University of Mississippi Medical Center

Jackson, Mississippi

The Starling forces, capillary pressure ($P_c$) plasma colloid osmotic pressure ($\pi_c$), tissue colloid osmotic pressure ($\pi_t$) and tissue fluid pressure ($P_t$) are related to the volume movement ($J_V$) across any capillary system by the relationship:

$$J_V = K_{FC} \left[(P_c - P_t) - \sigma_c (\pi_c - \pi_t)\right]; \qquad ...1$$

where $K_{F,C}$ is the filtration coefficient of the capillary bed (ml/min-mm Hg-100 gm) and $\sigma$ is the Staverman reflection coefficient of the plasma proteins ($\sigma$ of the protein is equal to 1 if the membrane is impermeable to the protein and is equal to 0 if the protein is as permeable as water in the membrane i.e. velocity of solute/velocity of water = 1). Obviously there is not just one $\sigma$ but a $\sigma$ for each of the various protein fractions in the body fluids ($\alpha_1$, $\alpha_2$ and $\beta$ globulins, albumin and $\gamma$ globulins); however, for practical purposes we can assume that $\sigma \cong 1$ for all plasma proteins and calculate total $\Delta\pi$ by the use of the Landis and Pappenheimer equation (1,2).

Normally, the sum of the forces on the right hand side of equation 1 are not equal to zero but a small net imbalance of forces exists that causes movement of fluid out of the capillaries into the interstitium. This slight filtration of fluid is what finally forms lymph.

When $P_c$ is elevated in equation 1, fluids will filter into the interstitium and if changes in the tissue forces, such as increased $P_t$, decreased $\pi_t$ and increased lymph flow are not sufficient to oppose the increase in $P_c$, then gross inter-alveolar edema will develop.

This paper evaluates the changes in one of these tissue forces, lymphatic protein osmotic pressure, during the formation of intra-alveolar edema.

## Methods

Whole dog lungs were isolated and perfused by methods developed earlier in this laboratory (3, 4). The lung was weighted continuously and arterial and venous pressures were measured using Statham strain gauges and the lung was respired with humidified air at 10 cycles/min with an average airway pressure of 2 mm Hg. Total plasma protein concentration (gm/100 ml) was measured using an American optical refractometer.

A pulmonary lymphatic was cannulated near the right duct and lymph was also analyzed for plasma proteins using the refractometer. Protein concentrations were then converted to colloid osmotic pressure using the equation developed by Lands and Pappenheimer ($\pi = 2.1\ C_P + 0.16\ C_P^2 + 0.009\ C_P^3$; where $C_P$ refers to total plasma proteins in gm/100 ml. (2)

## Results

Figure 1 is a typical experiment showing the decrease in lymph protein concentration after the capillary pressure was elevated 14.9 mm Hg. Control values for lymph protein concentration, lymph flow rate, and volume filtered were collected for 38 minutes before the capillary pressure was elevated. For this particular experiment the lymphatic protein osmotic pressure was decreased by 12.1 mm Hg below the control value.

Table 1 shows the results of 5 experiments for which the lymphatic colloid osmotic pressure decreased maximally. When capillary pressure increased from 6.3 to 23.9, a change of 17.6 mm Hg, $\pi$ across the capillary changed from 4 mm Hg to 18.9 mm Hg, or a difference of 14.9 mm Hg. The decrease in lymphatic proteins with increased filtration accounts for approximately 15 mm Hg of the filtration force change whereas other tissue forces account for only 3 mm Hg.

It is important to emphasize that these experiments represent the maximum washdown of lymphatic protein seen in our studies and that the lung was continuing to gain weight during the entire course of the experiment, i.e. the lung volume was not in a steady-state; but intra-alveolar edema was being formed.

## Discussion

These experiments illustrate that lymphatic colloid osmotic

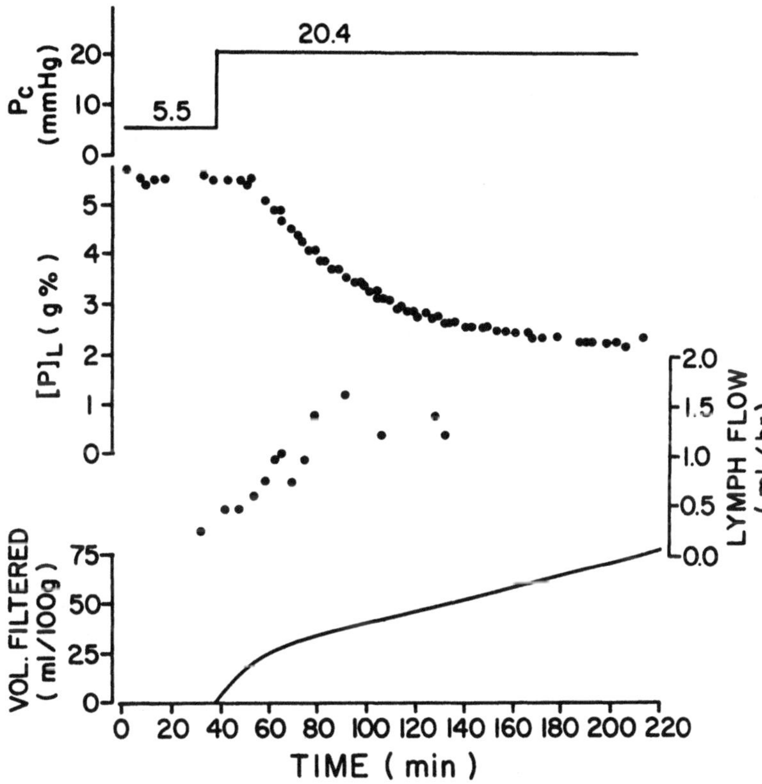


Figure 1. Plot of protein concentration of lymph, $[P]_L$ (gm%) lymph flow (ml/hr), and fluid volume filtered (ml/100 gm) for a typical normal Pc (5.5 mm Hg) and as Pc was elevated to 20.4 mm Hg. Note that the filtered volume was increasing at a rapid rate and intra-alveolar edema was present.

pressure can decrease drastically when capillary pressure is elevated to levels that cause intra-alveolar edema. The reported experiments represent the largest changes that are observed in lymph colloid osmotic pressure in over 18 lung preparations.

Many physiologists feel that lymphatic protein concentrations do not reflect tissue protein concentrations because there is a possibility that the fluid is concentrated within the lymphatics (Casley-Smith (5), Johnson and Richardson (7), Cuyton et al (6) Taylor and Gibson (8); but experimental proof of this possibility is lacking.

Since these experiments represent maximal changes in tissue proteins, the other tissue forces; lymph flow and increases in tissue pressure, must normally change to prevent excessive changes in lung interstitial fluid volumes for smaller changes in filtration pressures. Recent experiments from this laboratory indicate that tissue pressure changes by 6.8 mm Hg and that lymphatic protein concentration decreases by 2.1 - 12.1 mm Hg for isolated lungs that are near the critical point that intra-alveolar edema develops. The sum of these forces, the total edema safety factor, is 10.9 20.9 mm Hg which agrees quite well with earlier observations that pulmonary capillary pressures must be elevated by 18-20 mm Hg before the formation of intra-alveolar edema. (4, 9, 10).

The lar changes seen in lymphatic protein for these studies must reflect an alteration in the alveolar membrane that permits a greater wash down of tissue proteins than that seen maximally prior to the formation of inter-alveolar edema.

TABLE I. CAPILLARY PRESSURE, PLASMA AND LYMPH COLLOID OSMOTIC PRESSURE AT NORMAL AND ELEVATED CAPILLARY PRESSURES

| Exp.# | Capillary Pressure (mm Hg) | | Plasma Colloid Osmotic Pressure (mm Hg) | | Lymph Colloid Osmotic Pressure (mm Hg) | |
|---|---|---|---|---|---|---|
| | Initial | Final | Initial | Final | Initial | Final |
| 61 | 6.3 | 29.0 | 20.8 | 21.8 | 16.5 | 9.3 |
| 71 | 5.4 | 22.3 | 25.1 | 36.3 | 22.4 | 11.5 |
| 89 | 5.5 | 20.4 | 22.4 | 25.1 | 17.9 | 5.8 |
| 92 | 7.3 | 25.1 | 21.3 | 31.0 | 15.6 | 9.0 |
| 93 | 7.0 | 22.7 | 20.8 | 27.9 | 17.9 | 11.9 |
| (AV) | 6.3 | 23.9 | 22.1 | 28.4 | 18.1 | 9.5 |
| (SD) | ±1.7 | ±6.6 | ±1.9 | ±5.6 | ±2.6 | ±2.4 |

## References

1. Staverman, A.J. The theory of measurement of osmotic pressure. Rec. Trav. Chim. 70:344-352, 1951.

2. Landis, E.M., and J.R. Pappenheimer. Exchange of substance through capillary walls. In: Handbook of Physiology. Circulation. Washington, D.C.: Am. Physiol. Soc. 1963, sect. 2, vol. 2, chapt. 29, p. 961-1034.

3. Gaar, K.A., A.E.Taylor, L.J.Owens and A.C.Guyton. Effect of capillary pressure and plasma protein on development of pulmonary edema. Am. J. Physiol. 213:74-82, 1967.

4. Drake, R.E. and A.E.Taylor. Calculation of the edema safety factor in isolated dog lung. (abs.) Fed. Proc. 34:400, 1975.

5. Casley-Smith. A model of lymphatic concentrating ability. Microvascular Research. In Press.

6. Guyton, A.C., A.E.Taylor, R.E.Drake, H.I.Chen, and R.E.Brance. Physical and hemodynamic determinations of transcapillary exchange in the lungs. In: Krogh Symposium on Capillaries, Srinagar, Karhmir, India. Oct. 14, 1974.

7. Johnson, P.C. and D.R.Richardson. The influence of venous pressure on filtration forces in the intestine. Microvascular Research. 7:296-306, 1974.

8. Taylor, A.E. and H.Gibson. Concentrating ability of lymphatic vessels. Lymphology. In Press.

9. Staub, N.C. Pulmonary edema. Physiol. Rev. 54:678-811. 1974.

10. Guyton, A.C.,and A.W.Lindsey. Effect of elevated left arterial pressure and decreased plasma protein concentration on the development of pulmonary edema. Circulation Res. 7(4):649-657, 1959.

# LYMPH FLOW TRANSIENT FOLLOWING ELEVATION OF VENOUS PRESSURE IN THE DOG'S HIND PAW

H.I.Chen, H.J.Granger and A.E.Taylor

Department of Physiology and Biophysics
University of Mississippi School of Medicine
Jackson, Mississippi 39216 - U.S.A.

## Introduction

Steady-state lymph flows have been measured in numerous organs (1,2,6,8,9,10,11,12) for both normal and altered filtration pressure*. The steady-state measurement of lymph flow are very useful for measuring or calculating $P_C$, $P_T$, $\pi_L$ and the imbalance in Starling forces across the capillary membrane (8,9); however, this type of lymph flow measurement does not yield any information as to the mechanisms responsible for lymphatic propulsion.

The following paper discusses a transient analysis of lymph flow observed from small lymphatic vessels that drain the subcutaneous region of an isolated dog paw preparation during elevation of venous pressure to either 20 or 30 mm Hg. The time course of the lymphatic flow transients are then discussed relative to the relationship between capillary filtration and lymph flow.

---

*Filtration pressure is equal to the difference between capillary pressure and tissue pressure minus the difference between colloid osmotic pressure of the plasma and colloid osmotic pressure of the interstitial fluid or $FP = (P_C - P_T) - (\pi_C - \pi_T)$. $P_C$, $P_T$, $\pi_C$, $\pi_T$, and $\pi_L$ are defined as capillary hydrostatic pressure, tissue hydrostatic pressure, plasma colloid osmotic pressure, interstitial fluid colloid osmotic pressure and lymph colloid osmotic pressure respectively.

## Methods

A total of 8 mongrel dogs (18 - 23 kg) of either sex were used in the present study. In four dogs, five weeks prior to the experiment, a hollow polypropylene semispherical capsule of 20 mm diameter, with approximately 100 small holes, was implanted chronically into subcutaneous tissue of the dorsal hindpaw (4). The animals were anesthetized with intravenous sodium pentobarbital (30 mg/kg), the trachea intubated and the animal artificially ventilated with room air. To avoid irregular limb movement which alters lymph flow, 1 mg/kg gallamine (Flaxedil) was given intravenously. The animals were heparinized (5 mg/kg, iv), the right cranial tibial artery was cannulated and the hindpaw was perfused with autologous blood from the femoral artery (See Figure 1). Two T-tubes were inserted into the perfusion circuit, one was used for monitoring the perfusion pressure with a Stantham P23AC transducer and the other was connected to an arterial reservoir which was kept at a constant level in order to maintain the perfusion pressure at 100 mm Hg during the course of the experiment. The lateral saphenous vein was cannulated, connected to a venous reservoir and the venous pressure, which was monitored with a P23BC transducer, was set at the desired level by changing the height of the venous reservoir. All other small veins draining the paw were ligated. Approximately 4 - 6 weeks were allowed for tissue healing in the group of animals with implanted capsules. The animals were prepared in the same surgical fashion as described above and tissue pressure was measured in the following fashion. A 21 gauge hypodermic needle connected to a stiff catheter and the needle was inserted into the implanted capsule and pressure monitored with a P23BC transdurcer.

Two lymphatics on each side of the lateral saphenous vein were carefully dissected and cannulated with PE 90 tubing. The two catheters were then connected by a small Y-connector to another calibrated PE 90 tubing. Lymph flow was determined at one minute intervals using a ruler and a comparator, and the catheters were calibrated both before and after the experimental procedure. In all experiments, the venous pressure was initially set at 5 mm Hg. After the lymph flow became steady at this pressure, the lymph flow transients were obtained following sudden elevation of venous pressure to either 25 or 35 mm Hg for a 30 minute period.

## Results

At a venous pressure (VP) of 5 mm Hg, the baseline lymph flow (LF) was $3.3 \times 10^{-5} \pm 1.7$ ml/min and tissue pressure (TP) -6 mm Hg. Figures 1 and 2 depict typical changes of LF and TP (following elevation of VP to 25 (Figure 2) and 35 mm Hg (Figure

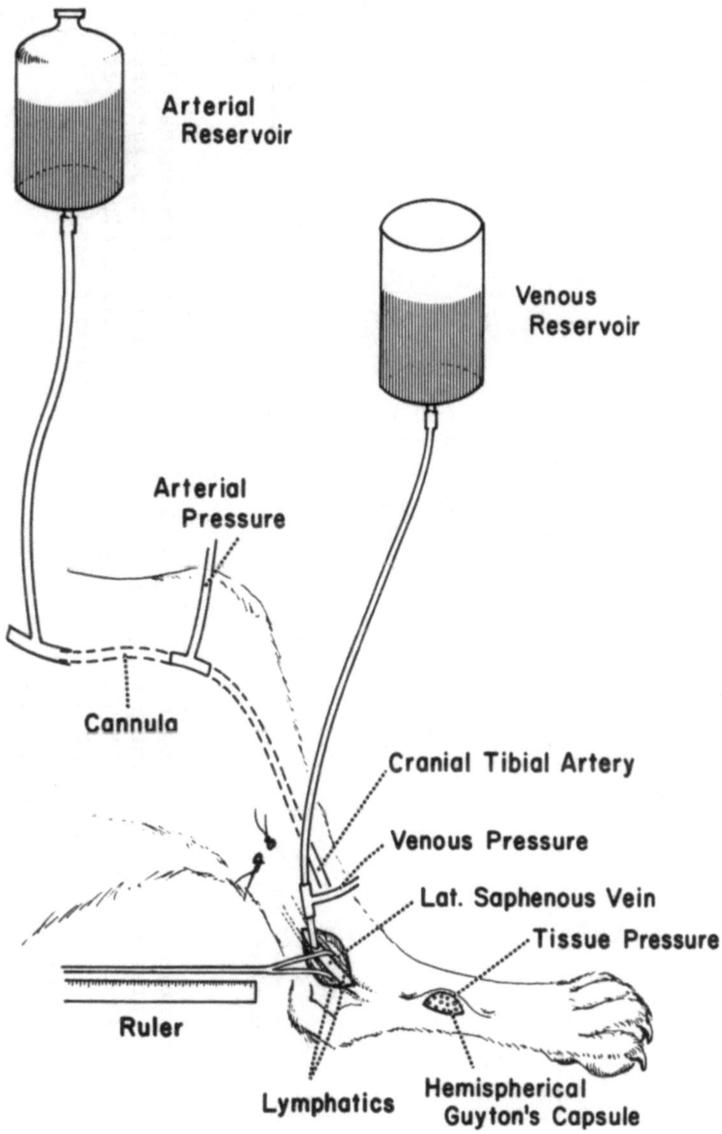


Figure 1. Schematic representation of experimental model.

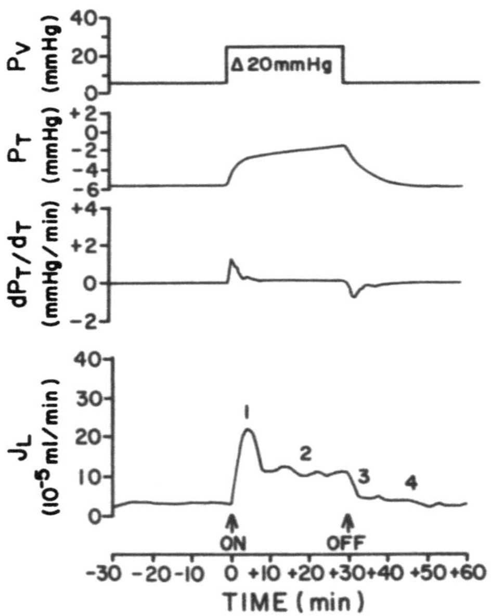


Figure 2. A typical experiment showing venous pressure ($P_V$), capsular pressure ($P_T$), change of capsular pressure as a function of time ($dP_T/dt$), and lymph flow ($J_L$). $P_V$ was elevated to 20 mm Hg and $P_T$, $dP_T/dt$ and $J_L$ were measured. Note the rapid elevation of lymph flow (phase 1), a plateau lymph flow (phase 2), and the rapid decrease in lymph flow seen when venous pressure was reduced to control values (phase 3) and the slow return of lymph flow to control values (phase 4).

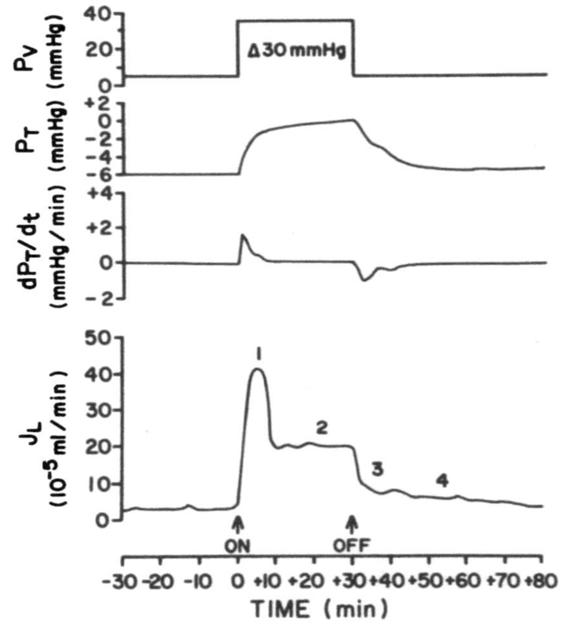


Figure 3. Plot of venous pressures ($P_V$), capsular pressure ($P_T$), rate of capsular pressure change ($dP_T/dt$) and lymph flow ($J_L$) for a change of 30 mm Hg in venous pressure.

3). Immediately following elevation of venous pressure, a rapid increase was observed for both TP and LF. Peak LF occurs at 3-5 minutes after elevation of VP (Phase 1). Thereafter, TP increased only slowly and LF decreased from the peak to a lower lymph flow state and reached a plateau (Phase 2). Table 1 summarizes the extent and time course of LF transients in all 8 animals. The peak and steady plateau LF for 20 mm Hg VP elevation were $32.5 \times 10^{-5} \pm 16.3$ ml/min (10-fold) and $18.6 \times 10^{-5} \pm 7.8$ (5.5-fold) respectively and $63.9 \times 10^{-5} \pm 16.3$ (18.1-fold) and 35.1 x $\times 10^{-5} \pm 9.9$ ml/min (9.8-fold) for 30 mm Hg VP elevation.

When VP was lowered to control levels, TP initially decreased rapidly; but then decreased only slowly. The LF decreased rapidly to one-half of the plateau level in 2 min (Phase 3), and gradually approached the baseline flow (Phase 4), requiring 26 and 46.5 min for VP elevation of 20 and 30 mm Hg, respectively. Both the on and off change of VP demonstrate both fast and slow components of TP and LF.

## Discussion

The baseline lymph flow (LF) obtained in the present experiment was approximately one thousandth of that obtained by Garlick and Renkin (3) from two lymphatics on both sides of the saphenous vein in the dog's two hindlegs. They cannulated the lymphatic vessels distal to the popliteal node---higher than the cannulation sites in this experiment. Obviously, the lymph collected from both legs and larger tissue mass from each leg would be greater than that observed in our preparation. In addition, they increased LF by moving the legs passively with a rotary device at 100 cycles/min which would also increase lymph flow. Also, the animals in our study received a neuromuscular blocker in order to prevent the irregular leg movement which will cause sudden increases in LF. Since the tissue motion in our preparation was reduced to a minimum, then the resting LF would be very low.

The data demonstrates that LF increases in proportion to the extent of venous pressure (VP), and that both the on and off changes in VP result in a fast and a slow component of LF changes. Gibson *et al*. (2,10) considered that the steady state lymph flow was a function of tissue pressure since elevations of venous pressure initiates increased capillary pressure and subsequently alters the tissue Starling forces. In the present study, approximately 5 min after venous pressure elevation, the TP had almost reached a new steady state, dTP/dt was 0.05 - 0.1 mm Hg/min (Figure 1 and 2). At VP = 25 mm Hg, TP ranged between -3 to -2 mm Hg and LF was 5.5 times control. At VP = 35 mm Hg, TP ranged from -1 to 0 mm Hg and LF was 10.4 times control.

Table 1. Lymph flow transients and time constants of the various components following 30 min elevations of venous pressure.

| Venous Pressure Elevatio[n] | Lymph Flow ($10^{-5}$ ml/min) | | | $LF/LF_C$ | | Time Course (min) | | | | | |
|---|---|---|---|---|---|---|---|---|---|---|---|
| | | | | | | On Transient | | | | Off Transient | |
| | Contro (C) | Peak (P) (1) | Steady Plateau (SP) (2) | P/C | SP/C | $t_{1/2}$ (C-P) (1) | Total Time (C-P) (1) | $t_{1/2}$ (P-SP) (2) | Total Time (P-SP) (2) | $t_{1/2}$ (SP-C) (3) | Total Time (SP-C) (4) |
| 20 mm Hg (n=8) | 3.2 ±1.6 | 32.5 ±11.6 | 18.6 ±7.9 | 10.4 ±2.0 | 5.5 ±0.7 | 1.4 ±0.8 | 5.3 ±1.8 | 1.8 ±0.9 | 9.3 ±3.7 | 1.8 ±0.6 | 26.0 ±4.7 |
| 30 mm Hg (n=8) | 3.3 ±1.7 | 63.9 ±16.3 | 35.1 ±9.9 | 18.1 ±4.5 | 9.8 ±1.8 | 1.3 ±0.8 | 5.3 ±1.5 | 2.0 ±0.9 | 8.6 ±2.0 | 2.1 ±0.5 | 46.5 ±11.6 |

This LF-TP relationship at steady state is in accordance with the earlier observations of Gibson _et al_. (2,10).

Several factors may contribute to the increased LF as TP rises:

1) increase in pressure gradient between tissues and lymphatic,

2) increase in amplitude and rate of lymphatic pump activity, which is stimulated by an increase in transmural lymphatic pressure (7), and

3) increases in tissue conductance as tissue volume expands.

The peak LF seen within the first 5 min following venous pressure elevation was related to the rate of TP increase (dTP/dt) instead of the absolute value of TP (See Figures 1 and 2). There was a rapid change in both TP and LF at this period of time. The fast component of increases in TP and LF implies that the lymphatics respond greater to the rate of change of Starling forces than they respond to the absolute value of pressure. The greater peak LF could not be attributed to increased pressure gradient between tissue and lymphatics, because TP was less than that observed at the steady plateau phase. We feel that the fast rate of change in TP causes a rapid increase in intrinsic pump activity. However, another simple mechanism could easily explain the rapid on-transient: a physical emptying of filled lymphatic vessels caused by the sudden venous expansion and restriction of lymphatic filling.

The rapid reverse off transients observed when VP was returned to control values may be explained in a similar fashion as the on transients. However, the difference between the return to base line flows is quite between 20 and 30 mm Hg elevations in VP. At thirty mm Hg, TP increased to a positive value; therefore, a longer time period was required for LF to return to control, because of the increased tissue compliance in the pressure region (5).

Since complex interactions and responses may occur in the vascular bed, capillary, interstitium and lymphatics, we have proposed many explanations for the various components of LF transients. Within the limit of our data, the most likely possibilities were discussed in this manuscript. The ultimate mechanism awaits further study. At any rate, the fast and greater increase in LF immediately following elevation of VP helps to remove more fluid and protein from the interstitium even when tissue pressure is still low. This priming effect provides a greater safety factor against elema in subcutaneous tissue.

## REFERENCES

1. Duffy, P.A., and A.E.Taylor. A mathematical analysis of the relationship between capillary dynamics and interstitial absorption. Proc. ACEMB 13:327, 1971.

2. Gibson, H., K.A.Gaar, Jr. Dynamics of the implanted capsule. Fed. Proc. 29:319, 1970.

3. Garlick, D.G., and E.M.Renkin. Transport of large molecules from plasma to interstitial fluid and lymph in dogs. Am. J. Physiol. 219:1595-1605, 1970.

4. Guyton, A.C. A concept of negative interstitial pressure based on pressures in implanted perforated capsules. Circ. Res. 12:399-414, 1963.

5. Guyton, A.C. Interstitial fluid pressure. II. Pressure-volume curves of interstitial space. Circ. Res. 16:452-460, 1965.

6. Korner, P.I., B.Morris, and F.C.Courtice. An analysis of factors affecting lymph flow and protein composition during gastric absorption of food and fluids and during intravenous infusion. Aust. J. Exp. Biol. Med. Sci. 32:301-320, 1954.

7. Mislin,H., and R.Schipp. Structural and functional relations of the mesenteric lymph vessels. In: Progress in Lymphology, ed. by A. Ruttiman. Hafner Publ. Co.: New York. 1967, pp. 360-365.

8. Mortillaro, N.A., and A.E.Taylor. Interaction of capillary and tissue forces in the cat small intestine. (In press).

9. Staub, N.C. Pulmonary edema. Physiol. Rev. 54:678-811, 1974.

10. Taylor, A.C., W.H.Gibson, H.J.Granger and A.C.Guyton. The Interaction between intracapillary and tissue forces in the overall regulation of interstitial fluid volume. Lymphology 6:192-208, 1973.

11. Uhley, H.N., S.E.Leads, J.J.Sampson and N.Friedman. Role of pulmonary lymphatics in chronic pulmonary edema. Circ. Res. 11:966-970, 1962.

12. Wasserman, K., and H.S.Mayerson. Mechanism of plasma protein changes following saline infusion. Am. J. Physiol. 170:1-10, 1952.

# LYMPHATIC REGENERATION AFTER SECOND DEGREE BURN

Sabine Godart, M.D.
Maître de Stage-Pediatric Surgery
Université Libre de Bruxelles and
Laboratorium Physical Therapy (Prof. Leduc)
Bruxelles, Belgium

## Introduction

Within a wider field of investigations on the lymphatic microcirculation in the burnt skin, special attention has been brought to the regeneration process which occurs after a second degree burn.

In previous studies on mice subjected to burns at various temperatures we have shown that a burn induced by a ten seconds contact with water preheated to 60° C, is comparable to a second degree burn in man (GODART 1973).

In the mouse, this type of burn does not lead to bleb formation so characteristic in man since its hairy skin does not permit epidermal separation. The fate of the skin, however, is comparable. Only superficial loss occurs and the skin will heal locally. When observed by vital microscopy, blood continues to flow into the burnt area during the first few hours. Platelet aggregation and sludge progressively impair local blood flow which soon comes to a complete settle in the smaller vessels (personal observation).

When observed after two or three days, the burnt skin appears avascular. In these second degree burns, however, by the 4th day there is reinvasion by newly grown blood vessels, sprouting from the convoluted and dilated vessels of the congested edges and in addition from the vessels coming from below along the perforating nerves. Consequently, the revascularized burnt skin will survive with only superficial loss.

The lymphatic vessels, as well as the blood vessels, disappear from the burnt skin between the first and second day. The purpose of this study was to investigate the regeneration of lymphatic vessels into the revascularized skin.

## Method

Under ether inhalation one hundred and twenty mice are scalded for ten seconds with water preheated to 60º C. on a surface approaching 1 $cm^2$.

At various intervals after the burn, the mouse is reanasthetized with urethane (2,5 gr./K.B.W. subcutaneously). By a mid incision the abdominal skin is opened and gently separated from the underlying muscles in order to observe the desper aspect of the burnt area. A minute amount of patent blue violet is injected intradermally, either into the burnt area, in order to show the local lymphatic resorption, or distally to show the main collector and the behaviour of lymph when approaching or passing the lesion.

## Results

During the first few hours, marked edema is observed. Interstitial fluid appears almost free not only at the level of the burnt skin but extended to the whole region.

At these early intervals blood microcirculation alterations are obvious: White masses, probably of aggregated platelets are seen to form and grow on the vessel wall; after some time they are detached to be removed with the blood flow. These big white masses are clearly seen flowing in contrast with the red cells. Red cell aggregation progressively occurs showing all the signs of sludging described by KNISELY: irregular flow, turbulence, backward flow, local settle etc... (KNISELY)

Injections of patent blue into the burnt area show local resorption of the dye by normal lymph vessels as well as venous resorption. Distal injections show considerably dilated lymph collectors passing the burnt area normally. Lymph flow is much faster than in the normal animal as seen by the spontaneous replacement of the dyed lymph by clear lymph, by the lymphatic wall contractions which flush lymph farther onwards and by the fast filling of the regional lymph node.

The venous vessels are highly permeable as shown by leakage of the dye along the vessel wall. This induces the increase of interstitial fluid formation.

After one day, edema is still present. At the burn level dermal blood capillaries are no longer seen: the deeper vessels still pass underneath with impaired blood flow. Lymph resorption still occurs in the burnt area. The regional lymph collector remains dilated with increased flow. Venous permeability continues to be increased.

After two and three days, the general edema has disappeared. Some edema remains at the burnt level. Convoluted blood vessels give a congested appearance to a ring surrounding the burnt skin. Some deep vessels still cross the burnt area. Blood flow at this level is very slow or settled. Injections in the burnt area show no more lymphatic resorption whereas the few veins which may fill by normal or reversed flow immediately leak the dye. The regional lymph collectors are still dilated and run, usually unchanged, under the lesion.

From the fourth day regenerated blood vessels begin to appear growing into the necrosed skin perpendicularly to the edges as quite thin and permeable comb like vessels. No lymphatic resorption occurs unless the dye reaches the edges. Distal injections show a wide lymph collector which becomes permeable when crossing the lesion, resuming its normal sharp appearance afterwards.

The following days the observations are similar to growing regenerated blood vessels until the seventh day when for the first time, in two out of 11 experiments the injected dye was resorbed by a lymphatic network (wide, irregular and highly permeable) which cannot be compared to the normal resorptive lymphatic capillaries. Distal injections still show a wide lymph collector. In one out of 11 experiments the collector gave birth to a network penetrating the burnt skin, another stopped at the burnt level, the lymph flowing by reverse flow into a very permeable collateral vessel along the lesion's edges.

During the following days, several lymph collectors were seen interrupted at the burnt level. Reflux occurred in collaterals running into the congested rim (shown in 12 out of 43 distal injections between the 8th and the 21st day). These collaterals are most permeable.

From the 12th day on lymphatic resorption occurs in all experiments. In half of the cases the dye fills a wide lymphatic network. These new lymphatic vessels are very permeable and immediately leak the just resorbed dye. The collector as shown by distal injections is usually dilated. It was interrupted at the level of the lesion in 7 out of 17 experiments and detoured the lesion by reflux into permeable collaterals.

In one experiment, after 15 days, budding of the collector is observed, giving an appearance of multiple hernias of its walls. In two other experiments the collector dilates and becomes permeable at the level of the burn.

After three weeks the regeneration process of the blood vessels seems to be completed. All burns give an almost normal macroscopic appearance. All congestion has disappeared. Lymphatic resorption occurs in all cases after local injection. A wide network appearance was still observed in 8 out of 17 experiments, half of these being permeable to the dye. In the other experiments, normal resorption occurred. Blood vessel permeability is still increased and the regional lymph collectors are still dilated.

## Discussion

Blood and lymph microcirculation should be investigated together. When at the first stage, during the hours following the injury, lymph resorption from the burnt area seems to occur normally, local blood microcirculation is progressively impaired by platelet and red cell aggregation. These phenomena induce a leakage of protein rich fluid giving rise to an exsudative edema which can only be evacuated through lymph vessels. The lymph collectors are seen considerably dilated, sometimes reaching the size of the main vein. The flow in them is much faster than under normal conditions when almost no spontaneous flow is observed. Intrinsic contractions, which are so rarely seen in the mouse in control experiments, are probably induced by the vessel dilatation. The amount of filtrated fluid probably surpasses the functional capacity of the lymphatic system although it is functioning much faster than under normal conditions. This explains the edema of the entire region drained by the same collector shich is overwhelmed.

After one day, the burnt dermis loses its blood supply. Consequently, no more fluid is delivered, nor can be lost at this level. The very active lymphatic system progressively empties the accumulated fluid of generalized edema which usually disappears after two days. Some edema remains in the necrotic area where lymphatic resorption no longer occurs.

To compensate for the blood vessels being interrupted at the level of the burn, dilatation and convolution of the surrounding collaterals and capillaries occur, giving an appearance of congested edges about the lesion. At this level, vascular permeability is highly abnormal and induces edema of the congested rim.

Second degree burnt skin does not remain unvascularized long. New capillaries invade the original skin as early as the 4th day. These new capillaries are very permeable and leak fluid into the burnt tissue.

A few days later, we observe a new lymphatic network, consisting of wide and irregular vessels. The appearance of this network

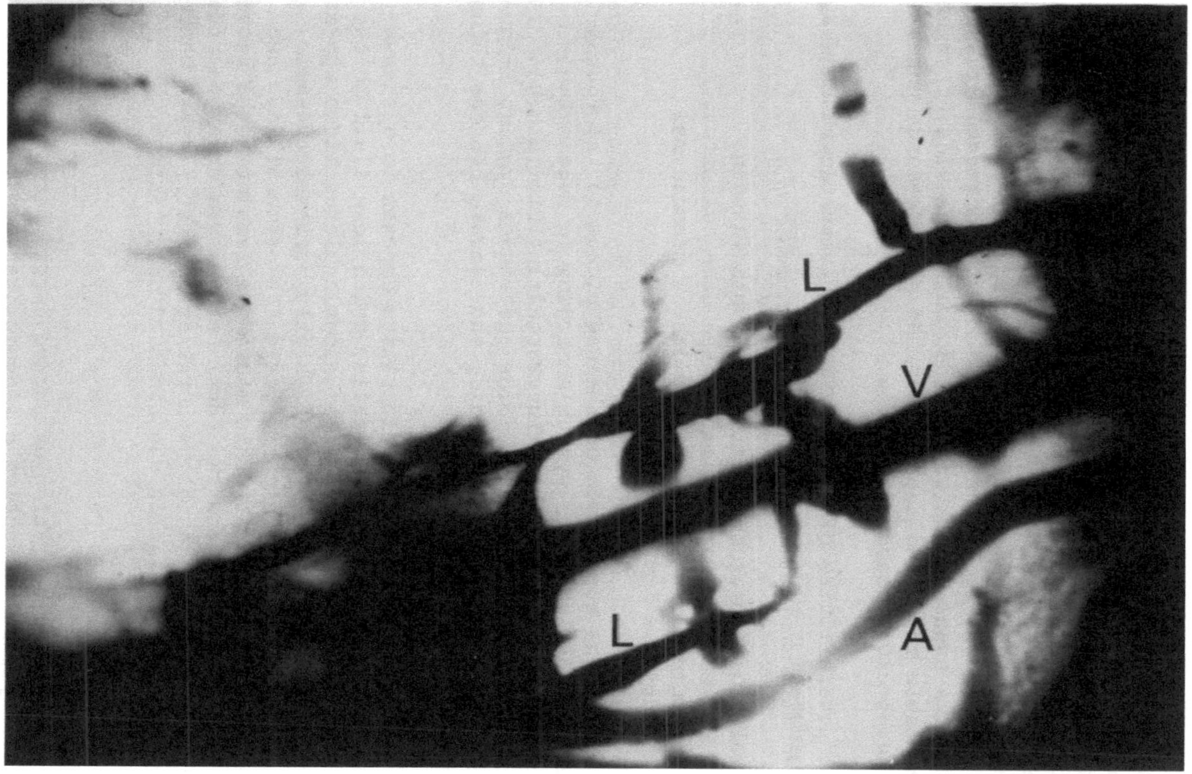


A : artery
V : vein
L : lymphatic hypodermic collectors with budding and new network

Fig. 1 - Lymphatic regeneration 14 days after a scald at 60° during 10 seconds

has little similarity with the normal dermal network. On the other hand, from the fourth day on, the lymphatic collector running underneath becomes permeable as it passes the level of the burnt tissue, resuming its normal appearance beyond the lesion. The deep collector may also be interrupted, reflux being observed in collateral lymphatics which run in the congested rim. These collaterals are very permeable (12 reflux out of 43 distal injections between the 8th and 21st days).

In six out of 59 distal injections performed after 7 days, we have noted collaterals leaving the collector and penetrating the burnt tissue. On two occasions, reflux from the collector in a lymphatic vessel similar to preexisting precollectors occurred (one after 9 days, the other after 19 days). In the other four, there seemed to be a budding of the lymphatic wall appearing as multiple hernias (7, 8, 15 and 21 days). With increased pressure of injection, a true network was filled, which was wide, irregular and so permeable that it disappeared after a few seconds under the shading of extravasated dye. (fig. 1)

Three possibilities of regeneration of lymphatic vessels are to be considered:

1) repermeabilization of original local lymph vessels,
2) budding and network formation from the deep collector,
3) local formation of a lymphatic network by mesenchymal differenciation.

We suggest the comparison of the new plexus to the foetal development of the lymphatic system according to Huntington's theory: disseminated slits with interstitial fluid join to form a wide network. When the latter joins the venous system, allowing the emptying of accumulated fluid, the network becomes thinner and thinner.

In the burn, the new lymphatic plexus appears in a tissue invaded by new permeable blood vessels, which lose fluid to the interstitial tissue. When the new lymphatic plexus first appears, it is very rich, consisting of wide, highly permeable vessels. Soon, this plexus becomes thinner, loses its permeability, and resumes a normal appearance. This mechanism remains to be proved. However, in our experiments, the local network was observed often: 22 out of 59 mice injected in the burnt area after 7 days, whereas budding of the deep collector was observed only 4 times.

Summary

The lymphatic circulation of second degree burns has been investigated. Lymphatic function disappears between 24 and 48 hours.

The first regeneration is observed after 7 days. Three mechanisms are suggested: the repermeabilization of previous lymphatics is possible but certainly not always the case; budding and network formation from the deep collector and local network formation in the burnt skin itself.

## Bibliography

GODART, Sabine & LEDUC, Albert, The lymphatic microcirculation after burns. 4th International Congress of Lymphology, Tucson, 1973, in press

HUNTINGTON, G.S., The anatomy and development of the systernic lymphatic vessels in the domestic cat. Philadelphia, 1911

KNISELY, Melvin H., ELIOT, Th. S. & BLOCH, Sludged blood in traumatic shock.

# EXPERIMENTAL METHODS TO EXAMINE SUBSTANCES AND PHARMACOLOGICAL POSSIBILITIES TO INFLUENCE THE PERMEABILITY OF THE BLOOD-LYMPH BARRIER

G. Vogel

Biologisches Institut Maclaus
Ostmerheimerstrasse 198
5 Kola-Merheim, West Germany

It is generally recognized that abnormalities of the permeability of the plasma-lymph barrier occur in certain diseases, for example rheumatic conditions, purpura and especially inflammatory states. These permeability abnormalities are connected with edema formation. There are various drugs which are claimed to be "capillary-active" in the sense that they can "seal" the plasma-lymph barrier or in other words that they can reduce excessive and abnormal permeability. This claim is, however, not so widely accepted. For the experimentalist, and in particular the pharmacologist, who wants to study the effects and the mechanism of action of these "capillary-active" drugs, there is an abundance of methods - too many for me to describe here. Because of the drawbacks of most methods we use the following technique. We cannulate the rat's thoracic duct and give the animal a continuous infusion of polyvinylpyrrolidone (PVP) of intermediate molecular weight. We then measure the rate of lymph flow and the PVP and protein concentrations in the plasma and the lymph and calculate the concentration ratios (Fig. 1). This procedure has certain disadvantages. Permeability is known to vary from one organ to another, but what we collect from the rat is mixed lymph from a variety of organs. Furthermore, we are working on the plasma-lymph barrier of an intact animal and the permeability situation is not necessarily representative of that existing in human disease. We have therefore gone over to rabbits and besides lymph from the thoracic duct we collect lymph separately from the kidneys, the liver and the muscles of the hind limb. There are, in fact, large differences in permeability, as you can see from the different filtration coefficients for PVP of different molecular weights - we used PVP with molecular weights ranging from 10,000 to 650,000. Whereas the plasma-lymph

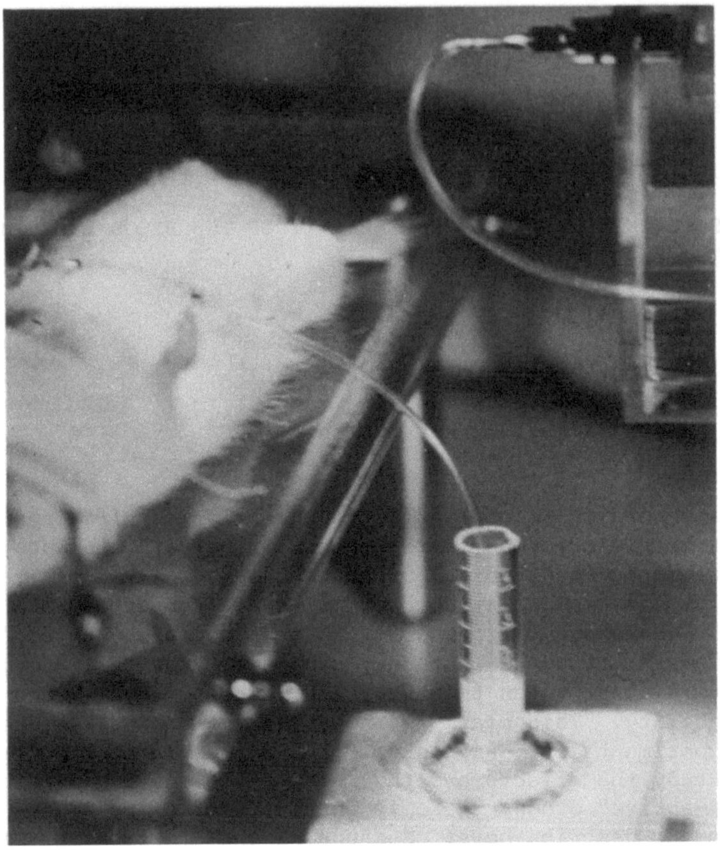

Fig. 1: Experimental arrangement for cannulation of the rat's thoracic duct. Above right: pump for continuous intravenous infusion of polyvinylpyrrolidone (PVP).

barrier of the hind limbs lets through only traces of PVP of molecular weight 38,000 (Fig. 2), the concentration of PVP 650,000 in liver lymph is 30% (Fig. 3) of the plasma level, and in lymph from the kidney it is as high as 40% (Fig. 4). This indicates that the plasma-lymph barrier in the liver and kidney must be "fenestrated". When we want to reproduce experimentally the permeability conditions existing in human inflammatory diseases we induce increased capillary permeability by systemic or local (intra-arterial) injection or infusion of the plasma kinins kallidin or bradykinin (Fig. 5 and 6). Normally this produces a 100% increase in lymph flow from the rat's thoracic duct and from the rabbit's thoracic duct or hind limb. However, this is not true of the rabbit's kidney or liver. In these organs the permeability of the plasma-lymph barrier is

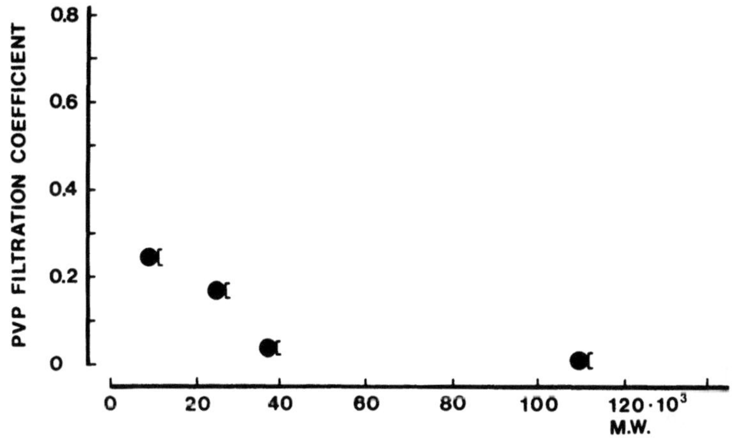


Fig. 2: Filtration coefficient of different batches of PVP of molecular weights 11,500, 25,000, 38,000, and 110,000 in the rabbit's hind limb. As only traces of PVP of molecular weight 38,000 and 110,000 were detected in the lymph, the filtration coefficient converges towards zero. Only PVP of molecular weight 11,500 and 25,000 is capable of penetrating the blood-lymph barrier in the hind limb.

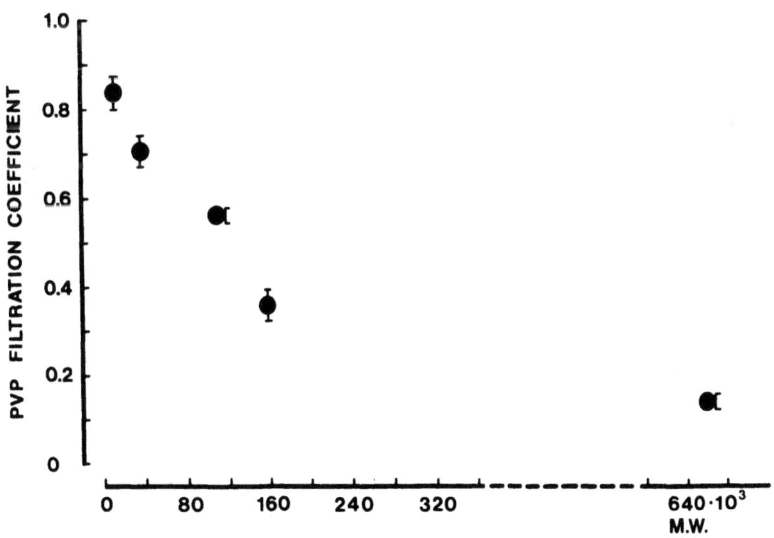


Fig. 3: Fig. 3 corresponds to Fig. 2. Determination of PVP filtration coefficient in the liver with supplementary measurements of the filtration coefficient of PVP of molecular weight 160,000 and 650,000. Low molecular weight PVP has a filtration coefficient of 0.7 to 0.8, but high molecular weight PVP - as shown by its filtration coefficient of 0.14 - also passes in measureable amounts through the blood-lymph barrier of the liver.

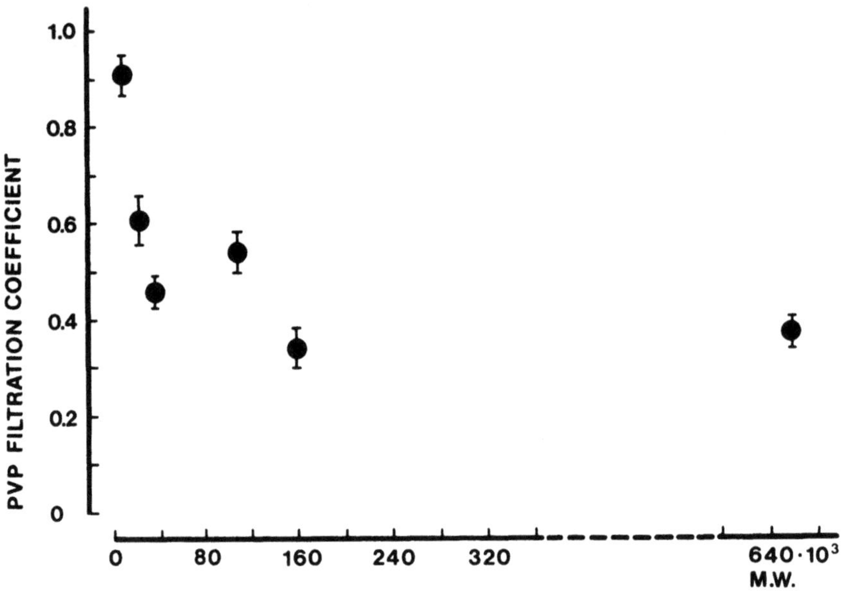


Fig. 4: Fig. 4 corresponds to Fig. 2. Determination of PVP filtration coefficient in the kidney. As shown by the experimentally high filtration coefficient of 0.37 for PVP of molecular weight 650,000, the permeability of the blood-lymph barrier in the kidney is even greater than in the liver.

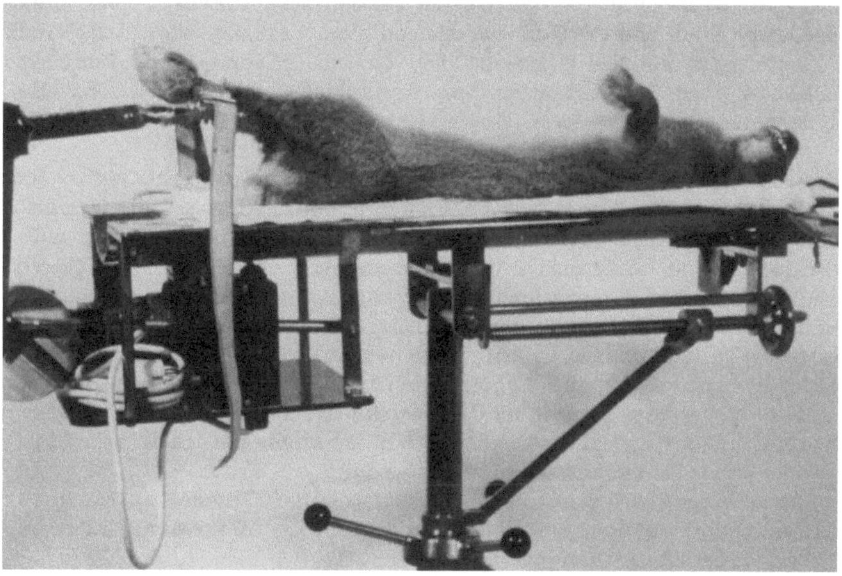

Fig. 5: Sight of the experimental arrangement for collecting lymph of the rabbit's hind limb. Passive movement of the hind limb because at rest lymph flow is too small.

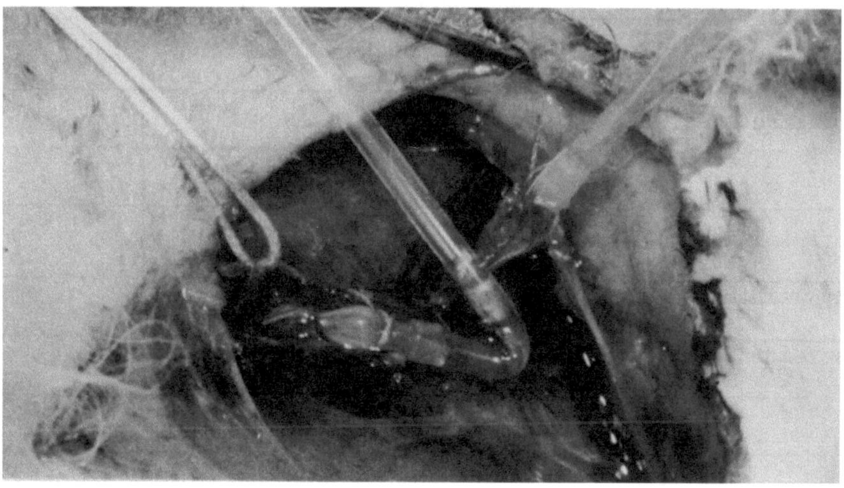

Fig. 6: Operating area for collecting lymph of the rabbit's hind limb. On the left: lymph vessel with cannula; on the right: cannula for intraarterial infusion of bradykinin.

evidently so high that it cannot be raised any further. We therefore believe that the method of choice for testing capillary-active drugs is to measure the permeability of the plasma-lymph barrier in the rabbit's hind leg after giving bradykinin to raise it to abnormal levels.

Bioflavonoids are often described as "capillary-active". When we measure lymph flow and PVP filtration coefficient in the rat's thoracic duct we find that bioflavonoids such as quercitrin and hyperoside have an intrinsic lymphagogue effect (Fig. 7). Quercitrin and naringin can antagonize the kallidin effect, but only in very high doses of 50 - 250 mg/kg (Fig. 8). Among the drugs which I have tested, the one with the most definite and pronounced "capillary-active" effect is the saponin escin extracted from horse-chestnuts. Even in doses as low as 0.3 mg/kg it largely neutralizes the lymphagogue effect of bradykinin, both in rats and rabbits (Fig. 9). When we remember that the molecular weight of escin - 1,184 - is nearly three times as great as that of the bioflavonoids in question, we realize that, molecule for molecule, escin is several hundred times more effective than they are.

| SUBSTANCE | Lymph Flow | | |
|---|---|---|---|
| | decreased | not altered | increased |
| Quercitrin | | | ++ |
| Quercetinrutinoside | | + | |
| Naringin | | + | |
| Hesperidinmethylchalcone | | + | |
| Diethylaminomethylrutin | | + | |
| Centaureidin | | + | |
| Hyperoside | | | + |

Fig. 7: Effects of various flavone glycosides on thoracic duct lymph flow in anaesthetized rats with an intact blood-lymph barrier.

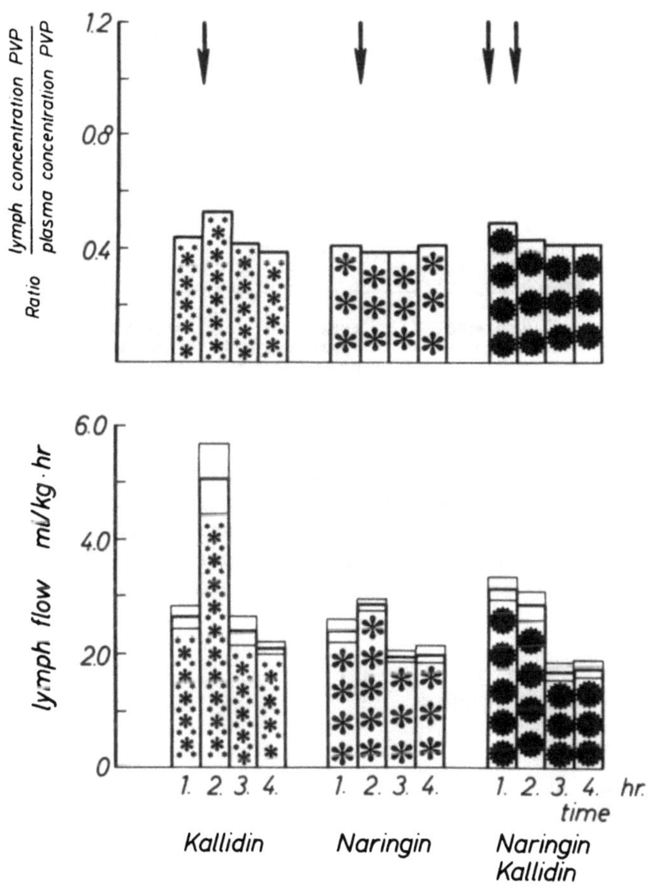


Fig. 8: Characteristic lymphogogue effect of kallidin as seen in the thoracic duct of anaesthetized rats (left-hand columns). Naringin has no significant effect on lymph flow or PVP filtration coefficients (middle columns). However, when naringin is given at the beginning of the experiment followed by an injection of kallidin 1 hour later (right-hand columns), the lymphagogue effect of kallidin fails to appear. Naringin has a quantitative antagonistic effect on kallidin.

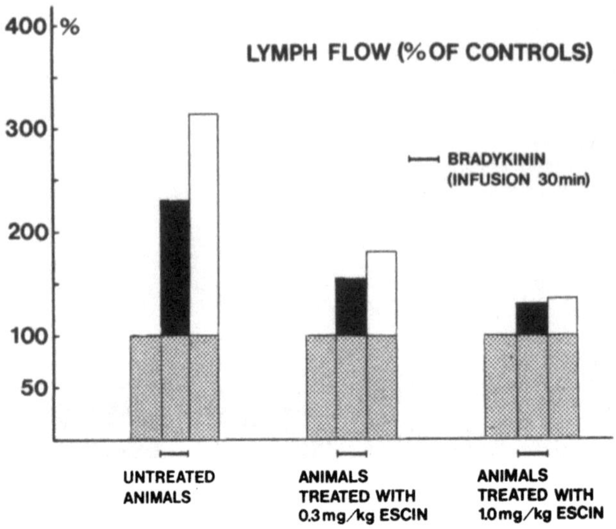


Fig. 9: Hind limb lymph flow in anaesthetized rabbits before, during and after intraarterial infusion of 100 mg/kg x min (periods of 30 minutes). Left-hand columns: untreated animals. Middle columns: animals pretreated intravenously with 0.3 mg/kg escin 1 hour before starting the experiment. Right-hand columns: animals pretreated intravenously with 1.0 mg/kg escin. Demonstration of the dose-dependent, antagonistic effect of escin on bradykinin.

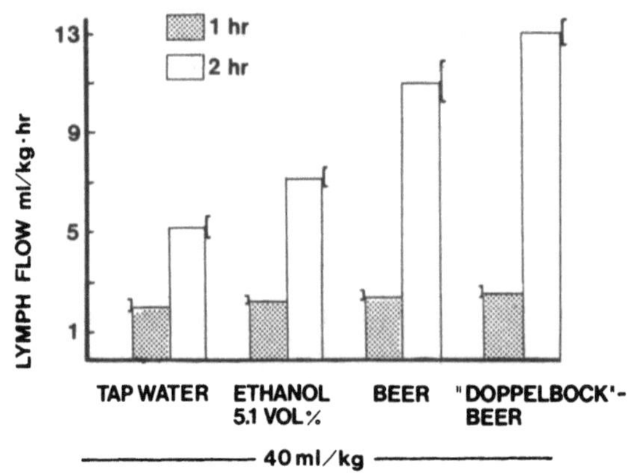


Fig. 10: Thoracic duct lymph flow in anaesthetized rats after intraduodenal administration of tap water, an ethanol/tap water mixture (with the same ethanol concentration as beer), Export-beer and Doppelbock-beer (a uniform dose of 40 ml/kg) over 1 and 2 hours. The power of beer to increase lymph flow is far greater than would be expected from its ethanol content. Beer must therefore contain one or more lymphagogue substances.

In conclusion let me draw your attention to a curious fact. Beer is a highly potent lymphagogue, and its effect is independent of its ethanol concent (Fig. 10). It is a first order lymphagogue in HEIDENHAIN's sense, in that it acts by increasing lymph production in the liver. Therefore, as convinced and faithful lymphologists you should abstain from whiskey and, if beer really cleanses the lymphatics of the liver, you will enjoy an entirely novel lymph sensation.

References

1. Vogel, G. und H. Strocker: Die Penetration von Polyvinylpyrrolidon durch die Plasma-Lymph-Schranke bei Ratten. Pflugers Arch. ges. Physiol. 279, 187 (1964)

2. Vogel, G. und H. Strocker: Uber eine neue Methode zur Beurteilung der Capillarpermeabilitat und deren Anderung durch Pharmaka - der Einflub von $Ca^{++}$ auf die Penetration von Polyvinylpyrrolidon durch die Plasma-Lymph-Schranke von Ratten. Naunyn-Schmiedebergs Arch. exp. Path. Pharmak. 247, 384 (1964)

3. Vogel, G. und H. Strocker: Gesteigerte Capillarpermeabilitat im tierexperimentellen Modell und ihre Beeinflussung durch Pharmaka. Naunyn-Schmiedebergs Arch. exp. Path. Pharmak. 251, 180 (1965)

4. Vogel, G., Lehmann, G., Meyering, E. und B. Wendt: Tierexperimentelle Untersuchungen zur lymphagogen, diuretischen und choleretischen Wirkung verschiedener Alkoholica. Arzneimittel-Forsch. 16, 673 (1966)

5. Vogel, G.: Uber eine bisher unbekannte biologische Wirkung von Bier - Steigerung der Produktion von Lymphe. Brauwissenschaft 19, 307 (1966)

6. Vogel, G.: Uber lymphagoge und andere Wirkungen verschiedener Alkoholica - experimentelle Untersuchungen an der weibem Laboratoriumsratte (Rattus rattus). Naunyn-Schmiedebergs Arch. Pharmak. exp. Path. 255, 88 (1966)

7. Vogel, G. und H. Strocker: Die Wirkung von Pharmaka - insbesondere von Flavonoiden und Aescin - auf den Lymphflub und die Permeabilitat der intakten Plasma-Lymph-Schranke von Ratten fur Flussigkeit und definierte Makromolekule. Arzneimittel-Forsch. 16, 1630 (1966)

8. Vogel, G. und H. Strocker: Regionale Unterschiede der Capillarpermeabilitat - Untersuchungen uber die Penetration von Polyvinylpyrrolidon und endogenen Proteinen aus dem Plasma in die Lymphe von Kaninchen. Pflugers Arch. ges. Physiol. 294, 119 (1967)

9. Vogel, G., Wendt, B. und H. Strocker: Versuche zur Wirkung von Pharmaka auf die Plasma-Lymph-Schranke von Ratten nach Einstellen eines Zustandes gesteigerter Kapillarpermeabilitat. Arzneimittel-Forsch. 17, 454 (1967)

10. Vogel, G.: Regionale Unterschiede der Capillarpermeabilitat - Untersuchungen uber die Penetration von Polyvinylpyrrolidon und endogenen Proteinen aus dem Plasma in die Lymphe von Kaninchen. Nauny-Schmiedebergs Arch. Pharmak. exp. Path. 257, 344 (1967)

11. Vogel, G. und M. Sass: Ein tierexperimentelles Modell gesteigerter Capillarpermeabilitat - Penetration von Polyvinylpyrrolidon durch die Plasma-Lymph-Schranke wacher Ratten im Dextran-Schock. Naunyn-Schmiedebergs Arch. Pharmak. Exp. Path. 258, 123 (1967)

12. Gartner, K., Vogel, G. und M. Ulbrich: Untersuchungen zur Penetration von Makromolekulen (Polyvinylpyrrolidon) durch glomerulare und postglomerulare Capillaren in den Harn und die Nierenlymphe und zur Grobe der extravasalen Umwalzung von $^{131}$J-Albumin im Interstitium der Niere. Pflugers Arch. ges. Physiol. 298, 305 (1968)

13. Vogel, G. und M. Ulbrich: Untersuchungen zur quantitativen Charakterisierung der Permeabilitat von Capillaren verschiedener Korperregionen des Kaninchens. Naunyn-Schmiedebergs Arch Pharmak. exp. Path. 260, 214 (1968)

14. Vogel, G., Ulbrich, M. und K. Gartner: Uber den Austausch des extravasalen Plasma-Albumins ($^{131}$J-Albumin) der Niere mit dem Blut und den Abflub von Makromolekulen (Polyvinylpyrrolidon) mit der Nierenlymphe bei normaler und durch Furosemid gehemmter tubularer Reabsorption. Pflugers Arch. 305, 47 (1969)

15. Vogel, G., Marek, M.-L. und R. Oertner: Untersuchungen zum Mechanismus der therapeutischen und toxischen Wirkung des Robkastanien-Saponins Aescin. Arzneimittel-Forsch. 20, 699 (1970)

16. Vogel, G.: Nachweis, dab zwischen Capillarfragilitat und -permeabilitat keine Korrelation besteht. Naunyn-Schmiedebergs Arch. Pharmak. 266, 471 (1970)

17. Vogel, G.: The effects of drugs of plant origin on capillary permeability and the lymphatic system. In: H. Wagner and L. Horhammer (Ed.) : Pharmacognosy and Phytochemistry, 1. Int. Cong. Munich 1970, p. 370. Springer, Berlin-Heidelberg-New York 1971

18. Vogel, G.: Gambrinologie - oder die Wissenschaft von den Wirkungen des Bieres. Bild der Wissenschaft 8, 228 (1971)

19. Vogel, G.: The pharmacology of the lymph and the lymphatic system. In: H. Meessen (Red.): Lymphgefass-System. Handbuch der allgemeinen Pathologie, Bd. III/6, p. 363. Springer, Berlin-Heidelberg-New York 1972

# THE EFFECT OF HYDERGINE® ON SPONTANEOUS AND BRADYKININ-STIMULATED LYMPH FLOW IN DOGS

E. Sturmer

Department of Pharmacology, Medical and Biological Research Division, Sandoz Ltd., Basle, Switzerland

By way of an introduction, I would first like to show you a scheme of the peripheral vasculature.

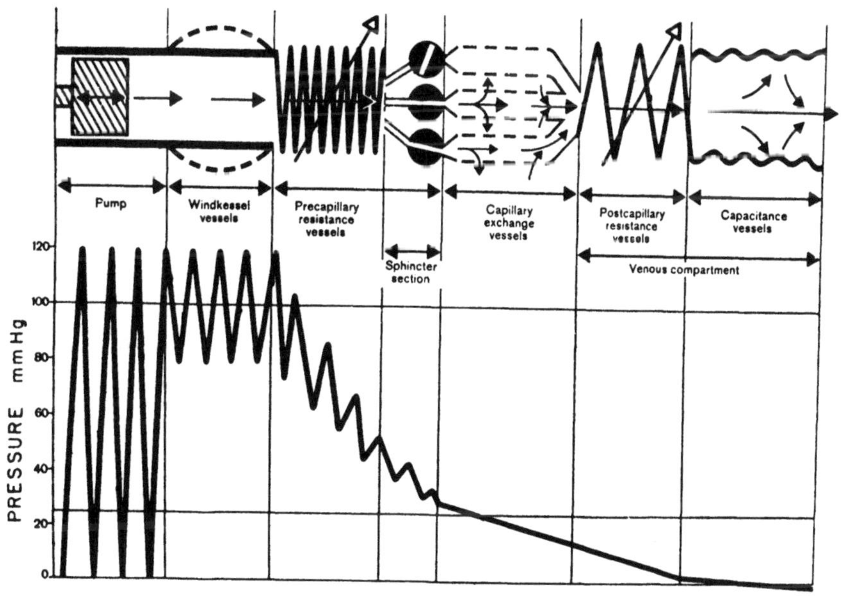


Fig. 1: Schematic illustration of the functionally differentiated consecutive sections of the vascular bed and the pressure profile along the circuit (from Mellander, S. and Johansson, B. {1968}).

You see the different consecutive functional sections beginning with the left ventricle, the Windkessel-vessels, the pre- and post-capillary resistance vessels, the capillary bed and the capacitance vessels. Each of the sections has a specialized function (see review by Mellander and Johansson, 1968). The effect of drugs on these different sections can be measured by use of a method described in 1960 by Mellander. Hydergine®, the dihydrogenated ergotoxine, displays, according to Owen and Sturmer, an unique pattern of activity:

It causes dose-dependent constriction of the capacitance vessels (Fig. 2), dose-dependent dilation of the pre-capillary sphincter vessels (Fig. 3) without significantly altering the tone of the resistance vessels (Tab. 1). These changes do not alter tissue blood flow, but increase the capillary surface area available for filtration and increase venous return to the heart.

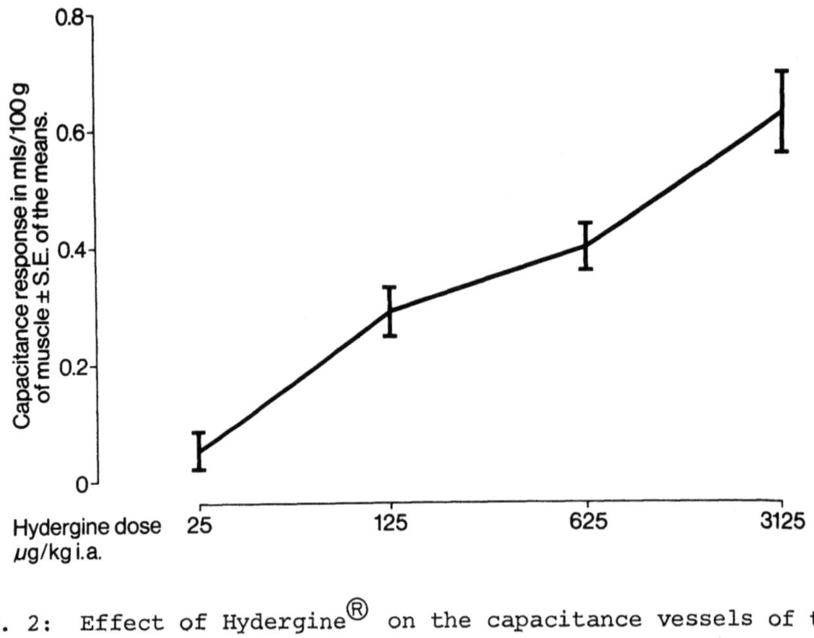


Fig. 2: Effect of Hydergine® on the capacitance vessels of the acutely denervated cat calf muscle. Abszissa: Hydergine dosage in µg/kg muscle (intra-arterial injection); ordinate: decrease in capacitance in mls/100 g muscle. Each point represents the mean value of 5 experiments ± S.E.

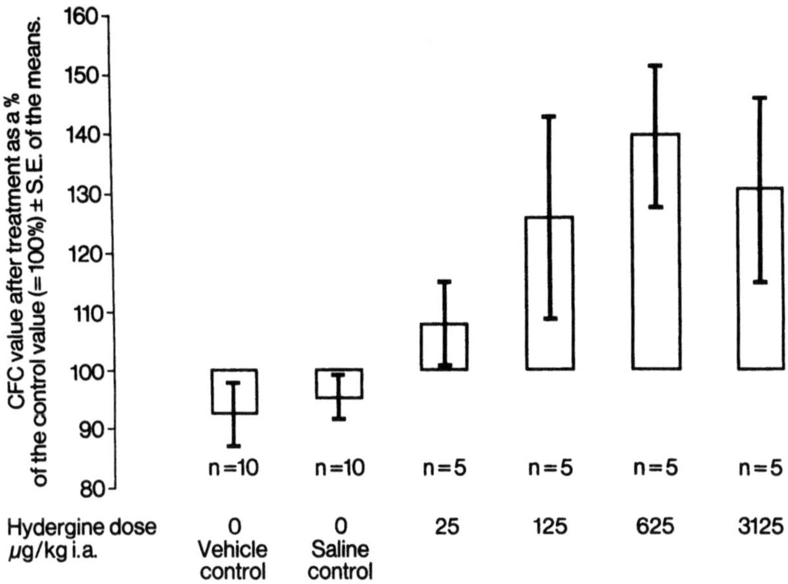


Fig. 3: Effect of Hydergine® on the precapillary filtration coefficient value (CFC). Hydergine® caused a dose-dependent increase in the CFC values i.e. the capillary area available for exchange was increased, indicating precapillary sphincter dilation. * = p<0,05: ** = p<0,01.

Table 1: Change in resistance of the denervated vascular bed of cat skeletal muscle after Hydrgine® and in control experiments with saline and with Hydrgine® vehicle.

| | *n* | Resistance response as a % of control resistance (= 100%) Mean ± S.E. | P |
|---|---|---|---|
| Saline 0.1 ml | 10 | 100.1 ± 0.3 | n.s. |
| Hydergine vehicle[a] | 10 | 101 ± 1.5 | --- |
| Hydergine | | | |
| 25 μg/kg | 5 | 104.8 ± 3.0 | n.s. |
| 125 μg/kg | 5 | 110 ± 4.1 | n.s. |
| 625 μg/kg | 5 | 108 ± 2.7 | <0.05 |
| 3125 μg/kg | 5 | 106.6 ± 3.2 | n.s. |

[a] Vehicle administered in the same volume as that given at the Hydergine 3125 μg/kg dose level.

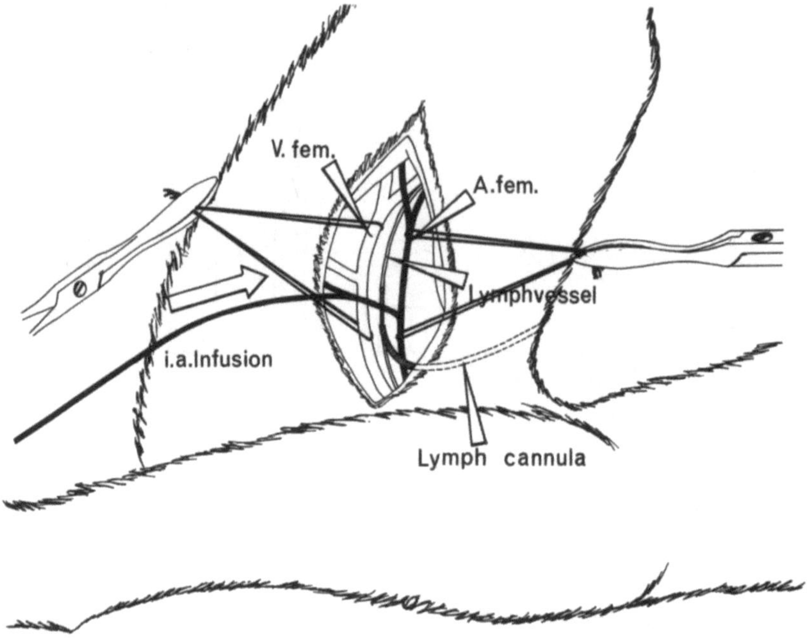


Fig. 4: Schematic illustration of the lymph vessels situated between femoral artery and vein in the fossa inguinalis of a dog.

An increase in capillary surface area would result in an increased lymph flow. We, therefore, investigated the effect of Hydergine® on lymph flow in dogs.

After the cannulation of a suitable lymph vessel, we carefully tied the remaining lymphatics in order to collect the lymph from the entire leg. All drugs were given by infusion into the first side branch of the femoral artery.

By cycling the leg by means of a rotating disc, a steady state of spontaneous lymph flow was achieved (Fig. 5). Furthermore, bradykinin-induced increase in lymph flow was both reproduceable and reversible. A typical experiment is shown in Fig. 6. The abscissa gives the sampling periods, each comprising 15 minutes, the ordinate the lymph flow in mg/min, and the black bars represent the intra-arterial infusions of bradykinin or normal saline over a

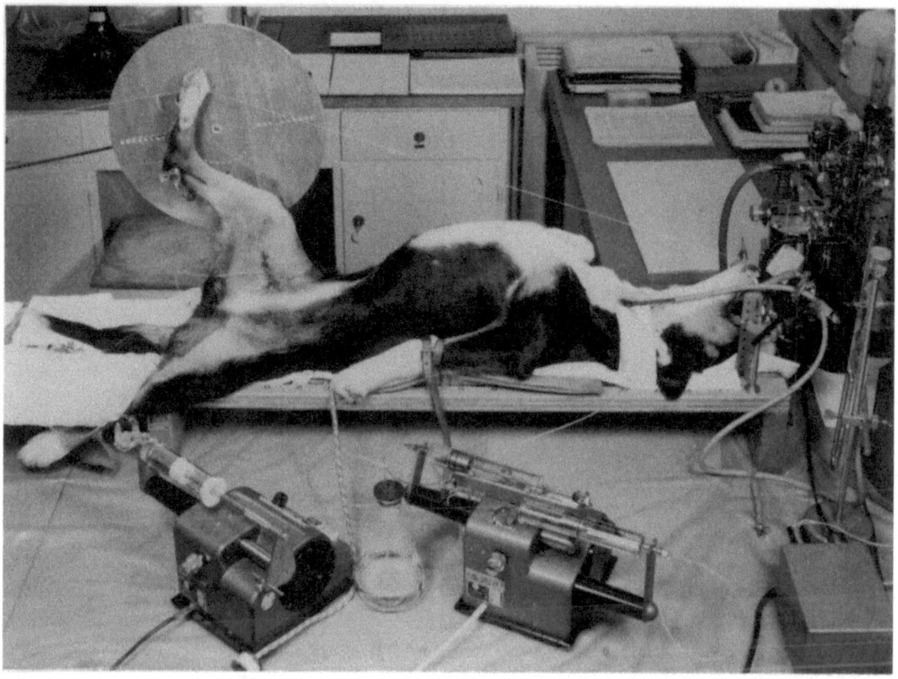

Fig. 5: The experimental set-up (notice the rotating disk cycling the leg).

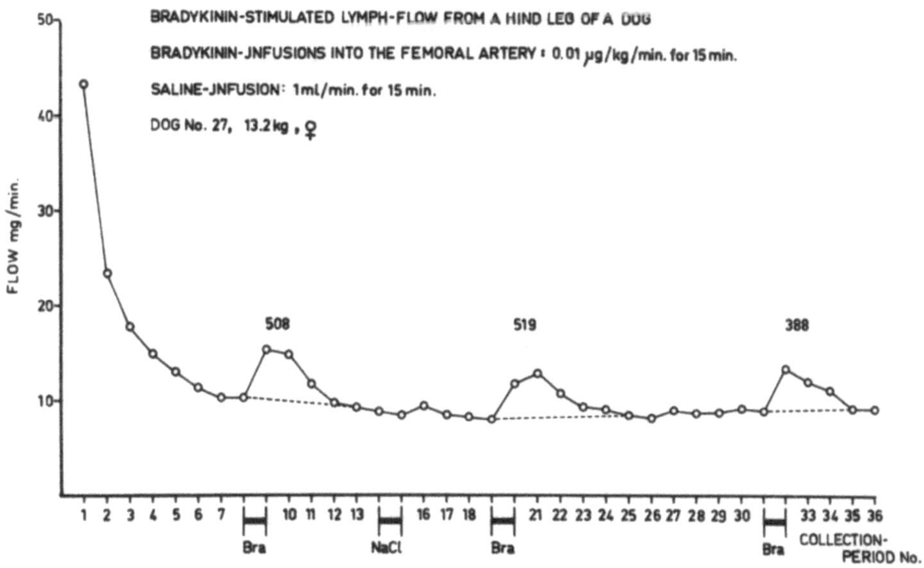


Fig. 6 : A typical experiment.

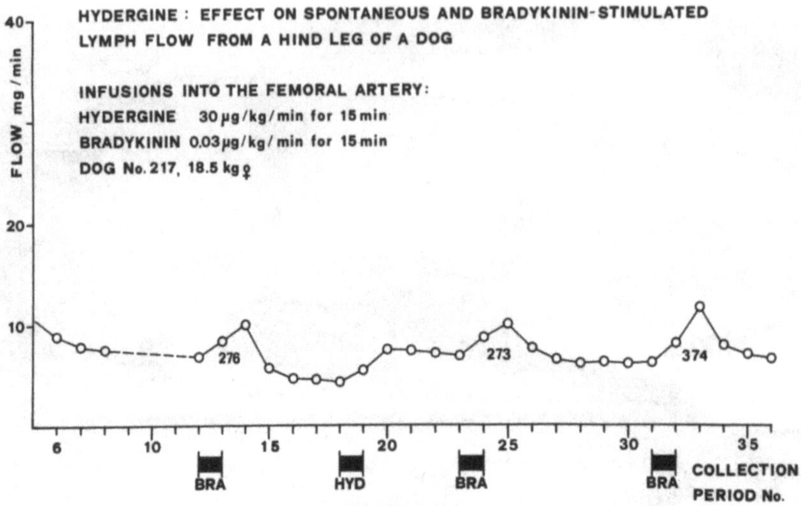


Fig. 7: A graph of a typical experiment. You see a fairly good steady state lymph flow, then the reversible increase after bradykinin infusions. And then comes the increase during and after the intra-arterial infusion of Hydergine®, which lasts more than 4 hours. The stimulating effect of bradykinin after Hydergine® administration is not significantly altered in that experiment.

15 minute-period. The figures represent the square area under the peaks (for details see Sturmer, E. and Cerletti, A., 1966).

What happens to spontaneous and bradykinin-stimulated lymphflow when we replace the saline-infusion by Hydergine®?

Table 2 shows that Hydergine® increases spontaneous lymph flow dose-dependently within a certain dose range. The threshold level lies between 0.1 and 5 µg Hydergine®/kg/min. A maximum is reached with 10 µg/kg/min, and increasing the dose further results in a decreasing effect which is probably due to the depressor effect of recirculating Hydergine®. The bradykinin-stimulated lymph flow is not altered significantly up to 5 µg/kg/min and after 30 µg/kg/min. Only after 10 µg/kg/min do we observe an increase which was statistically significant.

The reported results fit well into the picture of our present knowledge of the mode of action of Hydergine® on peripheral vasculature. If Hydergine® increases the capillary filtration area by decreasing the tone of precapillary sphincters without changing resistance as shown in the cat, it is expected to increase lymph flow.

Table 2: Hydergine® effect on spontaneous and bradykinin-stimulated lymph-flow from dog hind legs.

| Hydergine µg/kg/min for 15 min i.a. Infusion | Lymph Flow Δ% spontaneous | Δ % Bradykinin stimulated 60 min | 180 min |
|---|---|---|---|
| saline | +6 ±5 (6) | -14 ±34 (6) | -43 ±44 (6) |
| 0.1 | -8±35 (6) | -20 ±40 (6) | -6 ± 86 (5) |
| 5 | +31 ±12** (6) | -17 ±42 (5) | -22 ± 29 (3) |
| 10 | + 54 ±26*** (4) | +124±116* (4) | + 97 ± 74** (3) |
| 30 | +33 ±21*** (7) | - 39 ±45 (7) | +62±160 (3) |
| ( ) = n *p=<0.05 **p=<0.01 ***p=<0.001 | | | |

That that is the case is now shown in another species, the dog, using a different method. Increasing capillary surface area and lymph flow would improve tissue perfusion. The mean diffusion distance from the capillaries to the cells decreases together with blood flow velocity through the capillary bed leading to an increase in the time available for exchange processes.

It might be that the improvement of transcapillary exchange combined with the increased clearing of lymph contributes to the beneficial effects of Hydergine® in elderly patients.

References

1. Mellander, S.: Comparative studies on the adrenergic neurohormonal control of resistance and capacitance vessels in the cat. Acta physiol. scand. 50, suppl. 176, 1-86 (1960).

2. Mellander, S. and Johansson, B.: Control of resistance, exchange and capacitance functions in the peripheral circulation. Pharmacol. Rev. 20, 117-196 (1968).

3. Owen, D.A.A. and Sturmer, E.: The effects of Hydergine on acutely denervated cat skeletal muscle vasculature. Naunyn-Schmiedeberg's Arch. Pharmacol. 272, 395-401 (1972).

4. Sturmer, E. and Cerletti, A.: The effect of drugs on spontaneous and bradykinin-stimulated lymph flow in dogs. In: Intern. Symp. on Vasoactive Polypeptides: Bradykinin and Related Kinins (Rib. Preto, 1966), Edart, S. Paulo, 1967, pp. 73-80.

# LYMPHATIC DRAINAGE OF THE INNER EAR

C. V. Ilberg and W. Arnold

Universitat Hals-Nasen-Orenklinfk

6 Frankfurt/Main, West Germany

The sensory hearing organ is surrounded by two fluid compartments containing endolymph and perilymph. These fluids have different ionic composition and function. As we demonstrated recently, the perilymph space is connected with cerebrospinal fluid by different pathways.

1. aquaeductus cochleae
2. along the VIIIth. cranial nerve sheath

Consequently we were able to introduce in our experiments tracer substances into the closed fluid system of the inner ear, to study resorption and anatomical relation of its fluid spaces. As tracer substances we used indian ink, different dyes for histology and Thorium dioxyde for electronmicroscopy. The experimental animal was the guinea pig.

Within a few seconds after injection into the cisterna cerebellomedullaris all tracers were found in the perilymph space. This space includes the sensory organ itself. No tracer could enter the endolymphatic space. The tracer substances left the inner ear:

1. by micropinocytosis across the inner ear capillary endothelium,
2. along the round window membrane and spread out under the middle ear mucosa.

Here the tracer was taken up by the lymph vessels of the middle ear mucosa. After more than 30 minutes incubation, the tracer crosses the middle ear mucosa by cytopempsis and can be observed in the middle ear cavity.

Conclusion. 1) A close relationship between cerebrospinal fluid and perilymph spaces exists; 2) resorption of perilymph occurs not only at the level of the capillary system of the inner ear. A large amount of perilymph seems to leave inner ear spaces along the structures of the round window entering thus the submucosal space of the middle ear. Here the fluid is taken up by lymph vessels, which transport the tracer further to the lymph nodes of the neck. (As is described in the paper of Dr. Arnold: "Connections of the cerebrospinal fluid to the lymphatic system of head and neck") and 3) we have not obtained any information on reabsorption of endolymph as yet.

# THE CONNECTIONS OF THE CEREBROSPINAL FLUID (CSF) WITH THE LYMPHATIC SYSTEM OF HEAD AND NECK

W. Arnold and C. V. Ilberg

Johann Wolfgang Goethe Universitat

Frankfurt, West Germany

Numerous ear, nose and throat complaints indicate to the clinician that the lymphatic system of head and neck must depend to a certain degree on the cerebrospinal fluid - one need only think of the labyrinthine hydrops in Meniere's disease, of the various still completely unclear causes of spontaneous oto- and rhinoliquorrhea, of conducted otitis interna, or of Foldi's lymphogenic encephalopathy. We have therefore in animal experiments carried out morphological and kinetic investigations of the main connections between cerebrospinal fluid and the lymphatic system. The results were as follows: 3 minutes after intrathecal injection of 50 μl Thorotrast (applied completely without pressure), an x-ray of the skull of a guinea pig shows the spread of the contrast medium along the subarachnoidal space.

One however also finds that the CSF drains off the periphery in the olfactory region, in the region of the ear and along the optic nerve. Ten minutes later, one observes contrasting shadows on a lateral radiogram of the neck; these are lymph nodes.

If one injects trypan blue into the CSF, large areas of the olfactory mucous membrane, the perilymphatic basis of the cochlea and the mucous lining of the middle ear are immediately discolored.

The exposed situs of the neck of a living guinea pig shows increasing discoloration of the lymph vessels and lymph nodes 5 minutes after intrathecal application of a dilute colorant solution.

Histological sections reveal that the discolored CSF passes along the perineural spaces of the fila olfactoria and through the lamina cribriformis to under the olfactory mucous membrane and is absorbed into the lymph vessels from here. Shortly afterwards, it can be detected in all lymph vessels of the mucous lining of the nose and epipharynx.

The passage of the CSF through the inner ear is along the usually wide-open aquaeductus perlymphaticus sive cochleae and along the perineural space of the acoustic nerve, but also via the perineural space of the facial nerve to the perilymph spaces of the inner ear. From there, it drains via the lymph spaces of the round window membrane into the lymphatic system of the middle ear's mucous lining.

Cellular elements can also pass from CSF into the lymphatic system of the head and neck, although this occurs somewhat more slowly. One to 2 days after injection of Yoshida ascites tumor cells into the CSF, these can also be detected in the lymphatic system of the mucous linings of the middle ear and of the nose. In the perilymph spaces of the inner ear, they distribute themselves in the same way as the stain particles, in the scala tympani et vestibuli. Sarcomatous changes in the lymph nodes of the neck are detected after three days.

Our kinetic investigations with radioactive gold and dihydrostreptomycin show that the neck lymph nodes and the topographic regions through which the CSF drains contain the highest tissue concentrations of these substances. These concentrations are not reached after paraneural (intravenous or intramuscular) application. Finally, we made the detection of haemosiderin in the neck lymph nodes of patients who had died of recidivative subarachnoidal hemorrhage. In conjunction with the investigations of Key and Retzius, Yoffey, Courtice and Foldi, this should confirm that CSF drains very rapidly and without cellular control into the lymphatic system. Unfortunately, not enough clinicians are aware of these very important physiological facts, although it is apparent that they can play a considerable role in the pathogenesis of many neurotropic infectious diseases.

Curiously enough, Galenos, personal physician to Marcus Aurelius (160 B.C.), believed that the brain floats in a fluid which slowly drips away through the nose.

# LYMPHATIC TRANSPORT OF MELANOSOMES FROM THE TISSUE TO THE LYMPH NODE. AN ELECTRON MICROSCOPIC STUDY

Moriya Ohkuma

Electron Microscopic Laboratory, Department of Dermatology

Tokyo Medical and Dental University Yushima, Tokyo, Japan

Deposit of melanin-like particles in the lymph node of the healthy and diseased human as well as lipomelanic reticulosis of the lymph node associated with the various skin diseases have been reported by many investigators. This experiment was aimed to explain how the melanin reaches the lymph node from the connective tissue. However melanosomes were not put into the skin but into the abdominal cavity of the mice, because the former might injure the lymphatic capillary inducing its changed permeability (1).

Method. Melanosomal fraction was obtained by homogenizing and ultracentrifuging the Harding-Passey mouse melanoma after high density gradient centrifugation (2). And its suspension in saline solution was injected into the abdominal cavity of the mice, followed by an intraaortal perfusion fixation (3). The diaphragm and its regional lymph nodes were investigated by the light and electron microscope. Blood smears taken from the right atrium of the heart were stained with Giemsa. For the control saline solution alone was injected instead of melanosomes. The melanosome pellet was fixed in vitro and examined by the electron microscope, too.

Result and discussion. The melanosomes in the tissue were identified, because they appeared to be the same as those in the melanosomal pellet, and also because no control specimens showed any such particles in the tissue. The free melanosomes as well as intracellular melanosomes located in the phagosome of the macrophage were observed in the abdominal cavity, in the connective tissue area of the diaphragm and in the lumen of the diaphragmatic lymphatic capillary (Fig. 1, 2). The melanosomes were also detected in the phagosome of the diaphragmatic mesothelium, of the endothelium of the diaphragmatic lymphatic capillary (Fig. 2) and of the reticulum cell

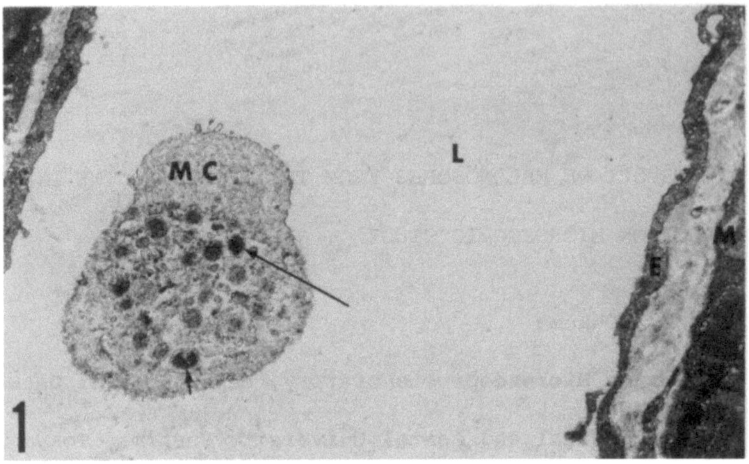


Fig. 1: Melanosomes are seen the phagosome of a macrophage found in the lymphatic lumen of the diaphragm. x 7,000 (MC: macrophage; L: lymphatic lumen; E: endothelium of the lymphatic capillary; M: muscle cell; and ↑: melanosome).

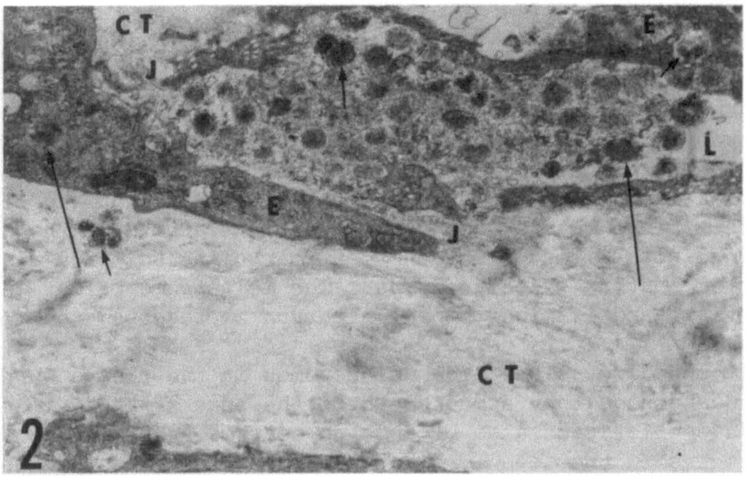


Fig. 2: A lymphatic capillary of the diaphragm with open junctions. The melanosomes are observed in the lymphatic lumen and endothelium as well as in the connective tissue area. x 10,500 (CT: connective tissue area; J: open endothelial junction; E: endothelium of the lymphatic capillary; L: lymphatic lumen; and ↑: melanosome).

of the lymph node. The manner by which the intralymphatic macrophage laden with melanin has entered from the connective tissue area of the diaphragm is not clear, although it is supposed to have entered through an open endothelial junction of the lymphatic capillary as Leak et al suggested (4). The melanin found in the lymph nodes and in the lymphatic lumina is considered to have reached there not by way of lymphatico-venous anastomosis via circulating blood, since blood smear has shown neither intra- nor extracellular melanin-like granules. The main pathway is thought to be the phagosome of the diaphragmatic lymphatic capillary, because no free melanosomes were located in the open endothelial junction, although it could happen, and also the melanin-laden macrophage occasionally found in the lymphatic lumen was not observed to be passing through the lymphatic wall.

Summary. Melanin in the connective tissue area is transported to the regional lymph nodes through the lymphatic channel as free melanosomes or melanin-laden macrophages. And its main pathway into the lymphatic capillary is the melanosome-containing phagosome of the lymphatic endothelium.

References

1. Ohkuma, M.: The fine structure and function of the injured lymphatic capillary after injection of saline solution. 3rd International Congress of Lymphology, Belgium, 1970.

2. Seiji, M., Shimao, K., Birbeck, M.S.C. and Fitzpatrick, T.B.: Subcellular localization of melanin biosynthesis. Annals of N.Y. Academy of Sciences, 100: 497, 1963.

3. Ohkuma, M.: Fine Structure and function of cutaneous and renal lymphatic capillary. Bullentin Tokyo Med. & Dent. Univ., 17: 103, 1970.

4. Leak, L.V. and Burke, J.F.: Electron microscopic study of lymphatic capillaries in the removal of connective tissue fluids and particulate substances. Lymphology, 1: 39, 1968.

# LYMPH AND TISSUE FLUID FLOW DEDUCED FROM MICROVASCULAR EXCHANGE PARAMETERS

M. Intaglietta

AMES-Bioengineering, University of California, San Diego

La Jolla, California 92037

Lymph is presumed to originate as a consequence of the imbalance between the filtration and absorptive mode of exchange at the level of blood capillaries. The factors which regulate this phenomenon are embodied in the so called Starling Hypothesis of fluid exchange. According to the commonly accepted interpretation of this theory exchange of fluid takes place at the level of blood capillaries, in such a fashion that at the arterial beginning, fluid filters out of the microcirculation, and is subsequently reabsorbed at the venous end by the osmotic effect caused by the plasma protein. According to this theory, therefore, the microcirculation has the functional properties of an osmometer. These concepts have been directly validated at the level of the microscopic exchange vessels of the frog by Landis (1927), and in mammals by Zweifach and Intaglietta (1968).

The major source of data on whether the dynamics of exchange processes described proceeds in such a fashion that capillary arterial filtration is balanced by venular reabsorption is provided by whole organ experiments, i.e. the so called isovolumetric and isogravimetric experiments. Neither in the microscopic, nor in the macroscopic experiments it has been attempted, to date, to characterize in quantitative terms what is the magnitude of the different exchange fluxes, and whether the filtration-absorption balance envisioned by Starling is compatible with the known rates of lymph flow.

The primary difficulty in attempting to quantitatively characterize exchange fluxes, is that these are intimately related to the amount of surface area available for exchange in the microcirculation. This parameter can only be unequivocally measured by means of direct intravital observations, and thus is only available from experiments where data is obtained directly at the microscopic level. Furthermore at the microscopic level, the exchange fluxes are not directly measurable, but must be inferred from measurements of related variables, such as the different pressures in the intraluminal compartments and the hydraulic conductivity of the capillary wall.

The necessary techniques and data have recently become available (see Intaglietta and Zweifach, 1973), and we are now in the position to relate exchange parameters to local quantitative geometrical properties. Furthermore, it is possible to translate observations in single capillaries to the functional behavior in whole organs by mathematical models (see Intaglietta and de Plomb, 1973).

One of the basic tenets of the hypothesis of fluid exchange is that the capillary hydraulic pressure is above colloid osmotic pressure in the arterial capillaries, and below, in the venular capillaries. To validate this concept we have made extensive surveys of pressure distribution in the mammalian microvasculature of the mesentery, omentum and skeletal muscle. These measurements, coupled with corresponding measurements of systemic blood plasma colloid osmotic pressure show that in more than 85 per cent of capillaries the hydraulic pressure of blood is higher than the plasma colloid osmotic pressure. As an example in the omentum of the rabbit, hyraulic and colloid osmotic pressures in capillaries are: 38-25, and 24-22 cm $H_2O$, respectively. In the cremaster muscle of the rat: 38-22 and 23-19 cm $H_2O$, respectively.

The capillary filtration coefficient has been functionally and quantitatively characterized by direct measurements in the microcirculation. Two basic facts emerge from these studies: 1) The capillary endothelium offers a comparatively high resistance to the passage of fluid; 2) There is a gradient of hydraulic conductivity, with increasing permeability towards the venous end. In fact, the conductivity of the venous endothelium is increased to the extent that plasma protein can leak through.

It is possible to summarize the above observations by defining an exchange perfusion parameter $R_{E/P}$ which relates the exchange flow in a capillary, i.e. the flux through the capillary due to the mechanism of exchange, to the local blood flow. The fluid filtered in a capillary where loss of fluid to the interstitium is the primary mode of exchange is given by the Landis-Zweifach relations:

$$m = \pi D\ L\ K\ \Delta P \qquad (1)$$

where m is the total fluid exchanged per unit time, D is the diameter. L is the capillary length, K is the permeability coefficient and $\Delta P$ is the net driving force for filtration (i.e. the average difference between hydraulic and colloid osmotic pressures, neglecting extravascular factors).

In the same capillary it is possible to either measure flow (see Wayland and Johnson, 1967) or to deduce it from the Poiseuille relation:

$$Q = \frac{\pi}{128} \frac{D^4}{L\mu} \Delta P^* \qquad (2)$$

where $\mu$ is the viscosity of blood and $\Delta P^*$ the net hyrostatic pressure difference between arterial and venous endings of the capillary. Dividing (1) by (2) and noting that $\Delta P^* \simeq 2\ \Delta P$ when the venous capillary pressure is approximately equal to the plasma colloid osmotic pressure, then the ratio (1) and (2) constitutes a dimensionless parameter: $R_{E/P}$ (termed exchange-perfusion parameter):

$$R_{E/P} = 64 \frac{K\mu L^2}{D^3} \qquad (3)$$

for muscle and omental capillaries this parameter is of the order of $3 \times 10^{-3}$. The significance of this value is that it indicates that plasma protein is not significantly concentrated due to the exchange processes in the microcirculation.

Combining the above finding with the results on direct capillary pressure measurements, and the fact that when filtration and absorption are tested directly in the capillaries absorption is seldom encountered (see Intaglietta and Zweifach, 1966), we are led to the possibility that venous capillary absorption is not a common fact in the microvascular beds investigated. Furthermore, it must be considered that this reabsorptive process is presumed to occur in the venous microcirculation, which is also believed to be the site of plasma protein leakage, and therefore is a region where in all probability the plasma proteins do not exert their full osmotic effect, thus further hindering the reabsorptive process.

The conclusion that can be drawn from the above considerations is that the methods of intravital microscopy do not validate the concept of venous capillary reabsorption of the fluid filtered in arterial microcirculation. As a consequence, since normal tissue is not aedematous, a major portion of the fluid which is filtered from the microcirculation must flow through the extravascular compartment and be collected by the lymphatic return.

The actual magnitude of this phenomenon can be estimated from the above given value of the $R_{E/P}$ parameter, namely that 0.3 per cent of the blood flowing through muscle and visceral tissue enters the lymphatic system, and presumably constitutes lymph flow.

References

1. Intaglietta, M. and Zweifach, B.W. (1966) Circulation Res. 19: 199.

2. Intaglietta, M. and de Plomb, E.P. (1973). Microvasc. Res

3. Intaglietta, M. and Zweifach, B.W. (1973). Adv. Med. Biol. Phys.

4. Landis, E.M. (1927). Amer. J. Physiol. 82: 217.

5. Wayland, H. and Johnson, P.C. (1967). J. Appl. Physiol. 22: 333.

6. Zweifach, B.W. and Intaglietta, M. (1968). Microvasc. Res. 1: 83.

REABSORPTION FROM THE RENAL PELVIS AND RENAL FUNCTION DURING TOTAL URETERAL OCCLUSION: AN EXPERIMENTAL STUDY IN DOGS

Kurt G. Naber and Paul O. Madsen

Section of Urology, Veterans Administration Hospital
and Department of Surgery, University of Wisconsin
Madison, Wisconsin

It has been clearly demonstrated that renal function, glomerular filtration as well as tubular secretion and reabsorption, continue following total obstruction of the ureter. It is postulated that continuing function is possible because of continuous reabsorption from the renal pelvis via lymph and/or blood vessels.

The reabsorption of various substances with low as well as high molecular weights, and even of bacteria has been demonstrated (1-5). No studies have, however, been carried out where two or more substances have been compared simultaneously in the same experiment. From such experiments, however, we could expect conclusions concerning the reabsorption mechanism and whether this mechanism is dependent upon physical or chemical properties. Since renal function during total ureteral occlusion and the reabsorption mechanism must be closely related, a method could be found to determine renal function during total ureteral obstruction.

Material and methods. Fourteen mongrel dogs were used in the first study. The left kidney was exposed through a flank incision and the ureter was tied off. The femoral artery and the renal vein was catheterized via the spermatic or ovarian vein. A hilar lymph vessel was cannulated with a 26 gauge needle connected to a silastic tubing. The renal pelvis was cannulated just below the ureteropelvic junction, but kept closed using a 3-way stopcock.

An accurately measured amount of urine (usually 1 ml) was removed from the renal pelvis and immediately replaced by the same volume of a known mixture of substances of varying molecular weights (Table 1). The concentration of these substances were followed at intervals in the artery, renal vein, lymph and urine. The urine

Table 1: Substances Compared in the Study

| Genertic Name | Trade Name | Manufacturer | Mol. Wt. |
|---|---|---|---|
| $^{99m}$Tc Pertechnetate | Technitium-99 | E.R. Squibb & Sons, New York, N.Y. | 163 |
| p-Aminohippurate | Sodium Aminohippurate | Merck, Sharp & Dohme, West Point, Pa. | 212 |
| Sulfamethoxazole | Gantanol | Hoffmann-LaRoche, Incl. Nutley, N.J. | 253 |
| $^{131}$I o-Iodohippurate | Hippuran-131 | Abbott La., North Chicago, Il. | 307 |
| Ampicillin | Omnipen-N | Wyeth La., Philadelphia, Pa. | 409 |
| Tobramycin | | Eli Lilly & Co., Indianapolis, Ind. | 519 |
| $^{125}$I Iothalamate | Glofil-125 | Abbott La., North Chicago, Il. | 583 |
| $^{169}$YbDTPA (diethylenetriamine Pentaacetic acid) | | Minn. Mining & Mfg. Co., St. Paul, Minn. | Approx. 600 |
| $^{99m}$Tc DTPA | Renotec | E.R. Squibb & Sons, New York, N.Y. | Approx. 600 |
| Inulin | | Arnas-Stone Lab., Inc., Mt. Prospect, Il. | Approx. 5000 |
| $^{131}$I Human Serum Albumin | RISA-131 | Abbott Lab., North Chicago, Il. | 69000 |
| $^{99m}$Tc Sulfur Colloid | Tesuloid | E.R. Squibb & Sons, New York, N.Y. | (50 to 150mμ) |

concentrations were measured by aspirating 0.3 ml of urine from the renal pelvis. In the last 9 experiments the urine in the renal pelvis was mixed immediately following the injection and again immediately before taking a sample by gently aspirating and replacing approximately 0.5 ml of urine with a tuberculin syringe. In all experiments but one, $^{125}I$ iothalamate was used as a reference substance and the concentration of this substance was compared to the other substances investigated.

Results and Discussion. In 10 out of 11 experiments the ratios between the concentrations of iothalamate in the renal vein and artery (Pv/Pa) were higher than one, sometimes only slightly but persistent. In 11 out of 13 experiments the ratios between the concentrations in the hilar lymph and the renal vein (L/Pv) were higher than one and less than one in 2 experiments.

Fig. 1 shows a representative example of an experiment comparing different substances of low molecular sizes. After the injection into the renal pelvis the rate of disappearance is very similar for all substances tested. After a second test injection the concentrations are almost equal to the ones following the first injection. The lymph concentrations are approximately 100 to 1000 times lower than the simultaneous urine concentrations, but approximately 10 times higher than the simultaneous plasma concentrations. The plasma concentrations in the renal vein are persistently higher than in the artery. The concentrations of all substances tested were found to be within the same range.

Fig. 2 shows an experiment comparing the absorption of iothalamate and $^{131}I$ albumin (RISA). A slightly higher rate of disappearance for RISA than that for iothalamate is remarkable. This phenomenon was observed in 3 further experiments and in experiments comparing iothalamate with $^{99m}Tc$ sulfur colloid. In order to trace this problem in 2 experiments $^{99m}Tc$ pertechnetate was injected into the renal pelvis in addition to the $^{125}I$ iothalamate and at the same time the dogs received a constant intravenous infusion of $^{131}I$ iothalamate. These two experiments showed that the difference of urine concentrations are caused by the different amount of recirculation of iothalamate with a high renal clearance and $^{99m}Tc$ pertechnetate with an almost negligible renal clearance under these circumstances.

From the simultaneous comparison of these substances of various molecular weights it can be concluded that all substances were absorbed from the renal pelvis at identical rates regardless of molecular sizes. A pyelovenous as well as a pyelolymphatic pathway, simultaneously active, could be demonstrated. Therefore, it can be concluded that there is a constant flow of urine leaving and entering the occluded renal pelvis.

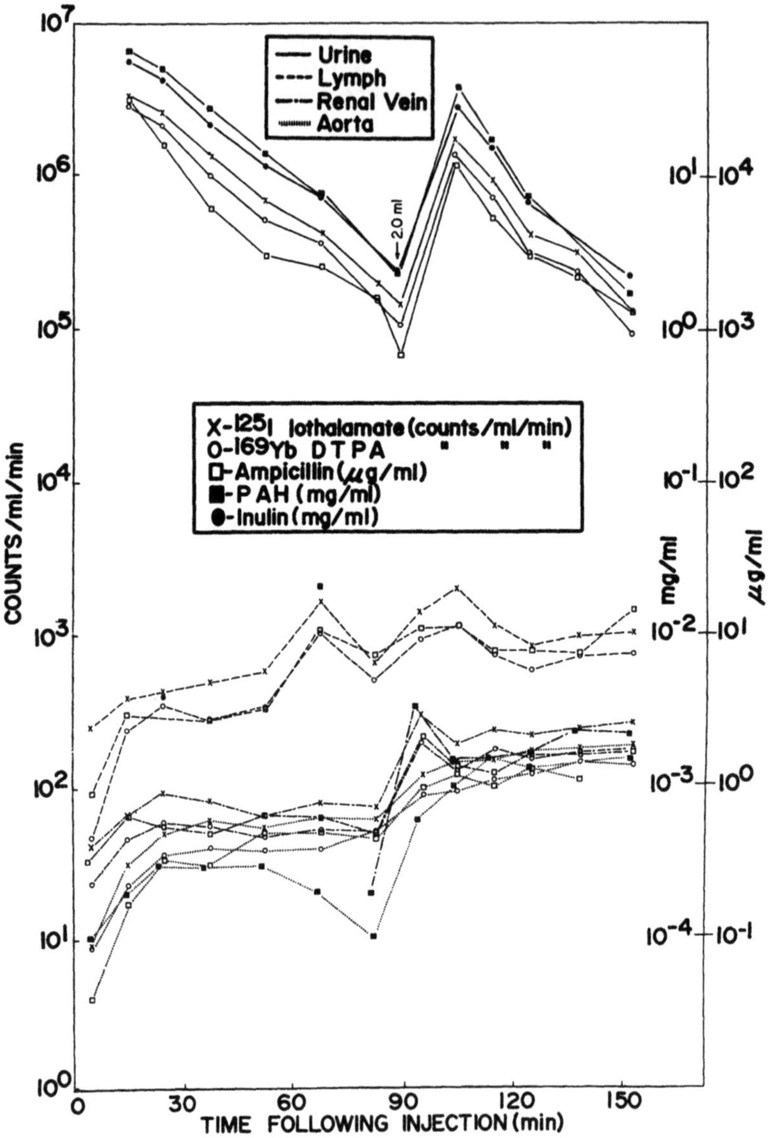


Fig. 1: Concentrations of various substances of low molecular weights in renal hilar lymph, renal vein and artery following injection of these substances into the occluded renal pelvis. The arrow indicates the second injection of the same amount.

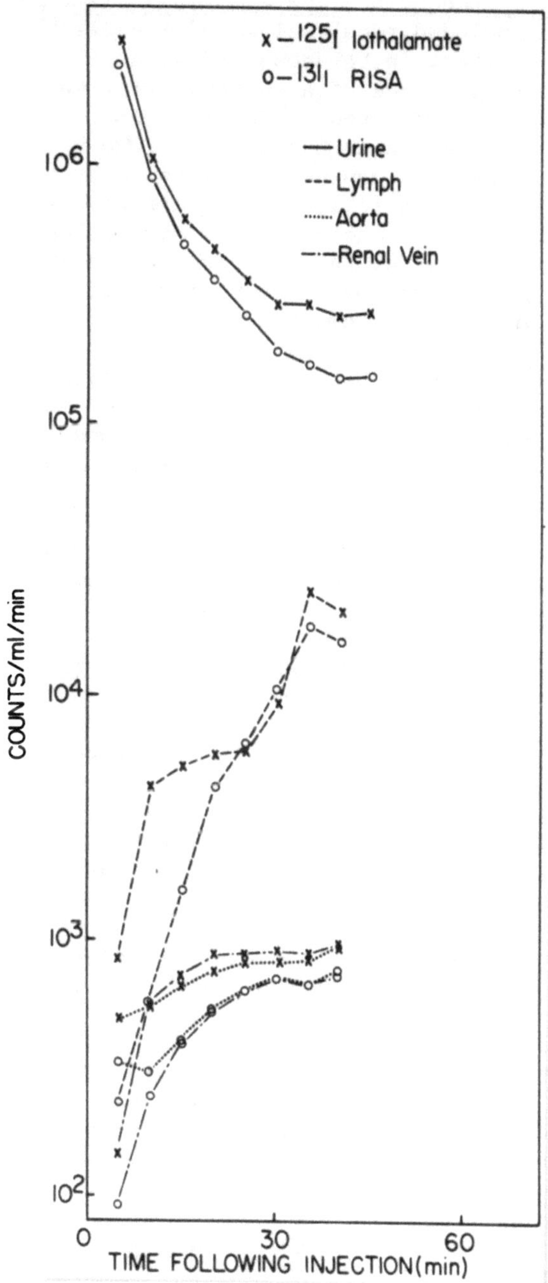


Fig. 2: Comparison of the absorption of $^{125}I$ iothalamate and $^{131}I$ serum albumin (RISA) following injection of these two substances into the occluded renal pelvis.

Calculation of the urine flow and renal clearance. The turnover rate in the occluded renal pelvis of any clearance substance administered by constant intravenous infusion can now be calculated by the rate of disappearance of a suitable test substance injected into the renal pelvis. We used $^{99m}Tc$ pertechnetate as test substance since its renal reexcretion is negligible. The urine concentration of the clearance substance can be determined from the same small urine sample necessary for following the disappearance of the injected test substance. The total volume of the renal pelvis can be considered as constant under these circumstances and can be measured from the distribution space of a known amount of a test substance injected and by direct measurement at the end of the experiment.

Material and Methods. We used this technique in 15 mongrel dogs in order to determine renal function during acute hydronephrosis The experiments were performed under steady state clearance conditions using $^{125}I$ iothalamate and $^{131}I$ o-iodohippurate as clearance substances.

The right kidney served as a control. Hilar and/or subcapsular lymph was collected from the left kidney continuously throughout the experiment. The left ureter was clamped after 6 control periods, each of 15 min. duration. The following 45 min. urine only from the right kidney was collected. After that, $^{99m}Tc$ pertechnetate was injected into the left renal pelvis and the urine concentrations were followed as mentioned above. Forty-five min. following the injection of the test substance 2 mg/kg of furosemide were administered intravenously and the procedure was continued for an additional 90 min. Three dogs received $^{99m}Tc$ pertechnetate intravenously by constant infusion together with the two other clearance substances in order to investigate the renal handling of $^{99m}Tc$ pertechnetate under these circumstances.

Results and discussion. The glomerular filtration rate as measured by the iothalamate clearance decreased in the occluded kidney to 13.7% and the effective renal plasma flow was measured by the o-iodohippurate clearance to 12.1%. The concentration ratio between urine and plasma (U/P) of iothalamate increased up to 125, indicating that 99.2% of the filtered fluid was reabsorbed. After intravenous injection of furosemide there was not only in the control but also in the obstructed kidney a reduction of tubular fluid reabsorption.

The total volume of the occluded renal pelvis was found to be on average 4.0 ml, the rate of turnover 1.4% of volume per minute and the urine flow 0.6 ml per minute.

The concentration of $^{99m}Tc$ pertechnetate injected into the occluded renal pelvis was far less than 1% of the urine concentration in hilar was well as in subcapsular lymph. The hilar lymph

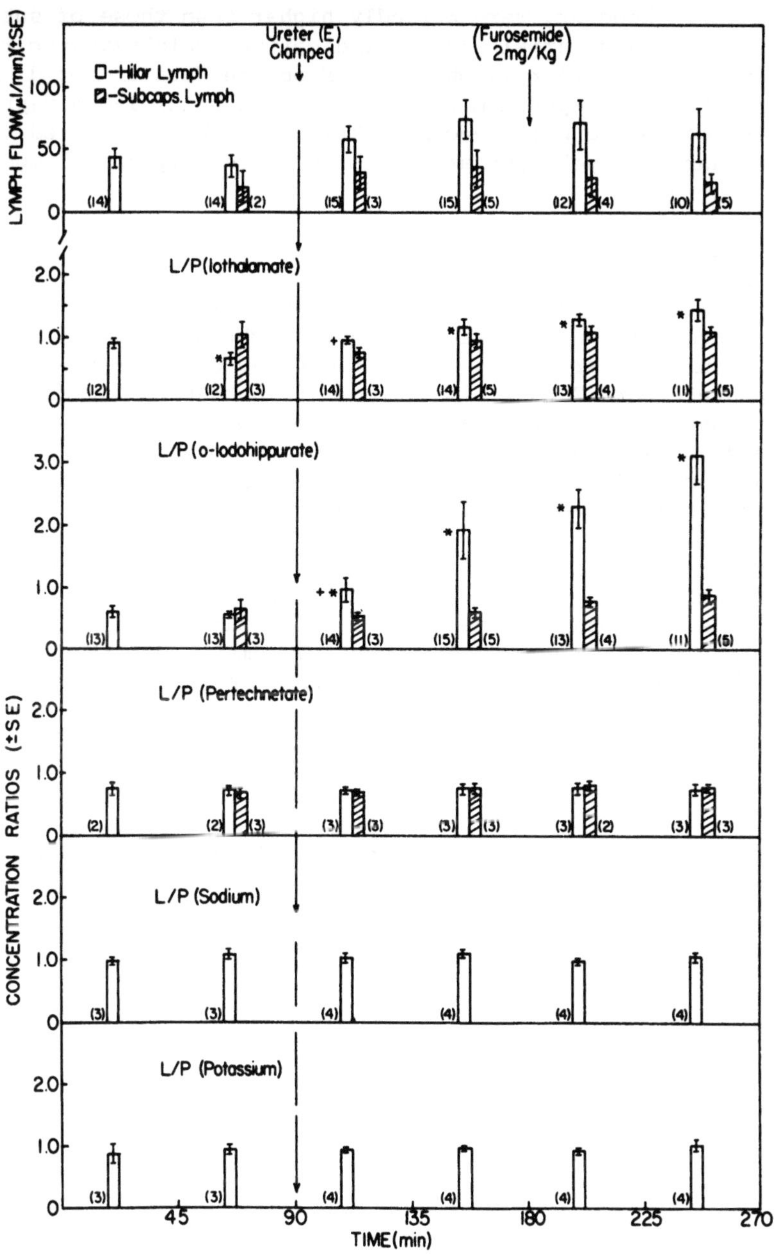


Fig. 3: Change in hilar and subcapsular lymph following acute total ureteral occlusion. L = lymph concentration, P = arterial plasma concentration. (n) = number of experiments, mean ± SE. * = significantly ($p < 0.05$) different from the control (first 45 min. value) + = significantly different from the preceding 45 min. period.

concentrations, however, were markedly higher than those of subcapsular lymph and arterial plasma, indicating pyelolymphatic reabsorption into the hilar lymphatics. From the data it could be calculated that only approximately 0.3% of the hilar lymph represents urine.* Therefore the pyelovenous backflow must be considered more effective than the pyelolymphatic, unless incredibly high lymph flow is assumed.

The effect of urine reabsorption into the hilar lymph can in addition be shown by the lymph concentrations of iothalamate and o-iodohippurate (Fig. 3). Following ureteral clamping there was a marked concentration increase of the two substances in hilar, but not in subcapsular lymph. Since the urine concentration of o-iodohippurate were 2 to 3 times higher than that of iothalamate, a sharper concnetration increase of o-iodohippurate in the hilar lymph could be expected. All substances with low urine concentrations, such as $^{99m}$Tc pertechnetate, sodium and potassium, did not show a significant change following ureteral occlusion.

In contrast to the hilar lymph no absorption of any substance from the renal pelvis into the subcapsular lymph could be demonstrated. The subcapsular lymph is therefore the only fluid compartment leaving the kidney under these circumstances without being influenced by the content of the renal pelvis.

*Similar results obtained by Heney et al (6) using a different technique.

References


1. Corriere, J.N., Jr., Lipschutz, L.I., Judson, F.N. and Murphy, J.J.: The use of $^{99m}Tc$ labeled sulfur colloid to study particle dynamics in the urinary tract. II. Routes of removal from the renal pelvis in normal and pyelonephritic kidneys. J. Urol (Baltimore) 103: 393, 1970.

2. Foldi, M., Papp, N. and Zoltan-Ors, Th.: Resorption von mit $J^{131}$ markiertem Serumalbumin aus dem Nierenbecken nach Ureterverschlub. Z. Ges. Exp. Med. 131: 440, 1959.

3. Goodwin, W.E. and Kaufman, J.J.: The renal lymphatics and hydronephrosis. Surg. Forum 6: 632, 1955.

4. Murphy, J.J. and Myint, M.K.: The renal lymphatics, II. Effect of increasing pressure in the renal pelvis upon absorption of substances of various molecular sizes. Surg. Forum 7: 661, 1956.

5. Rattner, W.H., Myint, M.K. and Murphy, J.J.: The route of transfer of bacteria from the renal pelvis to the circulating blood. Surgery 43: 298, 1958.

6. Heney, N.M., O'Morchoe, P.J. and O'Morchoe, C.C.C.: The renal lymphatic system during obstructed urine flow. J. Urol. (Baltimore) 106: 455, 1971.

# PROTEIN CONTENT OF GASTRIC LYMPH

T.M. Bruggeman

Department of Physiology, University of Michigan

Ann Arbor, Michigan 48104

Samples of pure gastric lymph have not been collected and analyzed previously for amount and type of protein (1). In the following experiments, a free hand micropuncture technique was used to obtain samples of canine gastric lymph which were analyzed for total protein and electrophoresed on both polyacrylamide and cellulose acetate systems.

Methods. Mongrel dogs were fasted overnight. Acepromazine 1 mg/kg body weight was given intramuscularly as a pre-anesthetic. The dogs were anesthetized with pentobarbitol given intravenously to effect.

Polyethylene catheters were inserted into the right femoral artery to obtain blood samples and into the right femoral vein to infuse drugs. In each dog, a tracheal cannula was inserted and the dog was artificially respirated.

The abdomen was opened by electric cautery and the greater curvature of the stomach was exposed. The diaphragm was cut to reduce the external forces causing movement of the stomach. Gastric lymphatics which run parallel to branches of the gastroepiploic artery were punctured. A siliconized micropipette with a sharpened beveled tip 75 microns inside diameter was inserted into the lymphatics between the point where they surface from the serosa of the stomach and the first lymph node.

Single lymph samples which ranged in size from .5 to 2 microliters were withdrawn by gentle suction. The total protein analysis was done on 75 nanoliters of lymph and plasma using a microadaptation of the Lowry method for total protein (2). To avoid the effects of evaporation of sample concentration, the lymph was collected in oil filled pipettes and the micropipetting during analysis was done under oil. A Beckman Microzone System was used for the cellulose acetate and polyacrylamide gel electrophoresis. Densitometry tracings of stained cellulose acetate patterns were quantitated by planimetry.

Results. In seven control studies the mean lymph protein concentration is 4.1 gm%, the mean plasma protein concentration is 6.2 gm%, giving a L/P ratio of .66. The standard deviations are shown in Figure 1.

The polyacrylamide gel electrophoresis of both lymph and plasma samples gives 12 discrete bands. Even with high resolution polyacrylamide gel electrophoresis, all the bands present in plasma are also present in gastric lymph.

The cellulose acetate electrophoresis gives 6 bands for plasma and lymph. Densitometry tracings of typical banding patterns of plasma and gastric lymph are shown in Figure 2. Table 1 gives the results of planimetry quantitation of cellulose acetate densitometry tracings in 4 dogs. The mean albumin concentration is 1.79 gm % in lymph and 2.32 gm % in plasma, giving a L/P ratio of .77 for the low molecular weight albumin. On the other hand, the mean fibrinogen concentration is .43 gm % in lymph and 1.26 gm % in plasma, giving a L/P ratio of .34. One would expect the difference in the albumin and fibrinogen L/P ratios on the basis of molecular sieving (3).

In four dogs, 50 μ histamine base/kg hr was infused intravenously. This dose and route of histamine administration causes maximal gastric secretion in dogs (4). We wished to test if gastric secretion affected the concentration of protin in gastric lymph. Figure 3 shows the results of analysis of individual samples. Samples from the same dog are connected by straight lines. Obtaining samples is still a limiting factor in these experiments, therefore there is not a sample at every time interval for every dog. No single pattern of change in protein concentration in lymph discernible. Histamine infusion causes an increased blood flow, to the gastric mucosa (5). The decrease in lymph protein concentration may be due to an increased filtration associated with increased blood flow, vasodilation and increased capillary pressure. On the other hand, gastric secretion is in essence the movement of a relatively protein free fluid into the lumen of the stomach (6). The increase in protein concentration in the lymph may be the direct result of gastric secretion decreasing the interstial volume.

Summary. In summary, pure gastric lymph samples have been collected. The mean total protein concentration in gastric lymph is 4.2 gm % with a L/P ratio of .66. When separated by polyacrlyamide

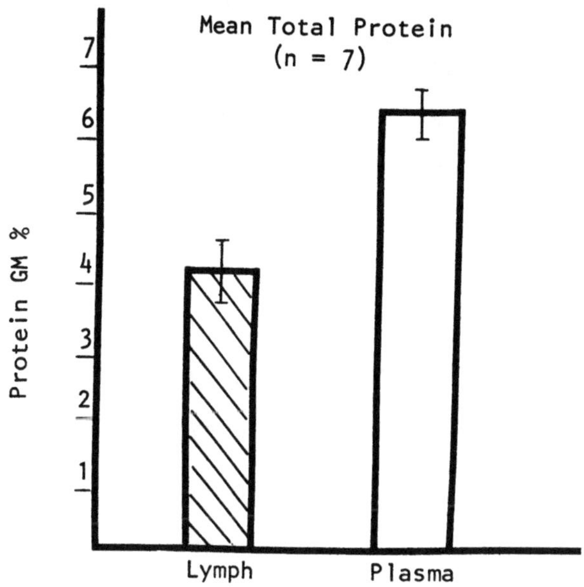


Fig. 1: Protein concentration in control gastric lymph and plasma. Standard deviations shown.

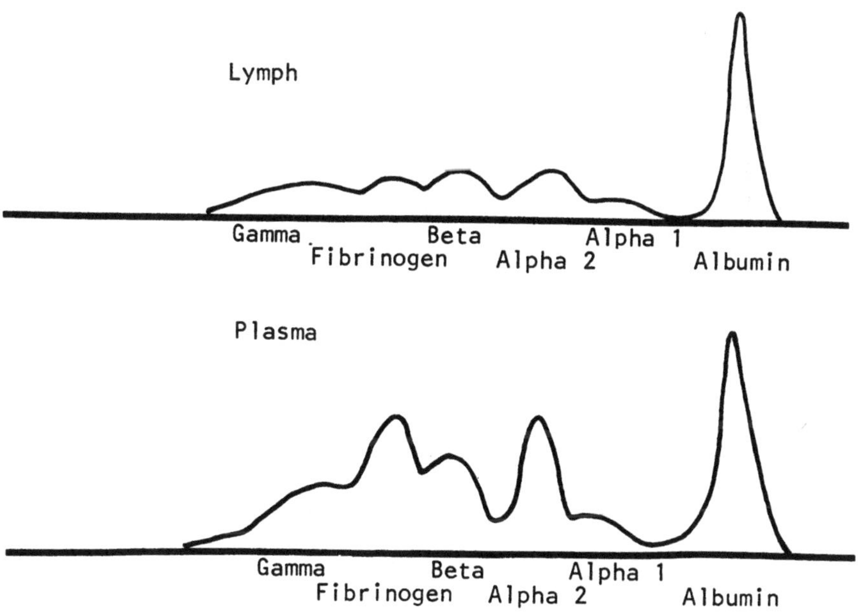


Fig. 2: Densitometry tracings of typical cellulose acetate banding patterns of control gastric lymph and plasma.

Table 1: Planimetry quantitation of cellulose acetate electrophoresis of control gastric lymph and plasma (n = 4)

| | Cellulose Acetate (n = 4) | | |
|---|---|---|---|
| Protein | Plasma gm% | Lymph gm% | L/P Ratio |
| Albumin | 2.32 | 1.79 | .78 |
| Alpha 1 | 0.26 | 0.15 | .60 |
| Alpha 2 | 0.69 | 0.60 | .88 |
| Beta | 1.02 | 0.57 | .56 |
| Fibrinogen | 1.26 | 0.43 | .34 |
| Gamma | 0.85 | 0.49 | .58 |

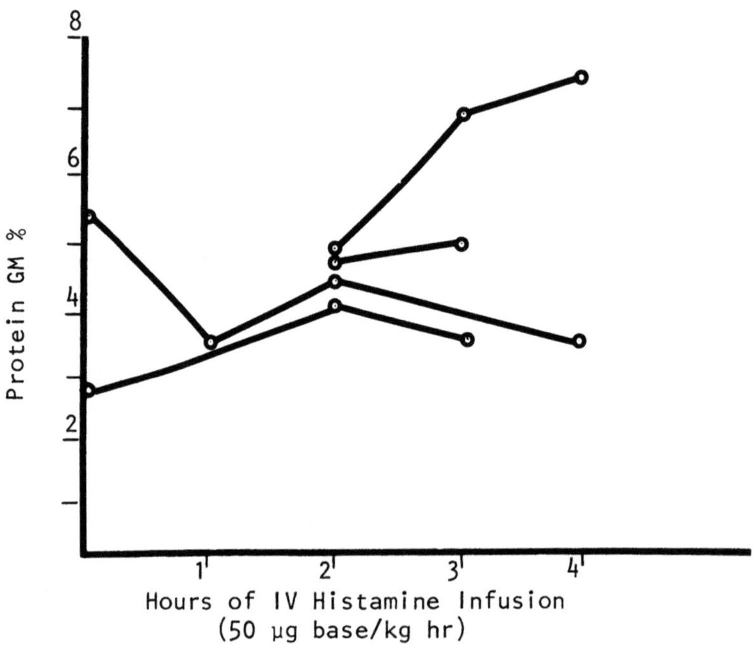


Fig. 3: Protein concentration in gastric lymph during administration of IV histamine 50 μg base/kg hr.

gel electrophoresis, all proteins presented in plasma are present in gastric lymph. The relative amounts of albumin and fibrinogen in gastric lymph are indicative of molecular sieving. The preliminary results with IV histamine which causes maximal gastric secretion indicate that both filtration and secretion may affect the concentration of protein in gastric lymph.

## References

1. Yoffey, J. and F. Courtice: Lymphatics, Lymph and the Lymphomyeloid Complex (New York: Academic Press, 1970), p. 209.

2. Lowry, O., N. Rosenbrough, A. Farr, R. Randall: Protein measurement with the folin phenol reagent. J. Biol. Chem. 193: 265-273, 1951.

3. Landis, E.M. and J.R. Pappenheimer: Exchange of substances through capillary walls, in Hamilton, W. and P. Dow (ed): Handbook of Physiology: Sec. 2 Circulation, Vol. 2 (Washington, D.C.: American Physiological Society, 1963), p. 961-1034.

4. Hanson, M.E., M.I. Grossman, A.C. Ivy: Doses of histamine producing minimal and maximal gastric secretory responses in dogs and man. Am. J. of Physiol. 153: 242-258, 1948.

5. Jacobson, E., K. Swan, M. Grossman: Blood flow and secretion in the stomach. Gastroenterology 52: 414-420, 1967.

6. Davenport, H.W.: Fluid produced by gastric mucosa during damage by acetic and salicylic acids. Gastroenterology 50: 487-499, 1966.

MODEL OF FLUID TRANSPORT IN THE SMALL INTESTINE: EFFECT OF VENOUS PRESSURE ELEVATION ON FLUID TRANSPORT

N. A. Mortillaro and Aubrey E. Taylor

Department of Physiology and Biophysics
University of Mississippi Medical Center
Jackson, Mississippi 39216

The intestine transports large volumes of fluid daily, approximately 9 liters, and this transported volume must not only traverse the mucosal epithelial cells, but the fluid must flow through the interstitium and finally enter either the lymphatics or capillaries. Figure 1 is a schematic, idealized representation of the mucosal membrane, intestinal interstitium and capillary. There are two possible flows across the mucosa: 1) The volume flow associated with the active transport ($J_{V,MA}$) and a passive volume flow ($J_{V,MP}$) that is related to the Starling forces operating across the mucosal membrane:

$$J_{V,M} = J_{V,MA} - J_{V,MP};$$

and

$$= J_{V,MA} - \left[K_{F,M}(P_T - P_M - \sigma_M(\pi_T - \pi_M)\right], \qquad \ldots(1)$$

where $J_{V,M}$ is the net volume movement across the mucosal membrane, $K_{F,M}$ is the filtration coefficient of the mucosal membrane (ml/min/mm Hg/100 gm), $P_T$ is the tissue fluid pressure, $P_M$ is the mucosal pressure, $\pi_T$ is the tissue colloid osmotic pressure, $\pi_M$ is the mucosal colloid osmotic pressure and $\sigma_M$ is the reflection coefficient of the mucosal membrane ($\sigma = 1$ if the membrane is impermeable to the plasma proteins and is equal to 0 if the proteins are freely permeable).

The change in interstitial fluid volume (dV/dt) is:

$$\frac{dV}{dt} = J_{V,C} + J_{V,M} - J_{V,L}; \qquad \ldots(2)$$

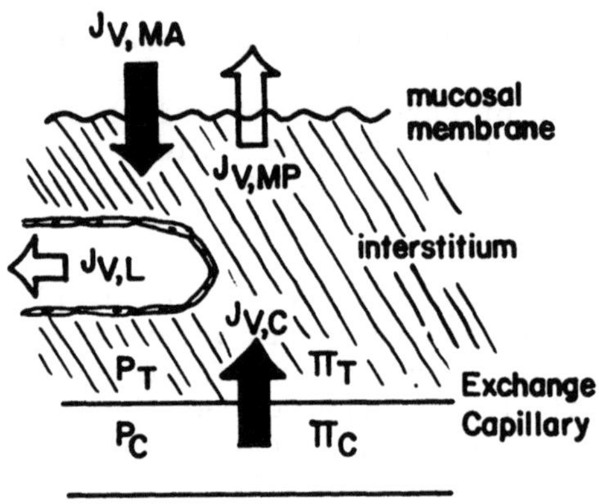


Figure 1

Schematic representation of the intestinal fluid exchange system demonstrating the mucosal membrane and the associated volume flows. The volume flow associated with active transport of solutes ($J_{V,MA}$) and a passive volume flow ($J_{V,MP}$) which is a result of the filtration properties of mucosal membrane and the Starling forces operative across the mucosal membrane. The flow into the tissue is a function of lymphatic removal ($J_{V,L}$) and capillary filtration ($J_{V,C}$) which is a function of the Starling forces acting across the capillary membrane (Courtesy of Taylor, A. E. and N. A. Mortillaro. Proc. of Summer Computer Simulation Conference, Houston, Texas, Vol. II, pp. 673-677, 1974.)

where $J_{V,C}$ is the capillary filtration and $J_{V,L}$ is the lymph flow. Now

$$J_{V,C} = K_{F,C}[(P_C - P_T) - \sigma_C(\pi_C - \pi_T)] ; \qquad \ldots (3)$$

where $K_{F,C}$ is the filtration coefficient of the capillary membrane, $P_C$ is capillary hydrostatic pressure, $P_T$ is tissue fluid pressure, $\pi_C$ is plasma colloid osmotic pressure, $_T$ is tissue colloid osmotic pressure and $\sigma_C$ is the reflection coefficient of the plasma proteins for the capillary membrane.

It is quite evident that interstitial fluid volume is a function not only of intestinal transport, but a function of lymph flow and capillary filtration. The purpose of this model was to evaluate how the tissue forces interact with the capillary forces and lymphatic flow to either enhance or oppose $J_{V,M}$.

## Materials and Methods

The functions relating venous pressure and lymph flow, tissue pressure and tissue volume, venous pressure and lymphatic protein concentrations, and $J_{V,MP}$ as a function of tissue pressure, were obtained in an isolated cat intestinal preparation by Mortillaro and Taylor (1,2). The basic equations were written and a PDP-9 digital computer was used to produce the model predictions.

## Results

Figure 2 shows the model's prediction of lymph flow (Δ), mucosal flow (O) and capillary filtration or absorption (x) as the venous pressure was elevated. The numbers in parenthesis above the abscissa are tissue pressures for the corresponding venous pressure (PV) At venous pressures less than 14 mm Hg, which corresponds to tissue pressures less than 4.0 mm Hg, both capillaries and lymphatics remove the transported volume. At 10 mm Hg venous pressure, the two systems remove equal volumes of the transported fluid which agrees quite well with the experimental studies of Lee ( 3). However, at experimental $P_V$'s greater than 14 mm Hg the capillary does not absorb and, in fact, becomes a filtering capillary (below the zero line). The lymphatic now must carry away both the filtration and the transported volume. As capillary filtration proceeds, the lymphatic system is overwhelmed (4) and the intestine now begins to secrete at 25 mm Hg venous pressure (5).

## Discussion

This model points out how tissue forces effect net volume movement across the mucosal membrane. For maximum transport, capillary pressure must be maintained low such that the capillary absorbs rather than filters. There are certainly many assumptions

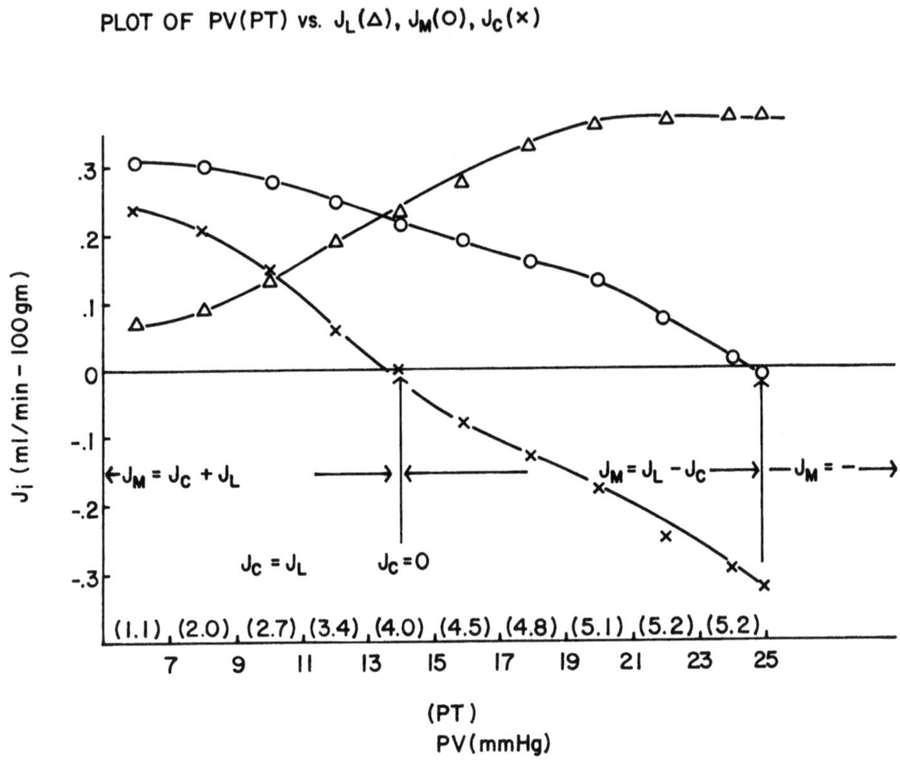


Figure 2

Plot of lymph flow (Δ), capillary volume movement (x) and net flow across the mucosal membrane (0) as a function of venous pressure (PV). The numbers in parenthesis above the abscissa are tissue pressures. Note that at $P_V$ = 14 mm Hg, the capillary is neither filtering nor absorbing, and at $P_V$ greater than 25 mm Hg net movement is seen to occur into the gut lumen across the mucosa (Courtesy of Taylo, A. E. and N. A. Mortillaro. Proc. of Summer Computer Simulation Conference, Houston, Texas, Vol. II, pp. 673-677, 1974).

that must be built into a model of this type; however, the positive results of such a model are extremely valuable in formulating new research projects and analyzing a complex system such as the intestine.

The Wittes (6) have demonstrated that tissue proteins can wash down to a greater extent with chronically elevated portal pressures than those observed in acute experiments from which this model was formulated. Obviously, some changes must take place in the tissue capillary exchange system for this to occur. Uhley et al. (7) have demonstrated a similar finding for chronic elevation of left atrial pressures relative to lung lymph flow. Perhaps the lymphatics proliferate and allow greater lymph flows with chronic elevations of portal pressures similar to the changes observed by Uhley et al. in lung tissue. But, the filtration coefficient may also decrease, $P_T$ may increase to values higher than normal, or the capillary protein permeability may decrease. Since Witte (6) has demonstrated that fat is still absorbed, even with chronically elevated venous pressures, then the transport systems are not altered by elevating venous pressure. Only the pressure induced backflux can be effected; therefore, chronically elevated portal pressures must cause an increase in lymphatic pumping capabilities which may also be coupled with the other changes in tissue forces and flows as mentioned above.

The model presented indicates that normal intestinal preparations will "secrete" when venous pressures are elevated to 25 mm Hg. The normal active transport systems are intact, but the pressure back flux exceeds the fluid movement propelled by the active systems such that fluid actively enters the lumen of the intestine. Basically, when tissue fluid pressure increases to values $>5$ mm Hg, the lymphatic and tissue systems are overwhelmed, the mucosal membranes are leakier (possibly pushing apart tight junctions), and fluid enters the gut lumen. Some pathological conditions, such as hypovolemic shock, will tend to accelerate the "secretory" process (8), i.e., the intestine will "secrete" at lower portal pressures because of tissue anoxia and epithelial cell sloughing.

## REFERENCES

1. Mortillaro, N.A., and A.E.Taylor. Interactions of the vascular, interstitial and lymphatic systems in the cat intestine. Cir. Res. Submitted.

2. Taylor, A.E., and N.A.Mortillaro. Reevaluation of the filtration hypothesis in intestine. Proc. of Summer Computer Simulation Conference, Houston, Vol. II:673-677, 1974.

3. Lee, J.S. Flows and pressures in lymphatic and blood vessels of intestine in water absorption. Am. J. Physiol. 200: 979, 1961.

4. Rusznyak, I., Foldi, M., and Szabo, G. Lymphatics and Lymph Circulation. Physiology and Pathology. Second Edition. Pergamon Press: Oxford, 1967.

5. Wilson, T.H. A modified method for study of intestinal absorption in vitro. J. Appl. Physiol. 9:137, 1955.

6. Witte, M.H. and C.L.Witte. Personal communication.

7. Uhley, H.N., S.E.Leeds, J.J. Sampson, N. Rudo, and M. Friedman. The temporal sequence of lymph flow in the right lymphatic duct in experimental chronic pulmonary edema. Am. Heart J. 72:214-217, 1966.

8. Cook, B.H., E.R.Wilson, Jr., and A.E.Taylor. Intestinal fluid loss in hemorrhagic shock. Am. J. Physiol. 221:1494-1498, 1971.

THE CYCLIC CHANCES OF THE LYMPH VESSELS IN THE UTERUS OF THE MOUSE WHICH HAS BEEN PREGNANT

G. Fabian

Department of Anatomy, Ruhr-University

Bochum, Germany

Attempts were made to visualise the cyclic behaviour of the lymph vessels in the uterus of animals which had been pregnant, using Patent blue violet and Japanese ink in a modified form adapted to the natural absorption possibilities of the uterus. Here also the mouse, an animal with a haemoendothelial type of placenta, is a particularly suitable experimental animal, because material can be obtained in a known phase without great expense of material and time.

## Materials and Methods

Patent blue violet was selected again because, as is well known, it has an affinity for the lymph vascular system (Suter, 1969; Byk-Gulden, 1970) and a particle size of 6 Å, and for the same reason, Japanese ink with a particle size of 10,8 Å (Harms,1965).

The investigations were carried out in healthy female mice 3 weeks (vaginal smear) or 7 weeks (application of dye) after their second pregnancy.

In conformity with Preuss's uniform comparative terminology (1959), a mouse which has been pregnant also passes through a sexual cycle of stages, as earlier investigations by Fabian (1973) and Nitschke and Fabian (1970) in nulliparous mice showed:

1. Oestrus
2. Early post-oestrus
3. Late post-oestrus
4. Inter-oestrus
5. Pre-oestrus

The investigation was carried out here also under technically difficult conditions:

1. The smallness of the objects. The uterine horn has a diameter of only 2.5 to 3.5 mm when fixed. It is here 1 mm more than with nulliparous mice.

2. The necessity of working very, very quickly when and after the dye is applied.

3. The photographs of the mm thick sections were made floating in oil of wintergreen, with the Zeiss Photomicroscope.

The dyes were applied to the anaesthetised animal and also post mortem.

As in earlier studies, the peritoneal cavity was opened and 0.5 ml 2.5 % Patent blue violet solution injected into cavity of the left uterine horn. The dye was removed rapidly within second. After 10 seconds, the lymph vessel in the mesometrium next to the utero-tubal vein are coloured blue, after 20 seconds the external iliac lymph node and after a further 10 - 20 seconds the lumbo-aortic lymph node and the thoracic duct also stained blue. The application of Japanese ink solution also shows lymphogenic removal, but this occurs rather more slowly.

An accurately recordable time course of the dye removal was obtained by dropping the dye directly on to the surface of the mucous membrane under the stereomicroscope, the uterine horn being opened somewhat to the mesometral side.

## Results

For all 5 phases of the cycle, the following is also true for mice which have been pregnant:

The application of dye to the uterine mucous membrane produces a black mark on the surface between the epithelia and subepithelially.

Similar findings were also obtained in the intestinal villi of the dog, in the mouse and in various gallinaceous birds (Fabian, 1972).

Starting from the surface of the uterine mucous membrane, a mesh of capillary lymphatic reticulum with a simple outline is formed subsequently. Button-shaped thickenings are found here repeatedly. They also have several very fine brush-like ramifications, which are still visible under the light microscope. Such a configuration could not be seen in similar visualisations in nulliparous mice. Also ink which has entered glandular orifices not filled with secretion, makes its way deep periglandularly just behind the orifice.

Animals which have been pregnant have lymph capillaries of a greater diameter and consequently fill much more rapidly than those of nulliparous animals.

The following findings were obtained in the individual phases of the cycle:

Oestrus

Also in mice which have been pregnant, the mucous membrane in oestrus is oedematous and loose and attains the maximum surface area.

The more or less typical picture in this phase, in the form of the sporadically varied and enormously developed lymph capillaries in nulliparous animals is also found here, but not in such a pronounced manner.

On the whole, however, the reticulum of lymph capillaries is distributed symmetrically over the entire oedematous mucous membrane.

Removal of the dye takes place form the base of the mucous membrane in the larger efferent lymph vessels which lead throughout the circular muscle layer into the vascular layer formed in the mouse.

Early post-oestrus

In the next phase of the cycle, early post-oestrus, lasting 30 hours, the stroma which was most extensively loosened in the previous stage has also become very consolidated in these animals which have been pregnant.

At the beginning of the phase, the lymph capillary reticulum is still wide meshed in the first third of the mucous membrane, but it narrows very greatly towards the middle of the cycle in the subsepithelial portion. Very fine branches run out from the mesh and form a fine reticulum of lymph capillaries in the middle and lower thirds of the mucosa.

During this time small protuberances are seen very clearly projecting into the lumen of the uterus, and these show a very dense network of lymph capillaries.

Here also the dye is transported away from the base of the mucous membrane in the larger afferent lymph vessels.

Late post-oestrus

In the late post-oestrus with a short duration of 12 hours, the stroma is just as intensely consolidated as in the previous phase.

A great development of the protuberances into the lumen which appeared in the previous stage is striking. These protuberances are also present in carnivores (Fabian and Preuss,1966) and pigs (Fabian,1961), and may be so strongly developed as to suggest the villi of the small intestine. If suitably incised, usually one and sometimes several lymph capillaries can be seen running in these structures. The glandular ducts running there are surrounded by ring shaped lymph capillaries.

The mucous membrane between these structures shows a dense network of lymph capillaries similar to those in nulliparous animals, where a consolidation between two neighbouring ring vessels is present. It is to be assumed that in pregnant animals in this stage of corpus luteum of pregnancy, there is a relationship between vascular architecture and the site of implantation, since the placentae lie between neighbouring arterial rings.

Here, too, no such marked lymph capillary reticulum is visible in the middle third of the mucosa, but a dense reticulum at the base. Efferent lymph vessels also run there.

Inter-oestrus

The relatively long inter-oestrus lasting 2 days also still shows a marked consolidation of the stroma. The mucosal structures directed towards the lumen in the previous phase have now almost completely regressed.

The middle and lower thirds of the mucous membrane shows a regularly arranged network of lymph capillaries. In the upper third, there are very fine lymph capillaries which begin subepithelially and empty into the network of lymph capillaries in the middle third of the mucosa.

As in the previous phase, the removal of the dye occurs through the vascular layer.

Pre-oestrus

The 5th and last phase of the cycle, pre-oestrus, also lasts only 12 hours, like the late post-oestrus.

In this phase, the mucous membrane is oedematous and loose, but still does not reach the peak of oestrus. The lymph vessels resemble the picture in the nulliparous mouse. They also begin here subendothelially and have a varied, sometimes even enormous calibre. The numerous very fine efferent branches measure up to 2 um.

The middle and lower thirds of the mucous membrane contain a regularly arranged reticulum of lymph capillaries resembling those in the previous phase and also those of the nulliparous mouse.

The dye is further removed in the larger lymph vessels through the vascular layer in the mesometrium, already mentioned, in addition to the utero-tubal vein. The lymph vessels here are often coiled up like a corkscrew in animals which have been pregnant and here they have the typical string of pearls appearance. Further removal occurs into the lymph nodes already mentioned and into the thoracic duct.

Summary

Finally, it may be said that the findings just mentioned in mice which have been pregnant are in agreement with the findings I have already obtained in nulliparous mice (Fabian,1973), and that the cyclic behaviour of the lymph vessels in the uterus is determined by natural laws, primarily by the change from oedema to dehydration of the mucous membrane, which measurements by Nitschke and Fabian (1970) have already shown.

## REFERENCES


1. Byk-Gulden: Personal Information (1970)
2. Fabian, G.: Zum zyklischen Verhalten vornehmlich der Höhne des Endometriums beim Schwein. Zbl.Vet.Med.8, 214-251 (1961)
3. Fabian, G.: Zur Aufnahme des Vitalfarbstoffes Patent-blau-Violett und von japanischer Tusche in die Lymphkapillaren der Darmzotte. Zbl.Vet.Med.A,19, 52-62 (1972)
4. Fabian, G.: Experimentelle Untersuchungen über die enterale Resorption des Vitalfarbstoffes Patenblau-Violett und von japanischer Tusche. Z.Angw.Zool., 59, 17-31 (1972).
5. Fabian, G.: The lymphatic vessels of the uterus during the sexual cycles of the mice. (In Press)
6. Fabian, G., and F. Preuss: Messungen am Uterus der Katze in den Zyklusphasen. Zbl.Vet.Med.,A,13, 337-351 (1966)
7. Harms, H.: Handbuch der Farbstoffe für die Mikroskopie. Staufen-Verlag, Kamp-Lintfort (1965)
8. Nitschke, Th., and G. Fabian: Messungen am Endometrium der Maus in den Zyklusphasen. Zbl.Vet.Med.,A,17, 216-229 (1970)
9. Preuss, F.: Zur vergleichenden Terminologie der Sexualzyklen. Berl.Münch.Tierärztl.Wschr. 72, 303-307 (1959)
10. Suter, P.: Die Lymphographie beim Hund, eine röntgenologische Methode zur Diagnose von Veränderungen am Lymphsystem. Habil-Schrift, Zürich (1969).

# HORMONAL INFLUENCE ON THE RECIRCULATION OF LYMPHOCYTES THROUGH THE REGIONAL LYMPH NODE AND REGIONAL TISSUES OF THE SHEEP

A. D. Shannon, J. W. Quin and F. C. Courtice

John Curtin School of Medical Research, Australian National University, Canberra, Australia

There is a large scale migration of lymphoid cells from the blood vascular system into lymphoid tissues and a return by way of the lymphatic system as described by Gowans and others (see reviews 1,2). Despite the magnitude of this recirculation process, as shown in Fig. 1, little is known of the factors controlling lymphocyte recirculation and, particularly, the action hormones may have on this process. With this aim in mind,the effects of relatively small doses of ACTH and hydrocortisone on the recirculation process at the level of the local lymph node and through peripheral tissues were investigated in the sheep. A more detailed report of earlier work in this area has been presented elsewhere (3).

An efferent popliteal lymphatic in each of 16 sheep and an efferent popliteal lymphatic in each of 6 sheep were cannulated and experiments carried out after a recovery period of 3-4 days. ACTH (Acthar, Armour Pharmaceutical Co., England) was administered intravenously in sterile 0.9% saline to 8 sheep with efferent lymphatic cannulations and 6 sheep with afferent lymphatic cannulations. Hydrocortisone-21-sodium succinate (Sigma, U.S.A.) was administered intravenously in sterile saline to 8 of the sheep with efferent lymphatic cannulations. The lymph flow and cell output in efferent and afferent lymph were continuously monitored in the conscious sheep before and after the administration of both exogenous hormones and the results obtained are summarised in Table 1. The administration of 20 iu ACTH resulted in a 25% reduction in lymph flow and a 67% reduction in cell output, beginning 60-90 minutes after injection. Lymph flow and cell output returned to preinjection levels some 7 hours after the administration of 20 iu ACTH. This action of ACTH was

TABLE 1. Showing the changes in lymph flow and output of cells in efferent popliteal lymph following the intravenous administration of 20 iu ACTH and 10 mg hydrocortisone. Similar changes in afferent popliteal lymph following the administration of 10 iu ACTH are also presented. Values shown are means ± standard errors with the number of animals in each group shown in brackets.

| | | | Base period (2 hr period prior to administration of hormone) | Response period (2-4 hr after administration of hormone) |
|---|---|---|---|---|
| EFFERENT POPLITEAL LYMPH | | | | |
| 20 iu ACTH | Lymph flow | (ml/hr) | 6.00 ± 0.35 | 4.50 ± 0.21 ** |
| (6) | Cell output | ($x10^6$/hr) | 85.90 ±10.27 | 28.55 ± 2.72 ** |
| 10 mg Hydrocortisone† | Lymph flow | (ml/hr) | 5.49 ± 0.34 | 7.06 ± 0.27 ** |
| (8) | Cell output | ($x10^6$/hr) | 68.33 ± 8.56 | 46.55 ± 6.57 * |
| AFFERENT POPLITEAL LYMPH | | | | 3-5 hr after hormone |
| 10 iu ACTH | Lymph flow | (ml/hr) | 1.40 ± 0.11 | 1.10 ± 0.10 * |
| (6) | Cell output | ($x10^6$/hr) | 0.586± 0.088 | 0.265± 0.032 ** |

† Hydrocortisone-21-sodium succinate

* $P < 0.05$     ** $P < 0.001$

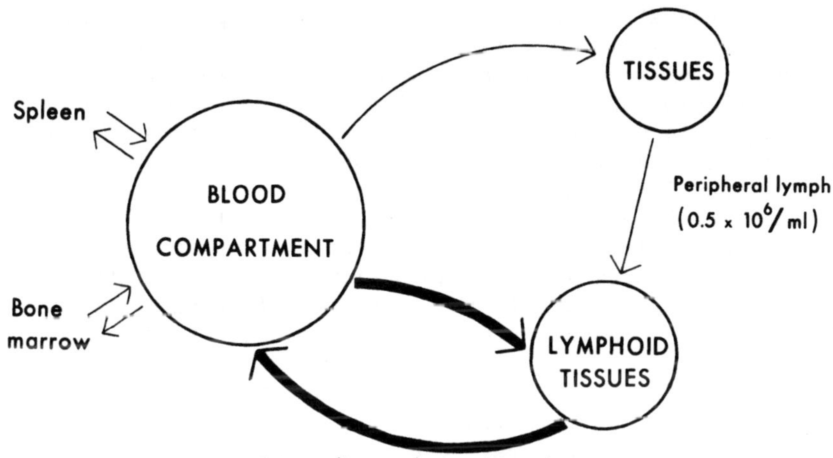


Diagramatic representation of the recirculation of lymphocytes in the sheep. The importance of re-circulation through the lymphoid tissues is reflected in the greater concentration of cells/ml in the intermediate and central lymph when compared to the concentration in peripheral lymph.

probably mediated through the release of endogenous hydrocortisone from the adrenal cortex of the sheep since the administration of exogenous hydrocortisone also resulted in a significant depression in cell output (Table 1), despite a rise in lymph flow. Concomitant with the fall in output in the efferent lymph following both ACTH and hydrocortisone, there was a rise in the number of total white cells in the blood. This finding ruled out the possibility that either of these hormones acted by destroying the lymphocytes.

The administration of 10 iu ACTH resulted in a 20% reduction in afferent popliteal lymph flow and a 55% reduction in the number of cells travelling from the tissues to the popliteal lymph node in afferent lymph (cf. Table 1). A similar reduction in the output of cells in afferent lymph was observed following the administration of small doses of exogenous hydrocortisone (2.5-5.0 mg). In view of the fact that these hormones had a similar effect in depressing cell output in both efferent and afferent lymph, it appears unlikely that there is a specific action blocking lymphocyte migration at the level of the postcapillary endothelium within the lymph node. Rather, the present findings are suggestive of an action on the lymphocyte surface membrane resulting in the alteration in recirculation pattern observed in both peripheral and lymphoid tissues.

It is concluded that corticotrophic and corticosteroid hormones influence the recirculation of lymphocytes in the sheep and that this action may have a bearing on the immunocompetence of stressed animals.

## REFERENCES

1. GOWANS,J.L.: Life-span, recirculation, and transformation of lymphocytes. Internat.Rev.exp.Path. 5 (1966) 1-24.

2. MORRIS,B.: The cells of lymph and their role in immunological reactions. In Handbuch Der Allgemeinen Pathologie. Lymph Vessel System (1972), ed. Meessen, H., Berlin, Heidelberg : Springer-Verlag. pp 405-456.

3. SHANNON,A.D., M.A.S.JONES : Influence of corticotrophic and corticosteroid hormones on the output of cells from the popliteal lymph node of the sheep. Aust. J. exp. Biol. med. Sci. 52 (1974) 515-525.

THE ORIGIN OF LIPOPROTEINS IN THE PERITONEAL FLUID OF THE RABBIT: PERMEABILITY OF THE MESOTHELIUM TO MACROMOLECULES

F. C. Courtice & D. C. K. Roberts

John Curtin School of Medical Research, Australian National University, Canberra, Australia

The perotoneal cavity usually contains a small amount of free fluid. In the present series of experiments the amount present in the normal rabbit was on average about 2ml. When cholesterol was added to the diet for 2 to 3 months to raise the level of plasma cholesterol to 1000 mg/100 ml, the free fluid in the peritoneal civity increased to an average of about 5 ml. This fluid is part of the extracellular fluid of the body throughout which macromolecules are continually moving. The main barrier to this movement resides in the walls of the small blood vessels; the walls of the small lymphatic vessels offer little resistance so that the composition of tissue fluid and lymph is approximately the same (1).

Peritoneal fluid is derived from adjacent submesothelial tissue fluid pools as shown in Fig 1. If we collect lymph draining these tissue fluid pools, then we can get a measure of the composition of the tissue fluid in the pools. The various tissue fluid pools that might contribute to the peritoneal fluid are depicted in Fig 2, and are as follows:

1. Parietal tissue fluid pools

(i) Diaphragm. The mesothelium covering the diaphragm is modified to aid absorption of fluid from the peritoneal cavity. There are stomata between the mesothelial cells, the basement membrane is poorly developed, the connective tissue layer consists only of a lattice-work of collagen fibres, and lymphatic capillaries in the form of lacunae come into close contact with the mesothelium. This modification of the mesothelium together with the rhythmic contraction and relaxation

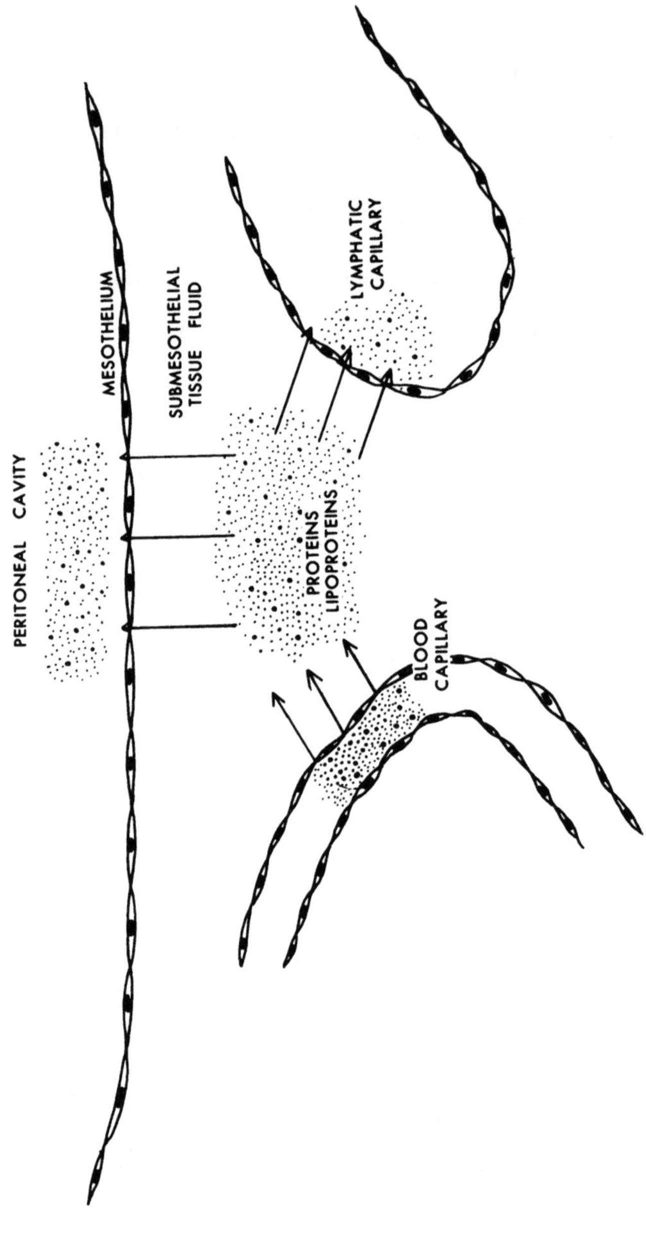


Fig. 1

Diagrammatic representation of the movement of macromolecules through the mesothelium into the peritoneal cavity.

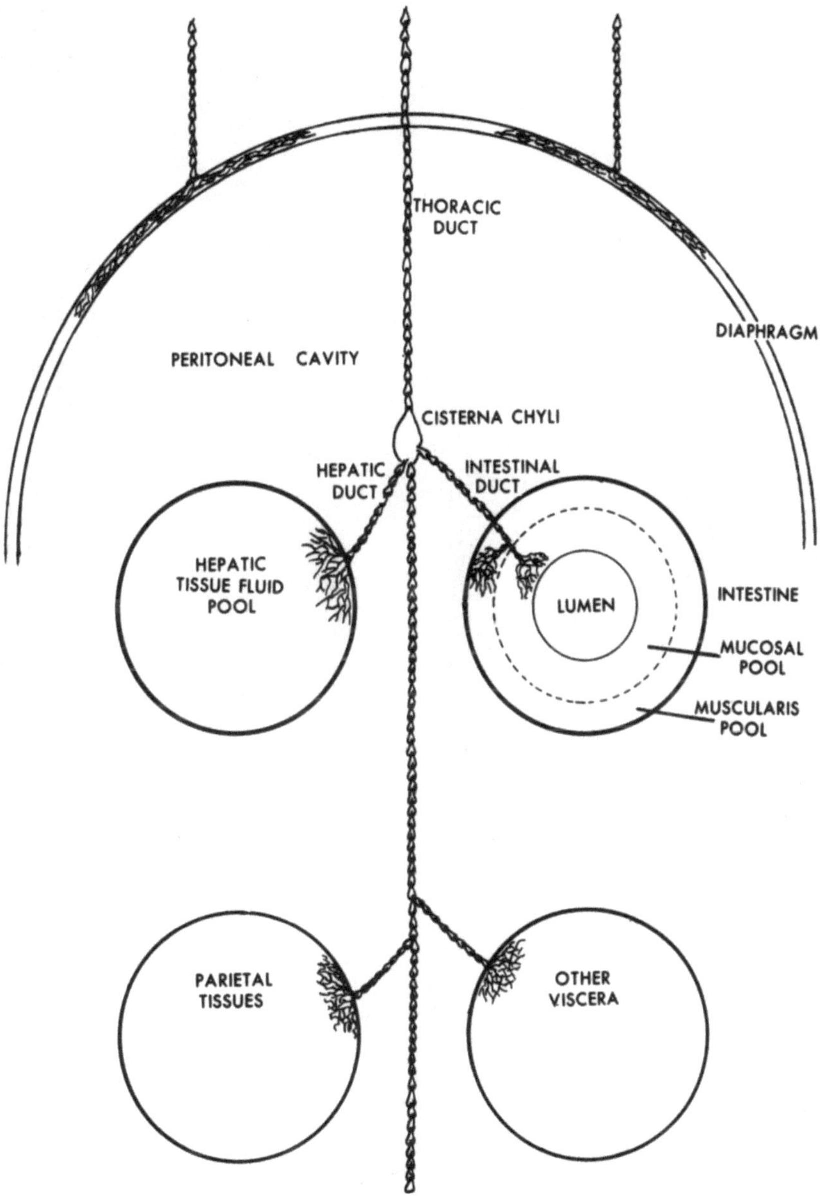


Fig. 2

Diagrammatic representation of the lymph drainage of the tissue fluid pools adjacent to the peritoneal cavity.

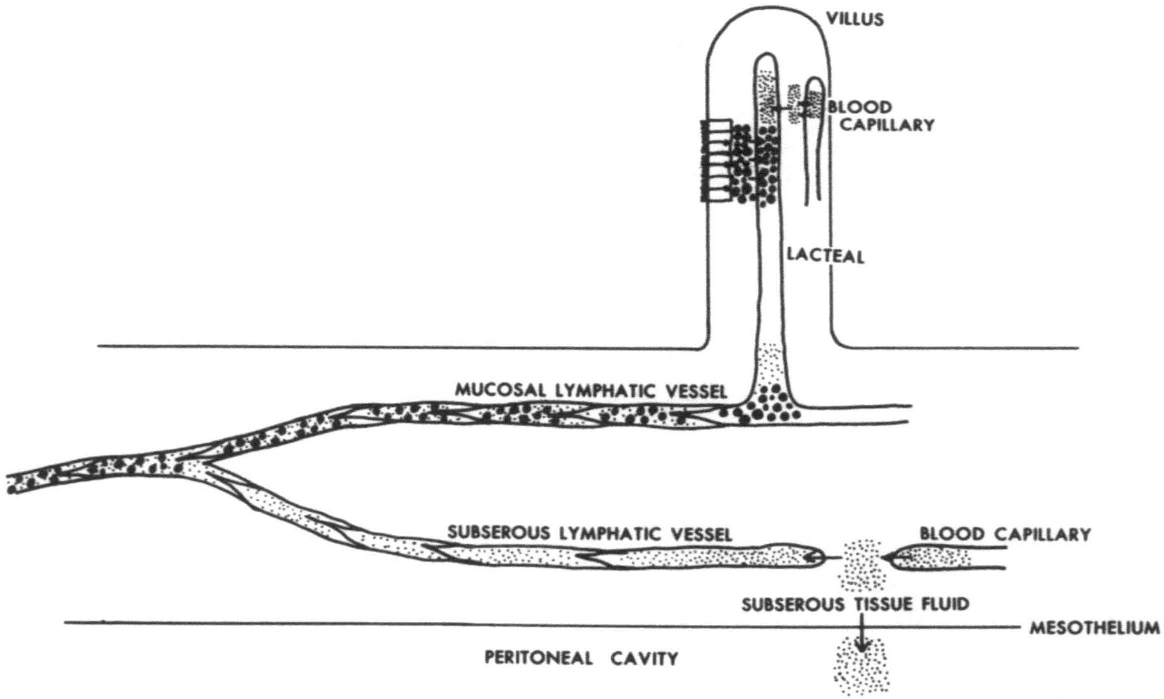


Fig. 3

Diagrammatic representation of the lipoproteins in intestinal lymph. The large chylomicrons and VLDL formed in the mucosal cells enter the lacteals, together with LDL and HDL that escape from the blood capillaries of the villi. In the subserous tissue fluid pool LDL and HDL from the blood may enter the subserous lymphatic vessels and the peritoneal cavity. Lymph from the mucosal lymphatic vessels does not enter the subserous tissue fluid pool, unless the valves become incompetent.

of the diaphragm aids the rapid absorption of macromolecules and particles from the peritoneal cavity into the diaphragmatic lymphatic vessels (see 2). Even when the lymphatic vessels draining the diaphragm are ligated, lymph from the diaphragm does not spill over into the peritoneal cavity; instead, fluid in the peritoneal cavity is absorbed into the lymphatics but then spills over into the pleural cavity (3). It is, therefore, unlikely that the tissue fluid of the diaphragm would normally contribute to the peritoneal fluid, even though the mesothelium in the region is freely permeable.

(ii) Parietal tissue fluid pool other than diaphragm. In the parietal region other than the diaphragm, the mesothelium is supported by a relatively dense layer of connective tissue. The composition of the tissue fluid in this region is not known, but it seems possible that it would resemble that of the tissue fluid pool of leg. Lymph from the leg has, therefore, been studied for comparison with the composition of peritoneal fluid.

2. Visceral tissue fluid pools

(i) Those supplied by the portal circulation, mainly gastrointestinal tract and liver.

(ii) Other viscera, mainly kidneys, uterus, bladder.

Of the visceral tissue fluid pools, attention has been focussed mainly on those tissues supplied by the portal circulation, because an increased intrahepatic portal pressure, as in cirrhosis of the liver or chronic heart failure, leads to a great increase in the amount of peritoneal fluid. In the present experiments we have collected lymph from the liver and from the thoracic duct to obtain a measure of the composition of the tissue fluid in these pools.

Lymph from the gastrointestinal tract reflects not only the movement of macromolecules from the blood stream into the tissue fluid, but also the absorption of lipid in the form of chylomicrons and VLDL from the intestinal lumen. The chylomicrons and VLDL are very much larger than the LDL and HDL or the main proteins present in the extracellular fluid. Within the small intestine there are probably two pools of tissue fluid which are quite separate - the mucosal pool and the muscularis and subserous pool. Because of valves it seems likely that the tissue fluid and lymph from the mucosal pool do not mix with the tissue fluid in the subserous pool, Fig 3.

Two groups of experiments were carried out. In the first, the plasma proteins — albumin, $\alpha$-, $\beta$- and $\gamma$ - globulins — and the concentrations of cholesterol and phospholipid were determined in plasma, peritoneal fluid, hepatic lymph and leg lymph. In all the latter three fluids the lymph: plasma ratio for albumin was statistically higher than that for the α-, β - and γ - globulins, which in turn was higher than that for TC + + PL which is a measure of the total liproprotein present, Table 1. These results also show that this ratio for any individual macromolecule was much higher for hepatic lymph than for peritoneal fluid and leg lymph.

In the second series of experiments the lipoproteins in plasma, peritoneal fluid, hepatic lymph and thoracic duct lymph were separated into four classes - $S_f$ >20, $S_f$ 12-20, $S_f$ 0-12 and HDL. The protein and lipid composition of each of these classes in these fluids was determined in two groups of animals, those fed the cholesterol diet only and those fed an additional supplement of corn-oil during the last week of the cholesterol diet. The additional corn-oil increased the amount of griglyceride in the thoracic duct lymph mainly in the $S_f$ >220 fraction.

The results in Table 2 show that the composition of each of the four lipoproteins is essentially the same in plasma, hepatic lymph and peritoneal fluid. In contrast to the results with hepatic lymph and peritoneal fluid, however, the composition of lipoproteins in the thoracic duct lymph, which reflects the absorption of fat from the gastrointestinal tract, differs considerably from that of plasma, especially in the cholesterol and triglyceride components of the $S_f$ > 20 and $S_f$ 12-20 fractions.

TABLE 1

The concentrations of albumin, α-, β- and γ- globulins and total cholesterol + phospholipid in hepatic lymph (HL), leg lymph (LL) and peritoneal fluid (PF) expressed as a percentage of the plasma (P) level, in 18 cholesterol-fed rabbits, together with standard errors of the means.

| | Albumin | α-globulin | β-globulin | γ-globulin | TC+PL |
|---|---|---|---|---|---|
| HL:P | 91.4 ±2.4 | 76.7 ±3.0 | 67.3 ±2.9 | 71.1 ±4.3 | 41.2 ±2.3 |
| LL:P | 48.1 ±2.0 | 38.6 ±3.0 | 30.3 ±3.0 | 36.7 ±3.3 | 14.9 ±1.2 |
| PF:P | 55.9 ±1.8 | 40.6 ±3.2 | 34.8 ±2.8 | 34.8 ±2.9 | 20.6 ±1.5 |

TABLE 2

The composition of lipoproteins in plasma (P), peritoneal fluid (PF), hepatic lymph (HL) and thoracic duct lymph (TDL), each component being expressed as a percentage of the lipoprotein concerned. Figures are means and standard errors of the means in 14 animals.

| | Protein | Phospholipid | Free cholesterol + cholesterol ester | Triglyceride |
|---|---|---|---|---|
| $S_f > 20$ | | | | |
| P | 8±0.6 | 21±1.7 | 60±3.2 | 11±2.1 |
| PF | 6±0.4 | 19±1.3 | 60±2.4 | 15±2.0 |
| HL | 8±0.6 | 20±1.1 | 57±2.2 | 15±1.9 |
| TDL | 4±0.6 | 15±1.4 | 26±5.7 | 56±7.5 |
| $S_f$ 12-20 | | | | |
| P | 15±1.1 | 23±0.9 | 56±1.8 | 6±1.0 |
| PF | 17±0.9 | 23±0.9 | 51±2.2 | 10±1.5 |
| HL | 15±0.6 | 22±0.6 | 58±0.8 | 5±0.4 |
| TDL | 14±1.4 | 26±2.1 | 40±4.4 | 19±6.5 |
| $S_f$ 0-12 | | | | |
| P | 23±1.6 | 24±1.5 | 47±2.3 | 7±0.9 |
| PF | 22±1.6 | 24±1.8 | 42±1.8 | 11±1.4 |
| HL | 25±1.5 | 27±1.4 | 42±1.5 | 5±0.5 |
| TDL | 21±0.8 | 37±1.6 | 28±2.5 | 13±2.0 |
| HDL | | | | |
| P | 47±2.5 | 23±1.4 | 24±1.7 | 5±0.6 |
| PF | 52±2.5 | 18±1.3 | 19±2.1 | 12±1.8 |
| HL | 46±4.3 | 23±2.5 | 26±2.4 | 5±0.9 |
| TDL | 48±3.1 | 26±2.0 | 15±2.8 | 11±1.3 |

In the $S_f > 20$ fraction, the percentages of protein and phospholipid are lower in thoracic duct lymph than in plasma suggesting that the complexes are larger in lymph. Adding corn-oil to the diet accentuated these differences as would be expected.

Since the composition of the lipoproteins in thoracic duct lymph differs from that of the corresponding fractions in plas-

TABLE 3

The amount of each lipoprotein in hepatic lymph (HDL), peritoneal fluid (PF) and leg lymph, (LL) expressed as a percentage of the corresponding levels in the plasma. Leg lymph values from (6).

| | $S_f > 20$ | $S_f$ 12-20 | $S_f$ 0-12 | HDL |
|---|---|---|---|---|
| HDL | 36.1±5.4 | 37.7±2.9 | 52.4±10.2 | 68.5±8.9 |
| PF | 14.7±3.0 | 15.4±1.8 | 21.6± 2.8 | 30.4±3.7 |
| LL | 7.1±0.7 | | 20.3±2.5 | 36.6±4.1 |

ma, the lymph:plasma ratio cannot be interpreted in the same way as the HL : P, PF : P and LL : P ratios. The results for these latter fluids show that the concentrations of each lipoprotein relative to the corresponding value in plasma varies inversely as the size of the lipoprotein complex, and that the values for peritoneal fluid and leg lymph are somewhat similar and much lower than the corresponding values for hepatic lymph, Table 3. These experiments indicate that peritoneal fluid is not derived from the mucosal lymph of the small intestine, but a proportion could be derived from the subserous tissue fluid pool. In chronic portal hypertension an increased amount of peritoneal fluid with a low protein content and no increased chylomicrons or VLDL could originate from the subserous tissue fluid pool of the small intestine (4,5). With obstruction of the thoracic duct, however, the valves of the lymphatic vessels of the wall of the small intestine will become incompetent and lymph from the intestinal mucosa will mix with the subserous lymph and ultimately spill over into the subserous tissue fluid pool and the peritoneal cavity to produce chylous ascites.

These experiments also suggest, although they do not prove conclusively, that the permeability of the mesothelium to macromolecules is similar to that of the lymphatic endothelium. This means that the amin barrier in the movement of macromolecules from the plasma to the peritoneal fluid resides in the walls of the small blood vessels in the tissues adjacent to the mesothelium.

REFERENCES

1. Courtice, F.C.: (1971) Lymph and plasma proteins: Barriers to their movement throughout the extracellular fluid. Lymphology, 4, 9-17.

2. Yoffey, J.M. and Courtice, F.C.: (1970) Lymphatics, lymph and the lymphomyeloid complex. Academic Press, London and New York.

3. Courtice, F.C. and Steinbeck, A.W.: (1951) The effects of lymphatic obstruction and of posture on the absorption of protein from the peritoneal cavity. Aust. J. exp. Biol. med. Sci. 29, 451-458.

4. Witte, C.L., Witte, M.H., Dumont, A.E., Frist, J. and Cole, W.R.: (1968) Lymph protein in hepatic cirrhosis and experimental hepatic and portal venous hypertension. Trans. Am. Surg. Assoc. 86, 256-266.

6. Witte, C.L., Chung, Y.C., Witte, M.H., Sterle, O.F. and Cole, W.R.: (1969) Observations on the origin of ascites from experimental extrahepatic portal congestion. Ann.Surg. 170, 1002-1015.

6. Courtice, F.C. and Carlick, D.G.: (1962) The permeability of the capillary wall to different plasma lipoproteins of the hypercholesterolaemic rabbit in relation to their size. Q. Jl exp. Physiol. 47, 221-227.

# BILIRUBIN IN AFFERENT AND EFFERENT LYMPH IN THE SHEEP

J. W. Quin, A. D. Shannon and F. C. Courtice

John Curtin School of Medical Research, Australian National University, Canberra, Australia

Efferent (postnodal) lymph in the conscious sheep is characterised by a distinctive yellow colour which contrasts sharply with the almost colourless appearance of afferent (prenodal) lymph. The yellow colour of efferent lymph was analysed qualitatively and quantitatively by biochemical methods and was shown to be due to bilirubin (1). Qualitative analysis demonstrating this association included a positive indirect Van den Bergh reaction and a similar Rf value to bilirubin standards on thin-layer chromatography. Quantitative analysis of the bilirubin content of both plasma and lymph was carried out using a modification of the alkaline diazo-coupling method described by Brodersen and Jacobsen (2).

The bilirubin concentrations observed in blood plasma and efferent and afferent lymph from 3 separate regions of the sheep are summarised in Table 1. The results showed that the total bilirubin concentration in efferent lymph was some 2-6 times higher than the corresponding concentrations in blood plasma. On the other hand, bilirubin concentrations in afferent lymph were considerably lower than those observed in the blood and accounted for the lack of colour in the prenodal sources of lymph. Similar results have been obtained for lymph from the prescapular, prefemoral and hepatic regions of the sheep (1).

The high bilirubin content of efferent lymph was shown to be protein bound, almost entirely to albumin. If the bilirubin in this source of lymph was entirely plasma derived, it could be expected that similar lymph : plasma ratios would be observed for both bilirubin and albumin. However, the

TABLE 1: Total bilirubin concentrations in blood plasma and various sources of efferent (postnodal) and afferent (prenodal) lymph of the sheep, together with their respective lymph : plasma ratios. Values presented are means $\pm$ standard errors with the number of animals in each group shown in brackets.

| | BILIRUBIN | |
|---|---|---|
| | Concentration (ug/ml) | Lymph : Plasma ratio |
| Plasma (32) | 0.89 ± 0.07 | |
| Lymph : | | |
| Efferent popliteal (15) | 3.72 ± 0.57 | 5.62 ± 0.89 |
| Efferent intestinal ( 7) | 2.00 ± 0.38 | 4.67 ± 1.74 |
| Efferent renal ( 2) | 1.82 ± 0.12 | 2.44 ± 0.44 |
| Afferent popliteal ( 9) | 0.37 ± 0.06 | 0.54 ± 0.12 |
| Afferent renal ( 3) | 0.42 ± 0.04 | 0.34 ± 0.14 |

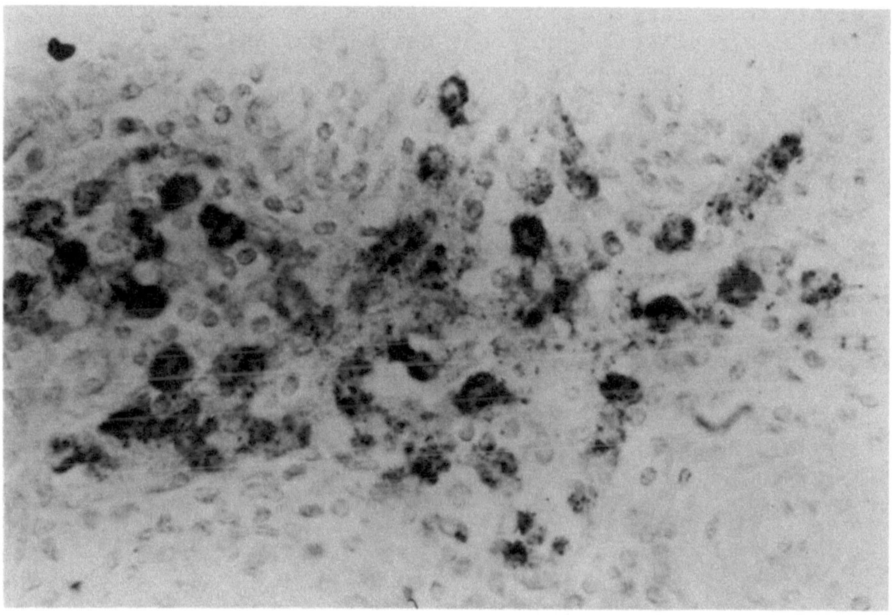

Fig. 1 - Section from a sheep popliteal lymph node stained for ferric iron. Specifically stained granules evident in cytoplasm of phagocytic cells adjacent to lymphatic sinuses. 450x.

lymph : plasma ratios for bilirubin were in all cases higher in efferent lymph than the corresponding values for albumin, indicating that bilirubin was being added to the lymph at the level of the lymph node.

Histological examination of popliteal, intestinal, prescapular and prefemoral lymph nodes of the sheep revealed the presence of whole red cells, free iron and specific bilirubin staining within the reticuloendothelial cells, particularly in the region of the lymphatic sinuses of the nodes (1). The presence of specifically-stained free iron within these large phagocytic cells in the lymphatic sinus area of a popliteal lymph node can be seen in Figure 1. This evidence points to the catabolism of extravascular red cells within lymph nodes in the sheep with the release of significant amounts of bilirubin into the postnodal lymph. Indeed, it can be computed from the bilirubin content of the various sources of lymph in the sheep that catabolism of red cells within the lymph nodes could account for approximately 5-10% of the total number of red cells catabolised per day in the whole animal. Further evidence for this hypothesis is provided by the observation that the injection of autologous red cells into a regional site drained by the popliteal lymph node increased bilirubin levels in the efferent popliteal lymph by some 200-300% at 3-5 hours after injection (1). This finding demonstrated the capacity of the lymph node to catabolise red cells.

## REFERENCES


1 - QUIN, J.W., A.D. SHANNON, : High concentration of bilirubin in post-nodal lymph associated with red blood cell catabolism in lymph nodes of the sheep. Lymphology (in press).

2 - BRODERSEN, R., J. JACOBSEN, : Separation and determination of bile pigments. Meth. biochem. Analysis 17 (1969) 31-54.

# THE EFFECT OF AN EXPERIMENTALLY INDUCED LYMPHOEDEMA ON THE COMPENSATORY HYPERTROPHY OF THE RAT KIDNEY FOLLOWING UNILATERAL NEPHRECTOMIA

M. Müller, H. Cremer and J. Tantow

Institute of Pathology, University of Bonn

Bonn, GFR

The observations in autopsy of patients with well functioned longterm kidney transplantation after total nephrectomia, which showed a smaller increase of the kidney wet weights as compared to those of patients after unilateral nephrectomia, induced us to examine whether the interruption of the lymph circulation alone besides surgical, nervous, therapeutical and other conditions influences the kidney wet weights.

First of all we therefore examined in our previous investigations the effects of an experimentally induced lymphoedema after thermocoagulation of the thoracic duct on the wet weights of the rat kidneys as well as on the nuclear surface areas of the proximal and distal convoluted tubular epithelia (CREMER et al. 1972).

For the planimetric measurements of the nuclear surface areas the proximal and distal convoluted tubules were photographed under high power field (hpf) by Agfapan film and yellow light. Then the pictures were enlarged 28 to 20 centimeters.

According to the planimeter technique of Ott the nuclear surface areas were measured and according to HINTZSCHE (1945) the values were statistically analysed and for each animal - three animals for each experimental day - the "Regelklassen" according to JACOBJ (1931) for the nuclear surface sizes were calculated, at least 300 nuclear surface areas of every animal were measured.

Thereby we were able to demonstrate for the animals with thermocoagulation of the thoracic duct alone that - after an initial increase of the wet weights - as a result of fluid storage in the perivascular spaces together with a filling of the lymphatic vessels in the renal hilus as it was obvious from our results of planimetric measurements of the perivascular spaces; in the longterm experiments of 1 year the renal wet weights stay behind those of the healthy control animals of the same age group. The kidney wet weights diminished about 24%.

These findings are confirmed by our measurements of the nuclear surface areas of the proximal and distal convoluted tubular epithelia which also showed a decrease of the nuclear surface areas (Fig. 1).

The question arose, whether this phenomenon - which is observed under steady state conditions - could also affect the compensatory hypertrophy of the rat kidneys as we could demonstrated at Part I of this congress for the regenerative capacity of the rat liver following subtotal hepatectomia.

Therefore we performed a left sided nephrectomia together with a thermoacoagulation of the thoracic duct before its entry into the left angle of junction at the base of the neck on 36 male and female Sprague Dawley rats for the following experimental days: 2,3,4,5, 6,8,12,16,20,30,60,90 and 360 days.

Unilateral hephrectomia but without thermocoagulation of the thoracic duct was performed on a second group of 33 rats. These rats served as controls for the determination of the wet weights of the right kidney as well as for the measurements of the nuclear surface areas. All animals were killed between 7-9 a.m. by decapitation during ether anesthesia. Then all animals were subjected to a complete autopsy. The wet weights of the kidneys were ascertained by an analytical balance. All organs were fixed in neutral formalin, embedded in paraplast, cut into 5 micron sections and stained for histological studies and prepared for the planimetric measurements.

The examination of the wet weights of the right kidney of successfully thermocoagulated rats after nephrectomia shows a statistically significant increase in the wet weights of the kidneys occur until the 8th day as compared to healthy controls. This is mainly due to the lymphoedema.

The wet weights of the right kidneys of rats, which survived up to 3 months and longer, were lower than those of the right kidneys of healthy rats of the same age group and of those rats in which only nephrectomia was performed without blockade of the thoracic duct. The differences of the values as compared to those of healthy controls are shown in the middle part of figure 2.

In the left side of this figure one can see the results for the liver wet weights of subtotal hepatectomized rats about which

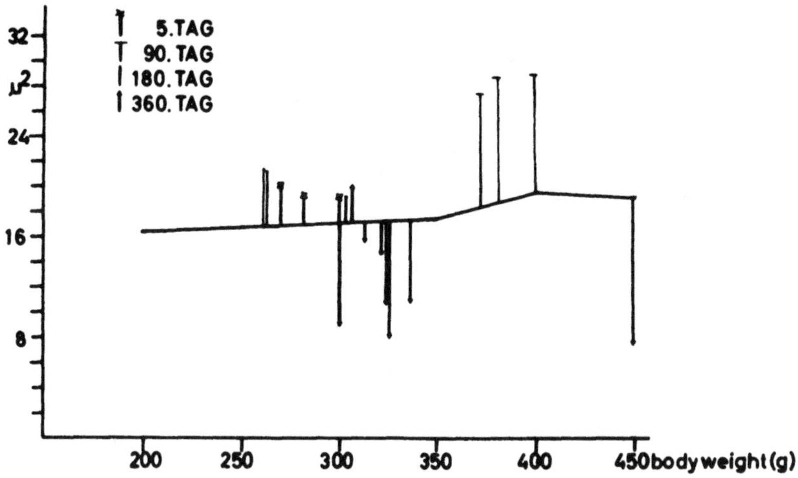


Figure 1

Nuclear surface areas of the proximal and distal convoluted tubules of thoracic duct operated rats as a function of time (5th - 360th day, vertical lines), plotted against those of healthy controls as a function of the body weight (200-450g, horizontal line).

| DAYS | 2/3 HEPATECTOMIA | | NEPHRECTOMIA | | CHRON. ART. HYPERTENSION | |
|---|---|---|---|---|---|---|
| | without | with | without | with | without | with |
| | Blockade of the Thoracic Duct | | Blockade of the Thoracic Duct | | Blockade of the Thoracic Duct | |
| 2-4 | -5,67 g | -3,30g | 0,076g | 0,138g | -0,04 g | -0,01g |
| 6-8 | -1,13g | -2,42g | 0,052g | 0,11g | -0,06g | -0,06g |
| 12-15 | -1,75g | -1,27g | 0,235g | 0,099g | | |
| 20-30 | -1,55g | -2,40g | 0,141 g | 0,238g | 0,04g | 0,01g |
| 60-90 | | | 0,469g | 0,379g | | |
| 360 | -5,19g | -8,88g | 1,44g | 0,90g | | |

Figure 2

Synopsis of wet weights of liver, right kidney and heart as compared to healthy controls after 2/3 hepatectomia, unilateral nephrectomia and chronic arterial hypertension with and without blockade of the thoracic duct in rats as a function of time.

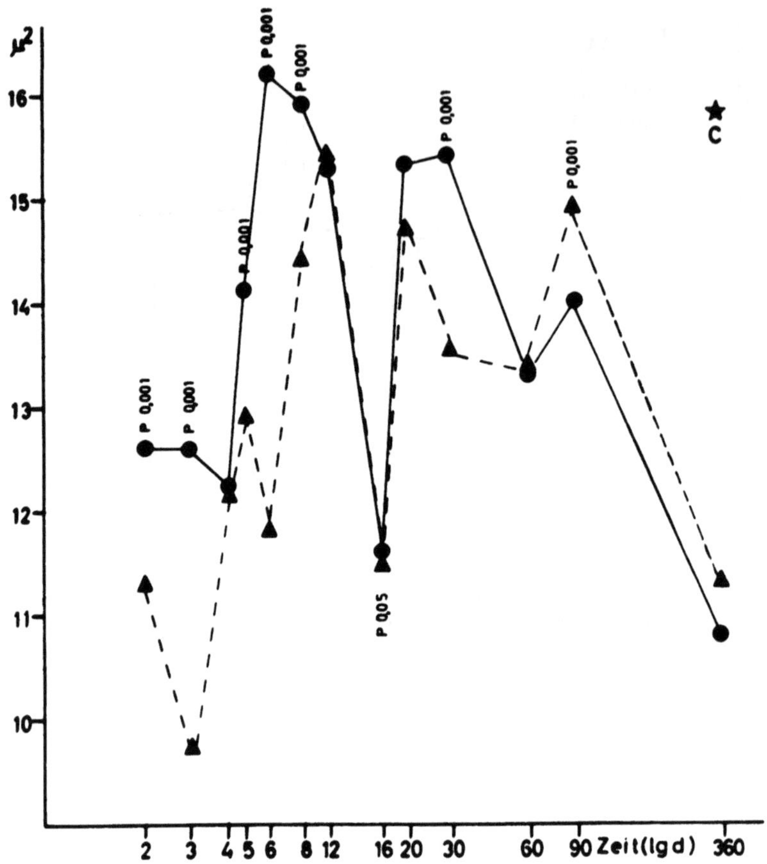


Figure 3

Nuclear surface areas of the proximal and distal convoluted tubules of rats with leftsided nephrectomia (▲- - - -▲) and of rats with leftsided nephrectomia together with thermocoagulation of the thoracic duct (●———●) as a function of time.
C = healthy control animals

we reported in Buenos Aires - Part I -, and which confirmed our results.

The nuclear surface area measurements corresponded to these differences in the wet weights of the right kidneys.

In figure 3 one can see the values of the "Regelklasse" K 1 according to JACOBJ (1931) i.e. the class of the highest frequency as a function of time.

For the first 30 postoperative days the influence of rhythmical proliferations in unilateral nephrectomized rats can be seen according to the investigations of HÜBNER (1967). The higher values in the animals with thermocoagulation of the thoracic duct may be due to lymphoedema.

But here are only of interest the variations after the 60th postoperative day. There is a decrease and after the 90th postoperative day there is a statistically significant decrease of the nuclear surface area values as compared to those of animals without thermocoagulation of the thoracic duct.

The correlation between the two groups for the 360th postoperative day shows as compared to the values of healthy control animals - point C in figure 3 - that there is an impressive decrease in the sizes of the nuclear surface areas.

To sum up, our experimental models might serve to emphasize the importance of the lymphatic vessels in the fields of human medicine and pathology, especially in cases of transplantation. But it is far to be clear, why the experimentally induced (chronic) lymphoedema due the organs'atrophy and decrease of nuclear surface areas which are confirmed by our measurements.

## References

CREMER, H. and MÜLLER, N.: Lichtmikroskopische Untersuchungen an Nieren sowie lipidchemische Untersuchungen im Serum nach Unterbindung des Ductus thoracicus bei Ratten. Virchows Arch. Abt. A Path. Anat. 357, 67-79 (1972)

HINTZSCHE, E.: Statistische Probleme aus der Kerngrössenforschung. Experientia (Basel) 1,103 (1945)

HÜBNER, K.: Kompensatorische Hypertrophie, Wachstum und Regeneration der Rattenniere. Ergebnisse der allg. Path. u. path. Anat., Bd 48, 1-80 (1967), Springer, Berlin-Heidelberg-New York

JACOBJ, W.: Volumetrische Untersuchung an den Zellkernen des Menschen und das allgemeine Problem der Zellkerngrösse. Anat. Anz. 72, 236 (1931)

# Lymphography

# A RATING SYSTEM AS AN AID TO LYMPHOGRAPHIC INTERPRETATION

M. Luening and K. Raab

Schumanstr - 20/21 Charitē/Roentgeninstitut

104 Berlin, GDR

The correctness of lymphographic diagnosis is largely determined by the wellknown limitations of this method although it is also dependent, to a considerable degree, on the experience and skill of the examiner. This, in turn, would account for the wide differences we find in the interpretation of lymphograms by different authors.

Thus, one way to improve the results of lymphographic diagnosis would be to elaborate a catalogue listing lymphographic criteria of metastases with an indication of their diagnostic value which might be as aid particularly to the inexperienced examiner in cases where problems of differential diagnosis have to be decided.

Moreover, for our research team a rating system for lymphographic criteria of metastases is needed for the work we do to standardize and optimize the method of lymphographic diagnosis by using computer techniques.

The use of computer techniques requires to have data on the clinical likelihood of the incidence of lymph node metastases and, additionally, to have data, expressed as mathematical terms, on the probability of the occurrence of criteria that are seen in an X-ray picture.

Rating systems have been worked out and tested for lymph node metastases in cases of malignant melanoma and testicular tumours. At the present time other tumours models are being elaborated.

Lymphograms of 251 patients with malignant melanomas and 147 patients with testicular tumours were analyzed. We found 62 cases of lymph node metastases in the first group, and 53 cases in the second.

As analysis of the frequency distribution of the criteria of 50 inguinal and 104 paraaortic metastatic lymph nodes and their lymph vessels was carried out by means of electronic data processing.

A comparative analysis was made of these criteria with those of 80 inguinal and 115 paraaortic non-metastatic lymph nodes. Subsequently, a statistical examination was made of the results obtained using the $\chi^2$ test. At the end of this, 10 criteria remained for both the malignant melanoma and for the testicular tumours that may be used as an indication for the occurrence of lymph node metastases (Table 1 and 2).

As could be expected, both tables show the 3 principal symptoms for the presence of metastases, though in a different order. These are: filling and storing defects, replacement and, enlargement of the lymph nodes.

We regarded the $\chi^2$ values as a measure for the diagnostic value of the individual criteria. On the basis of these a rating system was established and this rating system was used to evaluate all cases of normal and metastatic lymph nodes.

In this analysis an average number of 111.5 points was found for metastases in malignant melanomas, and of 13.6 points for non-metastatic lymph nodes. The difference is, statistically, highly significant.

The scale of the rating system was established as follows:

0 - 50 points : normal lymph node

51 - 80 points : uncertain

$>$ 80 points : metastatic lymph node

The average number of points found in cases of testicular tumours was 476 for metastatic lymph nodes and 52 for normal lymph nodes.

The rating system, in this case is:

0 - 180 points : normal lymph node

180 - 220 points : uncertain

$>$ 220 points : metastatic lymph node

TABLE 1: METASTASES IN MALIGNANT MELANOMAS

| Lymph nodes | | Points |
|---|---|---|
| Incomplete/complete Extinction | | 52 |
| Filling and Storing Defects | | 48 |
| Size | superior 2800 $mm^3$ | 42 |
| | Inferior 1250 $mm^3$ | 28 |
| Egg-cup-phenomenon/ rim sign | | 21 |
| Irregular structure | | 18 |
| Destroyed marginal sinus | | 9 |
| Spherical transformation | | 7 |
| Reduced intensity of contrast | | 6 |
| **Lymphatic vessels** | | |
| Displacement | | 14 |
| Collaterals | | 7 |

TABLE 2: METASTASES IN TESTICULAR TUMOURS

| Lymph nodes | Points |
|---|---|
| Filling and Storing Defects | 152 |
| Incomplete / complete Extinction | 143 |
| Considerable Enlargement | 142 |
| Egg-cup-phenomenon/ rim sign | 98 |
| Spherical transformation | 33 |
| **Lymphatic vessels** | |
| Displacement | 48 |
| Partial/ total Drainage blocking | 42 |
| Efferent vessels reduced | 32 |
| Afferent vessels reduced | 22 |
| Stasis of contrast medium | 27 |

In comparing the two systems one should not be confused by the different number points in the two rating systems as these result from the different number of lymph nodes examined for establishing the two tumour models. So the two ranges of points may be regarded as being roughly equivalent proportionally.

The Ranges of points established in this way will, inevitably include a certain rate of false diagnoses.

Thus, in the case of testicular tumours 4 lymph nodes, out of a number of 104 cases of paraaortic metastases were diagnosed as non-metastasis, i.e. a falsely negative evaluation was given while in 4 cases out of 115 cases of non-metastatic lymph nodes, a falsely positive estimation was given, i.e. 4 cases of non-metastatic lymph nodes were diagnosed as metastatic, and 8 cases were evaluated as uncertain.

In general, the correctness of this method is thus theoretically calculated to be 92.8%. This result is satisfactory particularly when seen from the point of views that the rate of false negative findings is only 1.8 %.

Analogous calculations were made for the lymph nodes in cases of malignant melanomas. In this analysis only two normal and one metastatic lymph nodes were found in this range considered as uncertain.

As a practical test, three roentgenologists, two of them experienced examiners, and one less experienced, were asked, independently, to evaluate 10 lymphograms of each tumour model system (with and without metastases).

There was no case where a wrong diagnosis was made on the basis of the above mentioned rating systems. Only slight differences in the number of points were observed between the 3 examiners.

In conclusion I should like to add a few remarks to explain why we are making such great efforts to establish separate rating systems for the different tumours.

Our own experience has shown that, on the one hand, peculiarities is the biological activity of different tumours may be reflected in the lymphogram while, on the other hand, regional peculiarities of the lymph nodes, i.e. the topographical anatomy of the tumour, have to be taken into account.

This means, an exact answer to this question can only be given if a sufficient number of rating systems for different kinds of tumours are available for comparison.

# CORRELATION OF HISTOLOGIC OVER LYMPHANGIOGRAPHIC FINDINGS IN LYMPHOEDEMA OF THE EXTREMITIES

P. Balas, M.D., J. Mauromatis, M.D., A. Theodosiou, M.D., P. Delikaris, M.D., and L. Nacopoulou, M.D.

First Department of Surgery
Athens University Medical School

Among the main diagnostic procedures for the investigation of lymphoedema of the extremities primary or secondary is lymphangiography. In addition, the classification according to Kinmonth[3], of different types of primary lymphoedema, is based on the lymphangiographic findings.

However, from previous works of Kaindl, et al. (1967)[2], Collard, et al., (1968)[1], and Olszewski, et al. (1972)[4] it was shown that the histologic examination of the lymphatic vessels of the extremities might change the traditional classification on one hand and help for the elucidation of the etiology of various types of lymphoedema on the other.

During the last three years in a series of 13 of our cases of lymphoedema of the extremities a correlation of the lymphangiographic to the histologic findings was attempted.

## Material and Method

Thirty eight cases of both sexes, with lymphoedema of the upper and lower extremities were studied (Table I).

The age of the patients varied from 15 to 50 years. The duration of symptoms extented from 1 to 15 years with an average of 5 years.

Of over one hundred cases of lymphoedema of the extremities seen during the last five years 38 cases were submitted to lymphangiography which was performed in 39 extremities. The lymphangiographic findings are shown on table II.

Table I

MATERIAL

38 Cases of Lymphoedema of the Extremities

| SEX | | EXTREMITIES | | CLINICAL CLASSIFICATION | |
|---|---|---|---|---|---|
| M | F | Upper | Lower | Primary | Secondary |
| 12 | 26 | 5 | 57 | 33 | 5 |

Table II

Lymphangiographic findings

| | |
|---|---|
| Normal | 8 |
| Aplasia | 5 |
| Hypoplasia | 8 |
| Solitary minute lymphatic vessels | 3 |
| Multiple minute vessels | 6 |
| Retrograde filling | 2 |
| Block of lymph nodes | 2 |
| Post-traumatic block | 1 |
| Total | 39 |
| No lymphangiography (Diffusion of patent blue) | 12 |

In 12 cases the attempt for lymphangiography failed because no lymphatic vessel was found on the dorsum of the foot or on the hand in spite of the intensive search. In these cases a diffusion of the injected patent blue was noticed. This was due to lymphatic aplasia or to the ectopic course of the lymphatics.

In 13 cases, after the completion of the lymphangiography and the removal of the canula, a segment of the efferent vessel about 5 or more mms was excised and was sent for histologic examination.

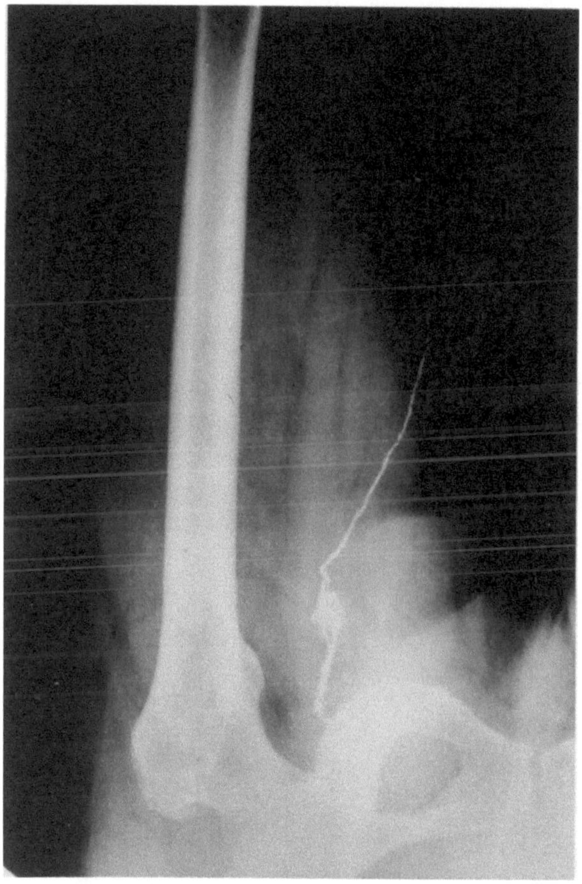

Fig. 1. Lymphangiogram showing solitary lymphatic vessel on the thigh on a patient with primary lymphoedema of the left leg. (Case 1)

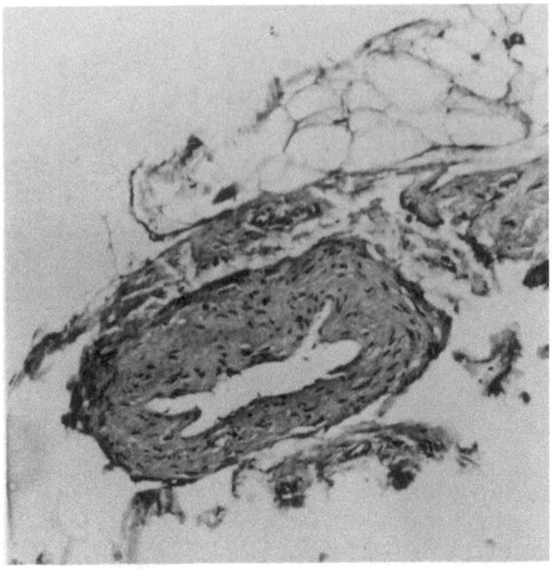

Fig. 2. Photomicrograph of normal lymphatic vessel (Hematoxyline - Eosine 1:120). (Case 1)

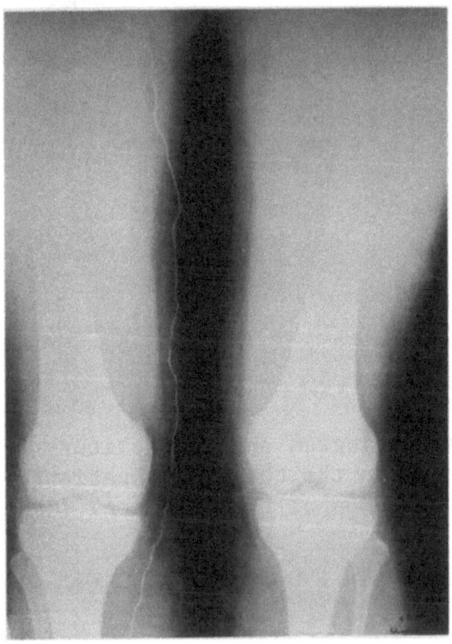

Fig. 3. Lymphangiogram showing solitary vessel on the right leg of a patient with primary lymphoedema of this extremity. (Case 2)

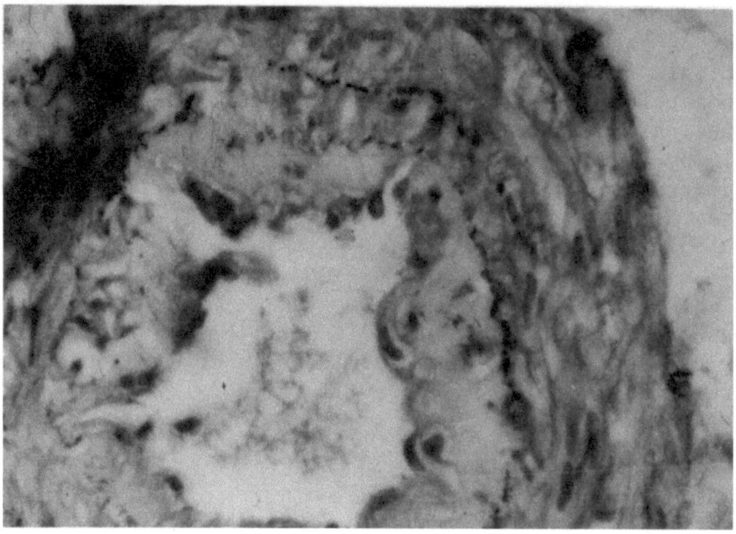

Fig. 4. Photomicrograph of lymphatic vessel showing intimal hyperplasia with duplication of the elastic internal lamina (Van Gieson - Orcein, 1:400). (Case 2)

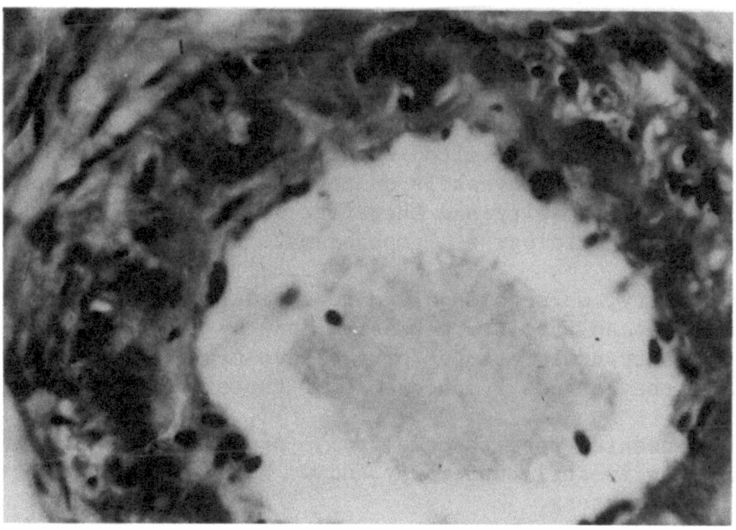

Fig. 5. Photomicrograph of lymphatic vessel showing deposits of P.A.S. positive substance (black homogeneous appearance) (Hyperiodic acid, 1:400). (Case 2)

The histologic specimens were reviewed by two pathologists separately. The first was without special experience on the histology of the lymphatic vessels and the other was an expert. No pathologic findings were noticed on the specimens except 1 in which a thickening of the intima with changes of hyalinosis were found, although the exact changes of the intima could be seen only by electron microscope. In figures 1,2,3,4,5 the lymphangiographic and the histologic findings of two cases are presented.

## DISCUSSION

Recently Kaindl, et al. (1967)[2] described characteristic histologic changes of the lymphatic vessels on lymphoedema of the extremities as shown in table III.

Table III

Histologic changes of lymphatic vessels (Kaindl, 1967)

Proliferative Thrombolymphangitis
Obliterative lymphangiopathy
Fibrotic lymphangiopathy
Lymphectasiae

However, from our limited experience the histologic examination of the lymphatic vessels on the affected extremities did not show any abnormality and therefore did not help for the elucidation of the etiology of lymphoedema.

In summary, we recommend a more extensive histologic investigation as an absolute necessity done by expert histologists using an electron microscope for the investigation of the lymphatic vessels in the various lymphoedemas of the extremities.

The presented results come from a preliminary study. Our investigation is still under way and we hope to bring more results to the next Congress.

Note: We are indebted to Professor Norman Browse and Dr.Whimster of St. Thomas' Hospital of London for their help in studying the histologic specimens of our cases.

## REFERENCES

1. Collard, M., Fievez, M.: Correlations radiologiques et anatomiques dans la pathologie tronculaire du lymphoedème. Phlebologie, 21:155, 1968.

2. Kaindl, F., Mannheimer, E., Pfleger, L., Thurnher, B.L Histology of lymphangiopathies. In A. Rüttimann: Progress in Lymphology, G. Thieme Verlag, Stuttgart, 1967.

3. Kinmonth, J.B.: The lymphatics. Edward Arnold, London, 1972.

4. Olszewski, W., Machowski, Z., Sokolowski, J. Sawicki, Z., Zerbino, D., Nielubowicz, J.: Primary Lymphedema of lower extremities. I. Lymphangiographic and histological studies of lymphatic vessels and lymph nodes in primary lymphedema. Polish Medical Journal, XI: 1564, 1972.

## REFERENCES

# LYMPHANGIOADENOGRAPHY IN FILARIASIS DUE TO WUCHERERIA BANCROFTI IN MEN

Sri Tinon Roesman Kromosoedirdjo, M.D., and
F. Partono, M.D.

Faculty of Medicine University of Indonesia
Jakarta, Selatan, Indonesia

## Introduction

Filariasis is widely distributed in Indonesia and Jakarta is endemic for Wuchereria bancrofti.

The aim of this study is:

1. To find out the possibilities for making a radiological diagnosis of elephantiasis caused by filarial infection.

2. To see what part of the lymph system is affected in selected bancroftian filarial infection and what changes could be found in early and late state.

3. To see whether there are morphological correlations with the clinical staging on its lymphangiographical features.

The classical description as found in most of the text books, the development of the disease can be divided into 4 stages:

1. The biological incubation period
2. The patent symptomless period
3. The acute stage
4. The chronic stage

During the biological incubation period no symptoms or one or more episodes of lymphangitis / lymphadenitis may occur in natives. In this stage no microfilariae could be found in the blood (11). The patent symptomless period, may last for many years or remain throughout life in native persons.

There are no symptoms although tissue changes could be found. The blood is positive for microfilariae (11).
Next comes the acute stage with the typical lymphadenitis, lymphangitis accompanied by fever (the filarial fever) which recurs periodically as frequent as once a month, some times accompanied by fatigue, headache or urticarial rash (11).

These attacks become less severe and may develop gradually into the chronic stage. The lymphatic vessels become hypertrophic. The worms become caught in this tissue, die off, degenerate and may cause inflammation again (11).

The recurrent inflammation attacks result in blockage of the lymph vessels causing dilatation of the distal parts, followed by lymphedema secondary infections and ending in elephantiasis (11).

It is generally accepted that the appearance of the acute symptoms is related to the presence of the adult worms in the lymphatic system (11).

## Method and Material

Polythene catheter is used to be inserted into the punctured part of the lymph vessel.

As contrast liquid, lipiodol ultrafluid 38% is used. About 10 cc contrast liquid is injected in each of the lower extremities in total a maximum of 25 cc.

The injection is done constantly and continually, propelled by electromotor.

By means of an acceleration box two conical rolls are propelled, so that it is possible to regulate the speed of the injection from 1 cc per 5 minute to 1 cc per 20 minute by means an adjustable transmission wheel.

Lymphangiogram are made of all parts of the retroperitoneal lymph system.

Twenty four hours after that, lymphadenograms are made of the lymph node part of the retroperitoneal lymph channels.

Thirty cases selected by the Department of Parasitology University of Indonesia are used, divided into three groups:

A. 10 patients which are: ( blood (+) for microfilaria
( clinically (-) without symptoms

B. 10 patients which are: ( blood (+) for microfilaria
( clinically (+) with symptoms

C. 10 patients which are: ( blood (-) for microfilaria
( clinically (+) with symptoms

## Results

Group A: 7 patients show: lymphangiographical pattern like dilatation on one or two vessels mostly unilateral. Lymphangiectasia could be also seen in one or two lymph vessels on one side, located around the kidney region para aortal $L_2$ - $L_3$, but also in the inguinal regions. 3 (three) cases show normal lymphangiographical features. No abnormalities are further to be seen.

Group B: Lymphangiographical features of 10 cases given important patterns.
2 (two) cases show normal lymphangiographical features, while 8 (eight) cases show variations in course, calibre and distribution.
The vessels revealed valvular incompetence (6,10).
Lymphatic pelvic fistulisation, type cystic and type semi circular according to Akisada 1968 were found (1).
The whole retroperitoneal lymph system shows dilated lymph channels (10).
The pattern of the retroperitoneal lymph vessels could be summerized as well as:

1. dilatation
2. tortuosity
3. stasis
4. leakage
5. Collaterals / anastomosis
6. Clear patterns in dilated afferent lymph vessel

The nodes were increased in size especially in the para aortic region and in the inguinal areas.
There was also generalized increase in the number of nodes. Both inguinal lymph nodulae are hypertrophic with discrete accentuation of the finaly pigmented structure of a normal node (7). Some times a with naked eye eight shape figure suspected to be that of an adult filaria worm are visible in one of the inguinal node.

Group C: In 9 cases no features of dilatation at all were found on the lymphangiographical findings. This is the important differences with the features as those in group B.
The pictures of the retroperitoneal lymph vessels have the same aspect, even without dilatation.

Very few locally rest-lymphangioectasia were found on one or both of the inguinal areas.
Characteristic are the collaterals and the anastomosis, a few fibrotic like patterns of lymph vessels are visible.
The pattern of the retroperitoneal lymph vessels could be summerized as well as:

1. collaterals / anastomosis
2. no dilatation
3. lymphatico pelvic fistulisation
4. fibrotic-like patterns

The nodes looks hypertrophic with discrete accentuation of the finaly pigmented structure of normal node.
Only in one case a normal lymphangiographical feature was found.

The following cases show the different features in the lymphangio-adenogram.

Case 1

Is a 28 years old Indonesian man, who complained of fatigue and recurrent fever of 3 years duration.
No other clinical sign were found.
The examination of night blood smear was positive for micro filarial bancrofti.
Lymphangiographical features showed: a few number of dilated lymphvessels on one side (unilateral) characteristic are the location of the lymph vessel dilatation: on the kidney region (figure 4), para aortal region $L_2$ - $L_3$.

Case 2

Is a thirty years old Indonesian man, who complained of fatigue and recurrent fever of five years duration.
No edema on both legs was found, but hydrocele present.
The examination of night blood smear was positive for micro filaria bancrofti.
Lymphangiographical features of the whole retroperitoneal lymph vessels show dilatation, tortuosity, stasis, leakage, collateral/anastomosis (figure 2).

In one of the left inguinal node, a with naked eye eight shape figure was visible, suspected to be of an adult filaria worm.
The retroperitoneal lymph nodulae shows localisations of hyperthrophic patterns.

Case 3

Is a thirty-two years old Indonesian man, who complained of fatigue and recurrent fever of eight years duration.

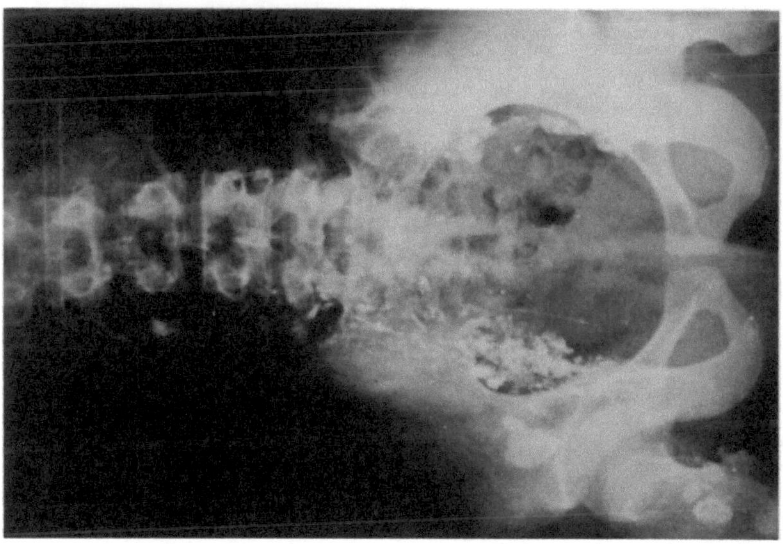

Fig. 1 - Lymphangiogram in bancroftian Filariasis

CHRONIC STAGE

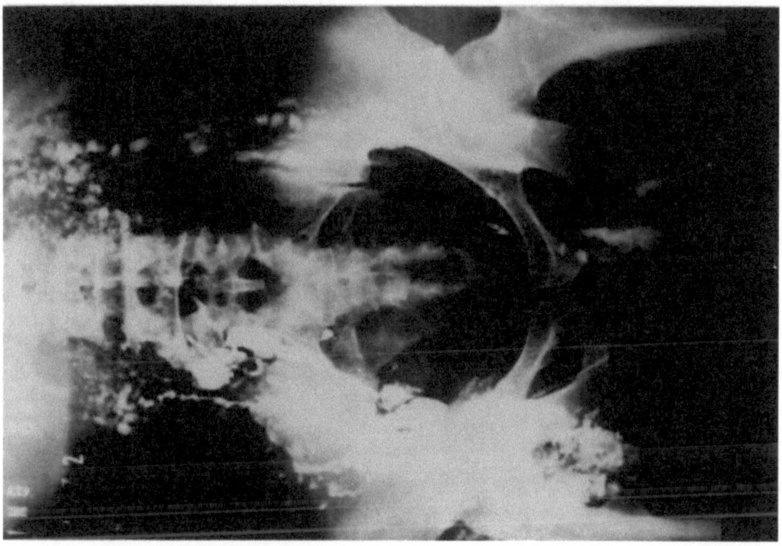

Fig. 2 - Lymphangiogram in bancroftian Filariasis.

ACUTE STAGE

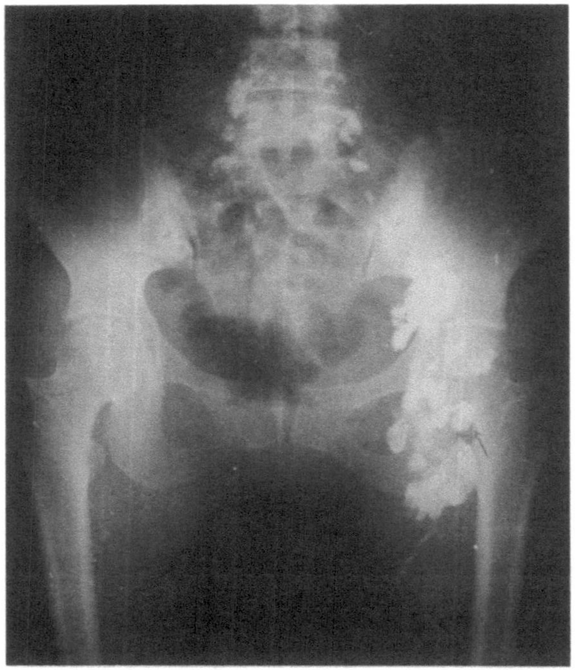

Fig. 3 - Lymphadenogram in Filariasis (W. bancrofti)

ACUTE STAGE

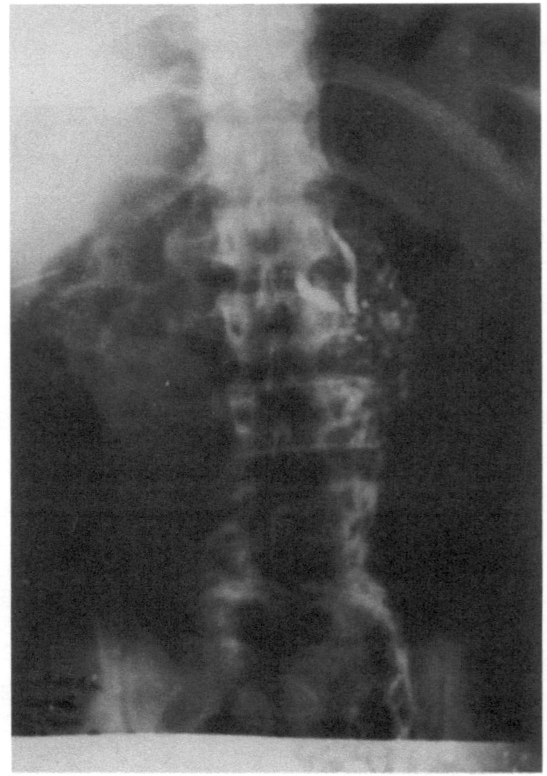

Fig. 4 - Lymphangiogram in Filariasis (W. bancrofti)

PATENT SYMPTOMLESS PERIOD

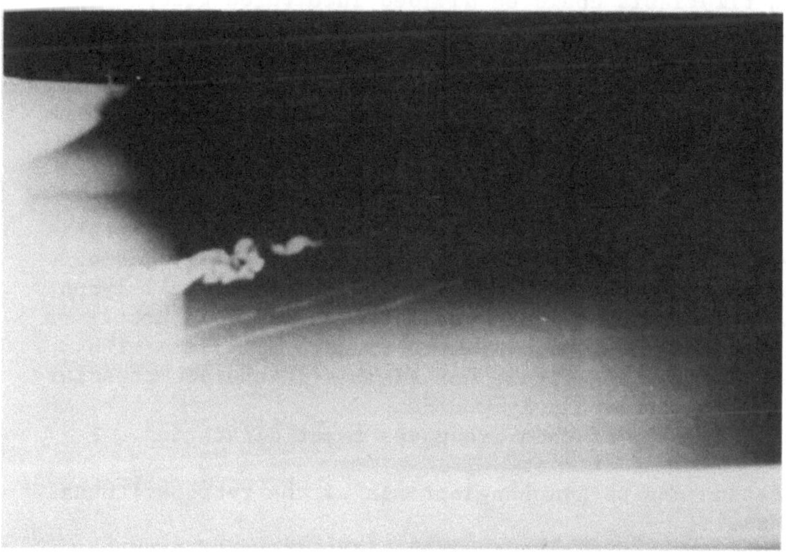

Fig. 5 - Lymphangiogram in bancroftian Filariasis - could also be in Malayan Filariasis
PATENT SYMPTOMLESS PERIOD

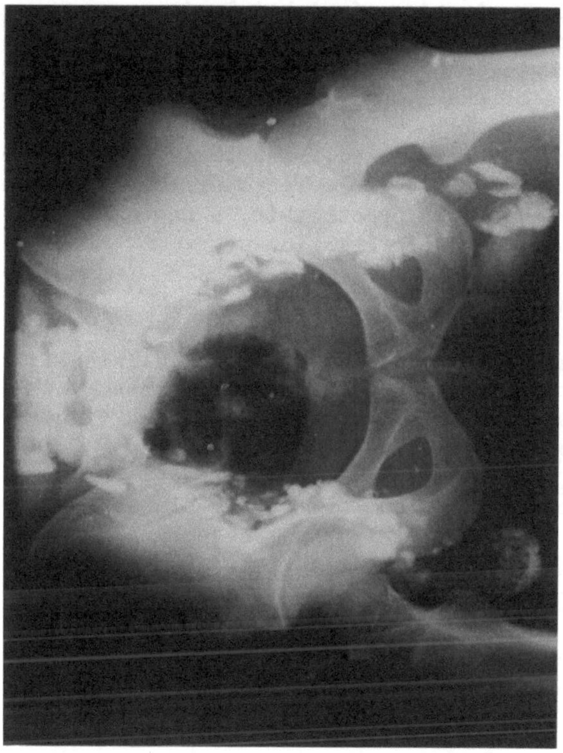

Fig. 6 - Lymphadenogram in Filariasis (W. bancrofti)
ACUTE STAGE

Slight edema on the right leg was found, hydrocele was also present. The examination of night blood smear was negative for microfilaria bancrofti.
The lymphangioadenographical features showed: collateral / anastomosis of the lymph vessels, also fibrotic features was visible (figure 1).
The most characteristic sign was found, exactly no dilatation shadows at all on the whole retroperitoneal channels.
The lymph node looks hypotrophic, a few node show calcified pattern, but no characteristic.

## Conclusion

Group A case with blood smear (+) and clinically (-), was called the patent symptomless period shows lymphangiographic features as was seen on figure four and five (figure 4,5) with description as was written in Group A.

Group B, case with blood smear (+), clinically (+): was called the acute stage, shows lymphangiographically as was seen on figure two, three and six (figure 2,3,6) with description as written in group B.

Group C, case with blood smear (-), clinically (+) was called the chronic stage, shows lymphangiographically as was seen on figure one with description as written on group C.

This diffuse injury of the human lymphatic system caused by bancroftian filariasis could be divided into three groups: namely: A,B and C.

A. A few dilatations and lymphangiectasia of the lymph vessels, characteristic on the kidney or inguinal regional during the patent symptomless period, unilateral but could be also bilateral.

B. Dilatation and lymphangiectasia, tortuosity, leakage, stasis, collaterals and lymphatico pelvic fistulisation (1) during the acute stage was seen of the whole retroperitoneal lymph vessels. Hypertrophic lymph nodulae localisation, mostly on both regions of the inguinal, were found. Sometimes with naked eye eight shape figure was visible in the sub capsular area of the hypertrophic lymphnode.
   The characteristic of this group was exact dilatation.

C. No dilatation and no lymphangiectasia of the retroperitoneal lymph vessels.
   But the aspect of the picture looks like those of group B without dilatation pattern.

CORRELATION BETWEEN CLINICAL FINDINGS AND LYMPHANGIOGRAPHICAL FEATURES IN HUMAN BANCROFTIAN FILARIASIS

| FILARIASIS DIVIDED INTO 3 STAGES | Clini-cal | Labor. Blood | LYMPHANGIOGRAM | LYMPHADENOGRAM |
|---|---|---|---|---|
| I.a. Biological in-cubation period | - | ± | Normal | Normal |
| b. Patent symp-tomless Group A | - | + | -Unilateral localized dilatation of lymph vessel on the renal re-gion/inguinal region<br>-Sometimes bilateral | Normal |
| II. Acute Stage Group B | + | + | -Dilatation of the lymphatics<br>-Tortuosity<br>-Stasis<br>-Leakage<br>-Colaterals/lymphatic anastomosis (type Akisada 1968)<br>-Clear patterns in dilated afferent lymph vessels | -Hypertrophy<br>-Eight shape figure suspected of adult filaria worm in the sub-capsular region of lymph node<br>-Sinus marginalis intact |
| III. Chronic Stage Group C | + | - | -Collaterals/lymphatic anasto-mosis (type Akisada 1968)<br>-No dilatation<br>-Fibrotic-like patterns<br>-Lymphatico pelvic fistulisation | -hypertrophy<br>-compact structure with calci-fication spots in the peri-lymphatic fat of the lymph node |

Localisation of fibrotic channels were visible with hypertrophic lymph nodulae, mostly on both regions of the inguinal. Also a few calcified small nodes were found during the chronic stage. Lymphatico pelvic fistulisation is also common to be seen, but characteristic are the collaterals and anastomosis of the lymph vessels without dilatation at all.

## Discussion

The results prove that injury of the lymphatic system is usually diffuse of a generalised lympho-ganglionar disease.
Dilatation of the lymphatic ducts with defects of the valvular function.
Only at the level of the kidneys that this valvular pathologic process is always observed in the course of chyluria (7).
This condition of Bancroftian filariasis could be seen on the lymphangiographical features of the acute stage and the patent symptomless period. (figures 2,3,4,5,6).

It is generally accepted that the appearance of the acute symptoms is related to the presence of the adult worms in the lymphatic system (11) figures 2,3).

The acute stage shows major disturbances, the circulatory stasis due to injury of the valvular mechanism (6,10) (figure 2).

Lymphangiography was done, on case with acute stage unilateral on the right side, peripheral up to the thoracic duct but this intralymphatic contrast medium comes back downward on the left side over kidney region into the marked dilated lymph vessels of the left enlarged scrotum. Dilated lymph vessels look like a wide loops with insufficient valve.

## Summary

Bancroftian filariasis cause an injury of the lymphatic system diffuse and generalized. It is a generalized lymphoganglionair disease. There exist an important alteration of the lymphatic system, the major disturbance being the circulatory stasis due to injury of the valvular mechanism. This general lymphatic injury caused by bancroftian filariasis could be divided into three groups lymphangiographically.
Table I shows correlation between clinical findings and lymphangiographical features. Confirmed by thirty selected bancroftian filarial cases from the Department of Parasitology University of Indonesia.
Six patients show normal lymphogram.

Acknowledgements

In the preparation of this paper I am indebted to Prof. Sjahriar Rasad. SEAMEO C.C.B. - member for Indonesia for his efforts in finding funds from C.C.B. for the implementation of this project. Also to Prof. Sri Oemijati Head Department of Parasitology University of Indonesia, for valuable advice.

## REFERENCES

1. Akisada M, Lymphaticopelvis fistulisation in filarial Chyluria, Progress in Lymphology II 1968, 125-126.
2. Akisada M, Tani S, Lymphographic study of 28 with Filarial (hemato) Chyluria, Progress in Lymphology I 1966,47-50.
3. Desprez-Curely J.P., Lymphographie dans le Chyluries Boerhave Cursus Radiologie, Leiden 82-97.
4. Gooneratne B.W.M., A Chronological lymphographic study of cats experimentally infected with Brugia Filariasis from 5 days to 5 years, Lymphology 6 (1973) 127-149.
5. Gooneratne, B.W.M., Lymphography - Clinical and experimental Butterworth 1974.
6. Kromosoedirdjo Roesman S.T., Technique of lymphography by Layden Method, Kongres Radiologi Nasional ke I, Jakarta 23-29 September 1969.
7. Picard J.D. Lymphographics in Chyluria Progress in Lymphology I, 1966, 43-46.
8. Roesman S.T. Lymphografi Retroperitoneal pada penderita Carcinoma Cervicis Uteri, M.K.I. 21-5 Jakarta 1971, 221-225.
9. Roesman S.T. Lymphographi, M.K.I. 23-1 Jakarta 1972, 1-11.
10. Roesman S.T. Lymphangio-adenografi in Filariasis, XIII International Congress of Radiology, Madrid, October 15-20, 1973.
11. Sri Oemijati, Clinical and immunological aspects of Filariasis proceedings of Seminar on Filariasis and immunology of parasitic infections, Singapore 1968.
12. Viamonte M, Lymphography in inflammatory conditions, Progress in Lymphology I, 1966, 148.

# PROGRESS ON THE LYMPHOGRAPHIC STUDY OF HEAD AND NECK

Dr. Federico J. Gruart

Calle Austria 2626

Buenos Aires, Argentina

Since we published our paper on the study of the lymphatic system of the head and neck (April 1967) by means of the perlingual injection of either Ethiodol or Ultrafluid Lypiodol and being able to obtain with it illustrative images of the main lymphatic groups in an important number of patients that carried different types of tumors we kept on using this lymphographic study based on what we consider interesting aspects of the same.

The radiological plates showed us a repetition of the lymphatic groups disposition in the different patients subjected to the study. As these groups are mainly the submental, submaxillary, subdigastric and the jugulocarotid chain which are usually the first stations affected by the cancer methastasis of oropharynx origin the possibility of visualizing the changes of the nodes morphology has a considerable value as a preoperative exploration as the palpation alone can not detect the same in a number of cases.

We applied this method in more than 200 patients in which a radical neck dissection was performed to do a postoperative control. With this useful means of investigation of the completness of the neck dissection we could prove in some cases the presence of residual lymph nodes that required further treatment.

As will be seen in the slides that are going to be projected later we also do the radiological study of the surgical specimens to certify the different concentration of the radiopaque substance in the lymphatic nodes and checking in this way with the pathological study that the radiological changes correspond to the cancer methastasis. We can state that we have a very small number of false positives.

In a percentage of cases (7% in a hundred) we could detect controlateral lymphatic nodes which proved to be methastatic. One aspect that is important to emphasize is the perfect tolerance that the tongue has to the radiopaque substance used to perform the study. We keep on using from 6 to 8 cc of it and divide it injecting one third in the anterior half of the tongue and two thirds in the posterior half.

Based in these previous considerations we have established a routine study of patients carrying tumors of the head and neck; a preoperative perlingual lymphography, a postoperative x-ray of the specimen and a week after an x ray of the neck to check that the operation has been complete. As part of the subsequent follow up we perform once a year another lymphography.

## Summary and Conclusions

Keeping on using the perlingual lymphography to study the head and neck patients lymphatic system have furnished us with useful results. As it shows the condition of the main neck lymphatic stations (submental, submaxillary, jugulodigastric chain) which most frequently methastasized it allow us to adjust our treatment.

Another point that is important to stress is the possibility of discovering a suspicious lymphatic node, that could have not been detected by palpation.

The postoperative follow-up of the patient can be easily done with this method.

It can finally be said that combining this perlingual lymphography with the scintigraphy we can achieve a more complete knowledge of the head and neck lymphatic system.

# LYMPHOGRAPHY AND SYSTEMIC LUPUS ERYTHEMATOSUS

G. Thibaut, G. Mayer, R. Herbeural

Clinique Medicale A

CHU 54000 Nancy, France

Lymphography is usually performed in hemopathies and lymphomas. It is also carried out in other diseases (sarcoidosis, tuberculosis, ...), but it is unusual in systemic lupus erythematosus. In this disease, clinically enlarged lymph nodes are present in some cases.

In two patients, lymphography demonstrated deep enlarged lymph nodes. The first case was a female aged 68, with fever, arthralgias, lymphocytosis, positive L.E. cells and antinuclear antibodies; lymphogram showed retroperitoneal tumoral lymph nodes. In the second case, a man aged 41, with arthralgias, lymphocytosis, positive L.E. cells, and antinuclear antibodies, lymphogram showed an identical aspect as seen in chronic lymphoid leukemia. The third patient was a female aged 53; the diagnosis for four years was chronic lymphoid leukemia. The lymphogram revealed deep nodes bulky, regularly enlarged. Subsequently, the patient had fever, thoracic pains and arthralgia. The new clinical data, hyperthermia, pericarditis arthralgia associated with biological alterations were consistent with the diagnosis of disseminated lupus erythematosus.

Lupus erythematosus is a polymorphic disorder characterized by multisystem involvement. Classically, arthralgia, hyperthermia, skin lesions, renal and cardiac abnormalities are usually found with variable frequency.

Adenopathies have been described during the course of acute dissemination lupus erythematosus. Different workers interested in this field of research do not agree about their frequency. The first description of enlarged lymph nodes in disseminated lupus erythematosus dates back to 1907 (Short). Fox and Rosham find localized or generalized adenopathies in 67% of 277 cases. Most workers consider that lymph node involvement is variable, ranging from 30-50% according to the cases. However, Dubois reports the presence of adenopathies in 58% of 520 cases, Jessar in 32% of 216 patients; Harvey in 50% cases, with 37% generalized enlarged lymph nodes and 13% cervical and axillary adenopathies. To our knowledge, the presence of deep adenopathies is never mentioned, though Pequignot recently showed the presence of bulky mediastinal lymph nodes in a patient with lupus. Our cases further demonstrate the existence of lymph node abnormalities in this disease. The first case showed a tumoral polycyclic ganglionic mass. The second case was more suggestive of chronic lymphoid leukemia with enlargement of lymph nodes, thought they remained delimited and homogenous. Finally, in the third case, lupus erythematosus developed in the course of chronic lymphoid leukemia and showed again a pattern suggesting chronic lymphoid leukemia. Undoubtedly, pathological lymph nodes may develop in the course of primary lupus, however the possible relationship between a disorder such as chronic lymphoid leukemia and lupus erythematosus must equally be considered.

It is well known that development of autoantibodies increases as a patient grows older. Such is the case for antinuclear antibodies. Moreover, certain disorders are accompanied by the production of autoantibodies, which are anti-organ, anti-platelet, anti-erythrocyte antibodies. These patients are more liable than other subjects to make auto-antibodies and it is not surprising to observe the formation of antinuclear antibodies. Antinuclear antibodies were thus found during the course of acute or chronic leukemia (Millier, Dreyfus, Bernard) of malignant lymphoma (Harvey, Cammarata), of Hodgkin's disease (Nilsen, Howqua). Numerous previous publications and ours demonstrate that immunologic abnormalities sometimes are associated with lymphoproliferative diseases which are in turn associated with lymphadenopathy and lymphographic abnormalities.

References

1. Andrew, V.C.: Systemic lupus erythematosus and neoplasia of the lymphooreticular system. Brit. J. Derm. 1968, 80, 503-508.

2. Deaton, J.G., Levin, C.: Systemic lupus erythematosus and acute myeloblastic leukemia. Arch. Int. Med. 1967, 120 345-353

3. Dubois, E.L.: Lupus erythematosus. Mac Graw Hill Book Co. New York 1966.

4. Howqua, J., Mackay, I.R.: L.E. cells in lymphoma. Blood 1963 22 191-198.

5. Kent-Smith, C., Cassidy, J.T., Bole, G.G.: Type I dysgammaglobulinemie, systemic lupus erythematosus and lymphoma. Amer. J. Med. 1970, 48, 113-119.

6. Miller, D.G.: Les desordres immunologriques au cours des leucemues de des hematosarcomes. Rev. Frang. etud. Clin. biol. 1962, 7, 1112-1125.

7. Nilsen, L.B.: Appearance of Hodgkin's disease in a patient with systemic lupus erythematosus. Cancer 1967 20, 1930-1933.

8. Pequignot, H., Liot, F., Schmit, G., Christoforov, B., Galian, A., Amouroux, J.: Adenopathies mediastinales resolutives au cours d'ure maladie lepique nevelee par des thomobosis venenses refetees. Ann. Med. Interne 1973, 123, 961-966.

9. Schaison, G., Najean, Y., Seligmann, M., Flandrin, G., Jacquillat, C., Weil, M., Cannat, A., Ripault, S., Dreyfus, B., Bernard, J.: Leucemie aigue a evolution proleugee et syndrome lupigue. Neuv. Rev. Franc. Heriat 1969, 9, 419-434.

# LYMPHOGRAPHIC INVESTIGATIONS ON RENAL CARCINOMA FOR CLASSIFICATION AND STAGING ACCORDING TO THE TNM-SYSTEM

J. Lissner, U. Klein, P. Carl, and W. Kroll

Klinik und Polklinik fur Radiologie der Universitat

Munchen, Munchen, Germany

Complete preoperative radiological diagnostics in cases of carcinoma serves - in addition to other clinical investigations - "to plan a special treatment, to establish a prognosis, to facilitate evaluation of treatment results and to encourage the exchange of experiences between research centres". (11)

Up to this day - and in spite of the claims of the "Union Contre le Cancer" - there is no preoperative classification of the renal carcinoma according to the TNM-System, except for one study of our Munich study group (3).

It was demonstrated in 142 patients with hypernephroidal renal carcinoma, who had undergone preoperative examination from May, 1969, up to October, 1972, that as a rule the prognostically relevant criteria are to be determined by angiographic examination, in opposition to, for instance, bladder and oesophagus carcinoma. Tumor size, capsule perforation and infiltration of tumor in the close environment, including liver and spleen have been determined by arteriographic means. Invasion of tumor into the renal vein and venacava caudalis has been traced by the cavo- and selective renal venography. Lymphography is a further angiographic method relevant for classification of a carcinoma. By the aid of lymphography it is possible to realize the primary stage of renal lymphatic nodes, for instance, the aortal and caval lymphatic nodes, and to recognize metastases (1). As a rule, the findings had been revised by operation and histological examination.

Since it is possible by means of the investigations under discussion to "determine the expansion of a tumor on the basis of precisely defined characteristics of quality (11)" - as it was recently confirmed by Lang (5) - we proposed the following classification for renal carcinoma according to the TNM-System (Table 1 and Table 2).

It is to be seen that we classified metastatic spread of a homolateral aortal or caval lymphatic node respectively as $N_1$, a contralateral metastatic spread as $N_2$.

Lymphography was performed on 92 patients with renal carcinoma, recruited from 42 female and 50 male patients. Eighty-two patients had undergone operation, and the lymphatic nodes were histologically examined.

While some authors, to some extent, have reported metastases on lymphography in up to 75% of patients (2,4,6,7), in our small number of patients, metastatic spread to the lymphatic nodes was demonstrated in only 21.7% (20 patients) in conformity with Staehler (10) and Robson (8). In 16 cases examined (80%) category $N_2$ and in 4 cases (20%) category $N_1$ was relevant. From these 20 patients showing metastases to the lymphatic nodes, 16 had undergone operation. In 4 cases (20%) operation was not indicated due to evident metastases in other regions and a very poor general condition, the cases being part of category $N_2$.

Evaluation of abdominally presentable lymphatic nodes raises special difficulty due to segmentation. So it is not surprising that in 15 patients examined (10.7%), interpretation of lymphatic nodes was doubtful. When histologically examined 3 patients of the above mentioned 15 patients had a positive diagnosis. 12 a negative one. On the other hand, in 5 cases under examination (6.1%) a false positive and in two cases (2.4%) a false negative was obtained.

The following results will show the prognostically important meaning of metastases to lymphatic nodes:

A tumor invasion into the renal vein or the vena cava caudalis respectively was traceable in 4 patients with metastases to lymphatic nodes. On the other hand no extrarenal vein invasion was evident in patients without metastatic spread to the lymphatic nodes.

Moreover, 11 cases with metastases to the lymphatic nodes were found to have metastases in other regions but only in one case without metastases to the lymphatic nodes. These observations underline the importance of preoperative lymphography in renal carcinoma. Lymphography is furthermore essential for planning the operation since in case of transthoraco-abdominal proceeding not only a radical tumor nephrectomy but also lymphadenectomy is feasible (9).

During the past 3 years 120 patients underwent operation in that

$T_1$ = Primary tumor < 5 cm Ø without infiltration into the pyelon or into the renal veins, without perforation through the fat capsule.

$T_2$ = Primary tumor 5-10 cm Ø with or without infiltration into the pyelon, without invasion into the main renal vein and without perforation through the fat capsule.

$T_3$ = Primary tumor 11-15 cm Ø or smaller, in combination with invasion into the main renal vein. Limitation of tumor to the fat capsule.

$T_4$ = Primary tumor > 15 cm Ø or smaller, in combination with cava invasion or cava occlusion respectively and/or infiltration into the surrounding and into neighboring organs.

$N_0$ = No tumor infiltration.

$N_1$ = Homolateral (para) aortal or (para) caval and iliacal infiltration of lymph nodes.

$N_2$ = Contralateral (para) aortal or (para) caval and iliacal infiltration of lymph nodes.

$N_x$ = Preoperatively no data to be given on lymph node infiltration.

M = Metastases to other regions.

Table 1: Classification of carcinoma of the renal parenchyma according to the TNM-System.

<table>
<tr><th></th><th>$T_1$</th><th>$T_2$</th><th>$T_3$</th><th>$T_4$</th></tr>
<tr><td>$N_0$</td><td>I</td><td>II</td><td></td><td rowspan="4"></td></tr>
<tr><td>$N_1$</td><td colspan="3">III a</td></tr>
<tr><td>$N_2$</td><td colspan="3">III b</td></tr>
<tr><td>M</td><td colspan="3">IV</td></tr>
</table>

Table 2: Staging of carcinoma of the renal parenchyma according to the TNM-System.

way however without laying down the time of survival.

We also make use of lymphography in cases of uncertain arteriographic interpretation of an intrarenal vessel process with suspicion of tumor. For instance, in the case of a 42-year-old patient, the vascular structure of the left-sided upper half of the kidney was uncertain. Lymphography demonstrated clear left-sided paraaortal metastases. Histological examination demonstrated a nephroblastoma with metastases to the lymph nodes.

Lymphographic evidence, however, is not always so well-defined. In the residual kidney of a 50-year-old female patient a poorly vascularized tumor suspicious of malignancy was observed. Lymphography showed enlarged left-sided paraaortal lymphatic nodes with well-defined storage defects interpreted to be metastases. Histological examination showed a renal cyst with reactively enlarged non-malignant lymphatic nodes.

It is our opinon that lymphography represents an essential preoperative method of examination in patients with renal carcinoma which is not only of importance for prognosis and thus for classification according to the TNM-System but also to elucidate for the surgeon the extent of metastatic invasion to the lymphatic nodes.

References

1. Fuchs, W.A., Davidson, J.W., Fischer, H.W.: Lymphography in Cancer. Springer Verlag, 1969.

2. von Keiser, D.: Renal tumours. In: Progress in Lymphology. George Thieme Verlag, Stuttgart 1967.

3. Klein, U., Heinze, H.G., Lissner, J., Eisenberg, F., Schmiedt, E.: Arteriographie, Cavographie, selektive Nierenvenographie und Lymphographie als Kriterien zur Stadieneinteilung (TNM-System) bei Nierentumoren. 2. Intern. Kongr. d. Europ. Ges. f. Radiologie, Amsterdam 1971.

4. Kunitsch, G., Holsten, D.R.: Erfahrungsbericht uber 428 Lymphographien bei Geschwulstkranken. Med. Welt 19 (1968) 239.

5. Lang, E.K.: Arteriographic Assessment and Staging of Renal Cell Carcinoma. Radiology 101 (1971) 17.

6. Ludvik, W., Zaunbauer, W.: Die Bedeutung der Lymphographie fur die chirurgischen Disziplinen. Fortschr. Rontgenstr. 105 (1966) 614.

7. MacDonald, J.S.: Discussion note Diseases of the Kidneys and Ureters. In: Progress in Lymphology II. Georg Thieme Verlag,

Stuttgart 1970.

8. Robson, C.J.: J. Urol. 89 (1963) 37.

9. Schmiedt, E., Heinze, H.G.: Nierentumoren. Operative und strahlentherapeutische Behandlung. Munch. Med. Wschr. 113 (1971) 973.

10. Staehler, W.: Klinik und Praxis der Urologie. Georg Thieme Verlag, Stuttgart 1959.

11. Union Internationale Contre le Cancer (UICC): Die Klassifizierung der malignen Tumoren nach dem TNM-System. Springer Verlag, Berlin 1970.

# ON THE PERSISTENCE OF AN OILY CONTRAST MEDIUM (LIPIODOL ULTRA-FLUID (R)) IN NORMAL AND ABNORMAL LYMPH NODES

H.-J. Teske and B. Kalkowsky

Universtate-Strahlenklinik

Hufelandstra, 55 West Germany

Patients having undergone lymphography who were followed up for a period of several years by x-ray controls showed marked differences in the decreasing rate of contrast medium (c.m.) according to time. There are few and contradictory reports in the literature on factors influencing the decrease of stored c.m. : Ruttiman found visible c.m. in lymph nodes (l.n.) up to 4-10 months. In normal nodes Viamonte observed the disappearance of the oily medium within 1-3 months. Abnormal nodes on the other hand retained the contrast material sometimes for years. In nodes with active inflammation Viamonte noticed disappearance within 48 hours. According to Fabion the c.m. persisted in the nodes for 5 to 34 months; 70% of the patients had c.m. sufficient for diagnosis at the end of 1 year, while in 12% it was still visible at the end of 2 years. Abnormal l.n. are thought to have a greater tendency to store than normal ones (Blaudow; Viamonte). There is however little information on the following factors: age, sex or mode of therapy.

Material and methods. From 1500 patients with lymphography 500 were selected, because only these had sufficient control films of the abdomen and the pelvis permitting detection of c.m. up to 42 months after the initial lymphography. There was a decrease in the number of available patients with increasing time after lymphography. After 24 months 30 out of 340 normal persons could be studied and after 42 months 10 persons (normal and abnormal) could be observed. The lymphography and control studies were done for clinical reasons and not for the purpose of prospective investigation. The patients under study were divided into 3 groups: 1) normal persons (340), by our definition patients free of malignant lymphoma or lymph node metastases below the diaphragma; 2) patients with malignant lymphoma only (100); and 3) patients with lymph node metastases below the diaphragma (60). Control studies of untreated patients without any further therapy were found only in the group of normal persons.

Calculation of the rate of the decreasing contrast medium was done defining the initial retention of c.m. on the film as 100%, the complete loss of c.m. as 0%; in between we defined intermediate categories of 80, 60, 40 and 20% respectively. By this the mean values for a group of patients at a given time permitted the drawing of curves describing the mode of disappearance of c.m. These curves are partly shown.

Our standard curve is the curve describing the rate of disappearance of c.m. in normal males and females.

Results. As shown in Fig. 1 there are no significant differences in the rate of decrease of c.m. in males (dashed line) and females (dotted line). Therefore the data on both sexes were used together in the standard curve (Fig. 2). When viewed according to the age there is a deviation from the mean values: we found a more rapid disappearance of c.m. in the age group below 20 years.

Extravasal c.m. disappears less rapidly than c.m. stored within the l.n. Furthermore c.m. accumulated in postoperative pseudocysts fades less rapidly. In Fig. 3 the curve of c.m. disappearance in 5 so-called second look lymphographies is plotted over a total of 12 months. Here the same rate of decrease as in primary lymphographies was noted. Then the effect of different modes of therapy was studied.

There was no significant change in patients undergoing radiotherapy (tumor killing doses), single or multiple chemotherapy or having both modes of treatment simultaneously (Fig. 4). This was also true for malignant lymphomas. Patients treated simultaneously with both, chemo- and radiotherapy showed slight increase in the rate of disappearance (Fig. 5). In patients with lymph node metastases undergoing radiotherapy alone or combined radio- and chemotherapy the curve is not changed (Fig. 6).

We also compared our material with these reports in the literature concerning the behavior of initially enlarged (non malignant) lymph nodes. As reported the original size was observed mainly after 3 weeks. However in some cases we found that this was true after 6 weeks. In rare instances we noted that there was still an increase in size 2-14 days after lymphography.

Discussion. Our own studies confirmed previous reports on the variable rate of decrease of c.m. in patients after lymphography. The mean values of c.m. disappearance showed little variation comparing the different groups of patients; there is, however, con-

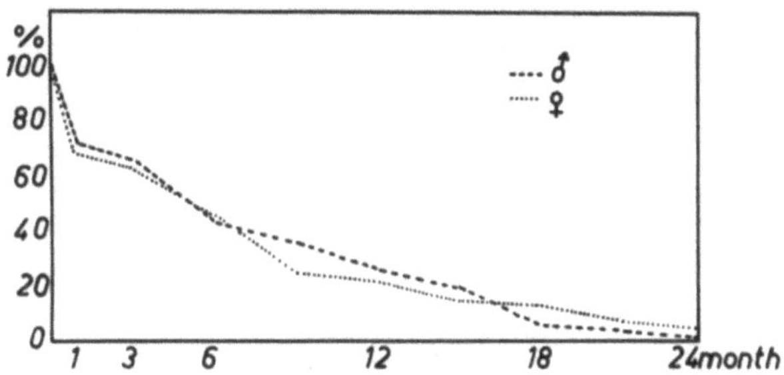


Fig. 1: Differences in the rate of decrease of contrast medium in males (dashed line) and females (dotted line).

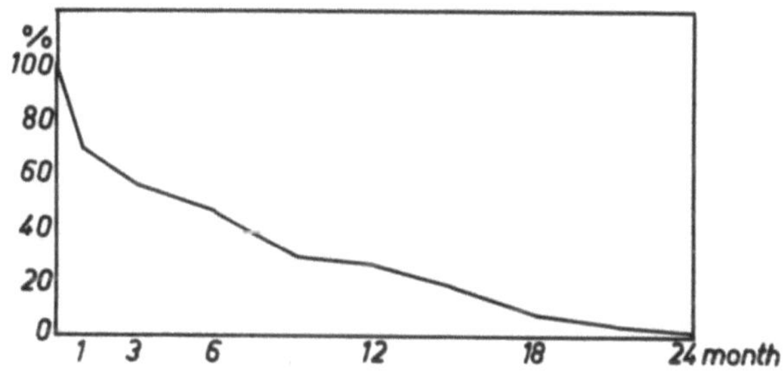


Fig. 2: Standard curve using data from both sexes.

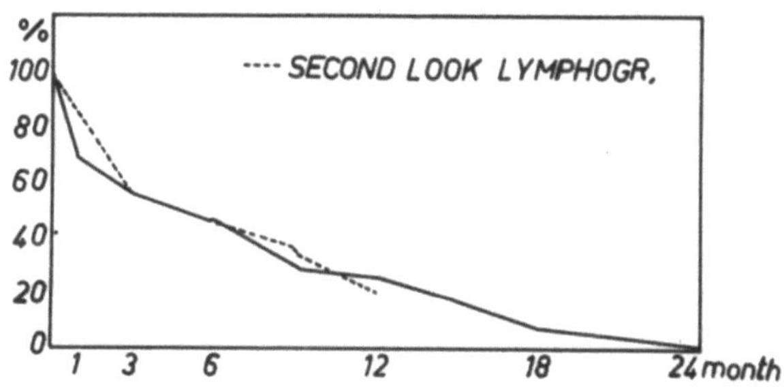


Fig. 3: Curve of contrast medium disappearance in five second look lymphographies plotted over a 12-month period.

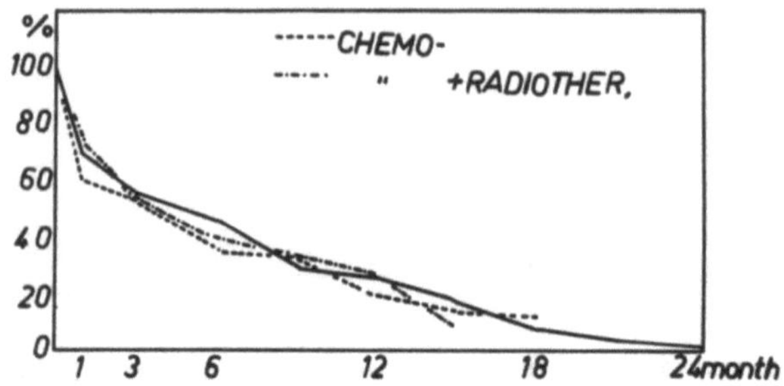


Fig. 4: Patients undergoing radio- and chemotherapy

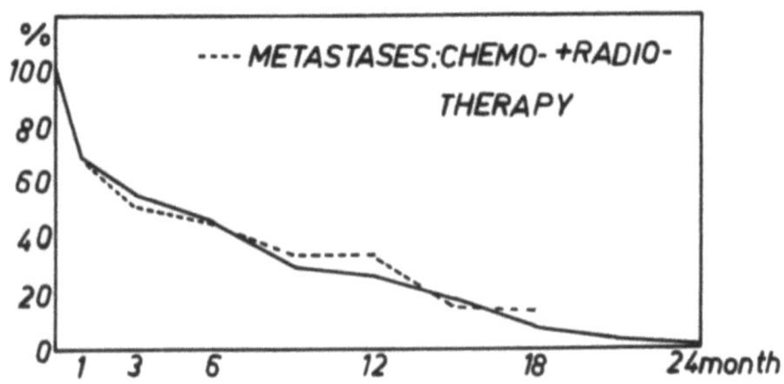


Fig. 5: Patients treated simultaneously with radio- and chemotherapy.

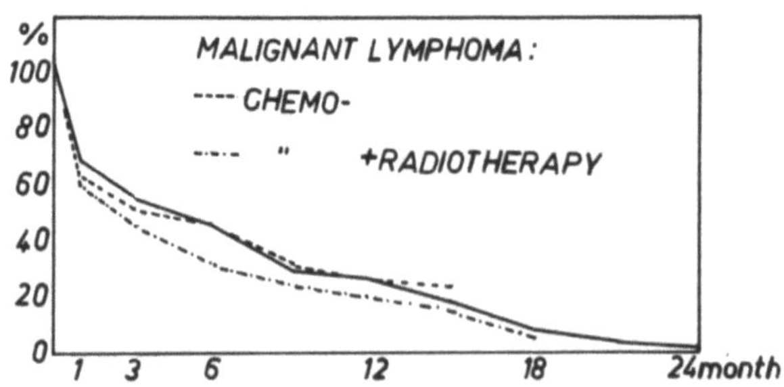


Fig. 6: Patients with lymph node metastases undergoing radiotherapy alone or combined radio- and chemotherapy.

siderable variation within single groups. A female patient, age 61, with collum carcinoma after operation and radiotherapy showed about 40% of the original c.m. still visible after 42 months. On the other hand we observed complete disappearance of c.m. after only 4 months. Disappearance of c.m. after a few days however could not be demonstrated in our material. This is in contrast to the observation of Viamonte. We could not confirm the statement of Viamonte and also of Blaudow, demonstrating a more prolonged storage of c.m. in abnormal l. n. as compared to normal l.n. Furthermore, we could not confirm the finding of Gerteis stating a more prolonged retention of c.m. in females. In our material there was no factor influencing c.m. storage which could be correlated to sex. Furthermore, the more rapid disappearance of c.m. in relymphography as noticed by Gerteis could not be observed in our material.

In summary these results indicate that one has to be very cautious not to overinterpret such factors as age, sex or mode of therapy in lymphography. In our findings only minimal correlation between the increased rate of disappearance of c.m. and very young age - below 20 years - was found.

References

1. Blaudow, K. and Banaschek, A.: Die Bedeutung der Lymphographie fur gynakologische Karzinome. Radiol. diagn. (Berl.) 9 (1968), 661-668.

2. Fabion, C.E., Nudelmann, E.J. and Abrahams, H.L.: Postlymphangiogram film as an indicator of tumor activity. Invest. Radiol. 1 (1966), 386-398.

3. Gerteis, W.: In: Handb. allg. Pathol. Springer, Berlin-Heidelberg-New York 1972, Bd 3, Teil 6, S. 595-656. Darstellungsmethoden des Lymphagefabsystems and praktische Lymphographie.

4. Teske, H.-J., Heissen, E., and Haller, J.: Lymphographische Verlaufskontrollen bei lymphatischen Systemerkrankungen. Munch. med. Wschr. 112 (1970), 1309-1316.

5. Viamonte, M.: In: Progress in Lymphology I. Thieme, Stuttgart 1967, page 168.

6. Weissleder, H., Renemann, H., and Baumeister, L.: Der diagnostische Wert lymphografischen Verlaufskontrollen. Fortschr. Rontgenstr. 104 (1966), 14-22.

7. Ruttimann, A., Del Buono, M.S.: In: Ergebnisse der medizinischen Strahlenforschung. Springer, Berlin-Heidelberg-New York 1964, Bd. I, S.248-318, Die Lymphographie.

# HYDROSTATIC PRESSURE IN PERIPHERAL LYMPHATICS - CORRELATION WITH LYMPHOGRAPHY AND CLINICAL DATA

A.R. Winterberger, B.Sc., M.D. and E.C. Jennings, M.D.

Roswell Park Memorial Institute

666 Elm Street, Buffalo, New York 14203

The measurement of hydrostatic pressure in human lymphatics has not previously been evaluated as a potential diagnostic modality. Szabo (1967) has measured pressures in various segments of the lymphatic system of dogs and has reported mean pressures in various vessels and trunks. He found the resting pressure in the extremities is close to zero. Drinker and Field (1933) also recorded near zero pressures in the dog leg at rest. Miller et al. (1963) found a mean pressure of 5 mmHg in the dog leg. Irisawa and Rushmer (1959) reported intralymphatic pressures in the dog leg slightly below corresponding venous pressures, i.e. between 2.5 - 12 cm of water.

Accurate data on the intraluminal lymphatic pressure in humans, recorded both in health and disease states, is virtually non-existent This lack of information is apparently due to the technical difficulties usually encountered in performing measurements of this type.

An attempt has been made to establish a procedure for the routine measurement of the hydrostatic pressure in peripheral lymphatic ducts and to determine its usefulness as an adjunctive diagnostic study.

Methods. Fifty-nine patients were studied in this series. Fifty-seven were lower extremity examinations and two were upper extremity measurements. A variety of clinical entities were included in the series, although the majority of the cases were lymphomas. None of the patients had significant electrolyte disturbances or plasma protein abnormalities. There were no cases of primary lymphedema included in the study. There were no patients with the fibrotic changes of chronic lymphedema.

The lymphatic ducts are identified and surgically exposed after the intracutaneous and subcutaneous injection of patent blue violet (Alphazurine 2 G. #217 Allied Chemical) in one or more of the web spaces of either the feet or hands. The lymphatics are intubated with 27 gauge cannulas, which are threaded cephalad up the duct for at least one centimeter. The cannula is anchored into the vessel with 4-0 silk suture. The system is tested for leaks with a syringe of heparinized normal saline and if no leaks are encountered, the lymphatic duct is connected to a standard venous pressure manometer filled with heparinized normal saline. Strain gauges with chart recorders offered no advantage over the simple manometer. The zero point in the leg is arbitrarily chosen as the level of the medial malleolus with the patient supine and at rest. In the arm the zero point used is the radial styloid with the forearm midway between pronation and supination and again with the patient supine and at rest. The system is allowed to reach equilibrium for at least one and one-half hours. At this time the manometer levels are recorded. A test for the validity of the measurement is then performed by applying a tourniquet below the knee to occlude venous return and actively exercising the toes. The lymphatic pressure will increase if the preparation is acceptable. If no increase is encountered, this data is discarded from the study.

Routine lymphography is then performed by injecting ethiodized oil (Ethiodol-Fourger) with a constant infusion pump.

Results. There were 114 pressure measurements performed on the 59 patients, two unilateral upper extremity measurements, two unilateral lower extremity studies, and fifty-five bilateral lower extremity examinations.

The data accumulated in the study is shown in Table 1.

It can be seen that there were no patients with disease whose peripheral lymphatic pressure was less than 10 cm. of water. There were six pressure measurements above 10 cm. of water in patients with apparently normal lymphography. Four of these measurements, however, were in two patients with mediastinal, liver and spleen involvement. There were only two elevated pressures in one apparently normal patient. It is also observed that the pressures were generally higher in patients with massive nodal involvement.

Discussion. The propulsion of lymph centripetally along a duct from one area to another is caused by the contraction of the vessel walls plus several extrinsic factors. Lymph pressure is not maintained by a constant flow in a closed system as it is in the venous circulation. It is the result of many forces acting on the lymphatic vessels. There are valves throughout the system except in the capillaries. These valves allow the lymph to flow from the periphery to the larger trunks. Among the most important extrinsic factors con-

Table 1: Tabulation of 114 pressure measurements in 59 patients.

| Range of Pressure in cm. of Water | Apparently Normal Lymphography | Abnormal Lymph Vessels with Normal or Unfilled Lymph Nodes | Abnormal Lymph Nodes with Normal Lymph Vessels | Abnormal Lymph Nodes and Lymph Vessels |
|---|---|---|---|---|
| Over 20 cm. | 5 | 14 | 14 | 33 |
| 10-20 cm. | 1 | 16 | 9 | 16 |
| less than 10 cm. | 6 | 0 | 0 | 0 |

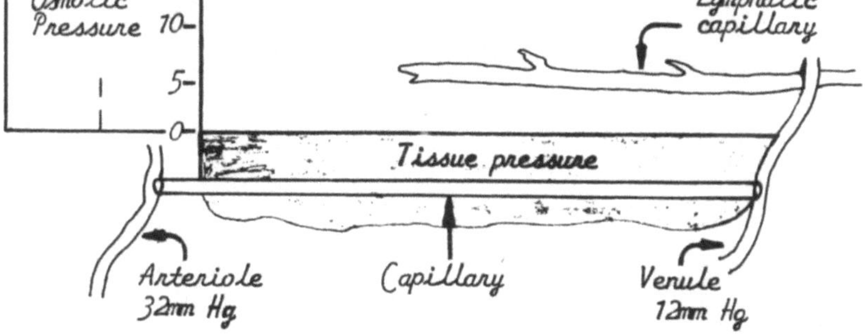


Fig. 1: Diagram of Starling's Hypothesis

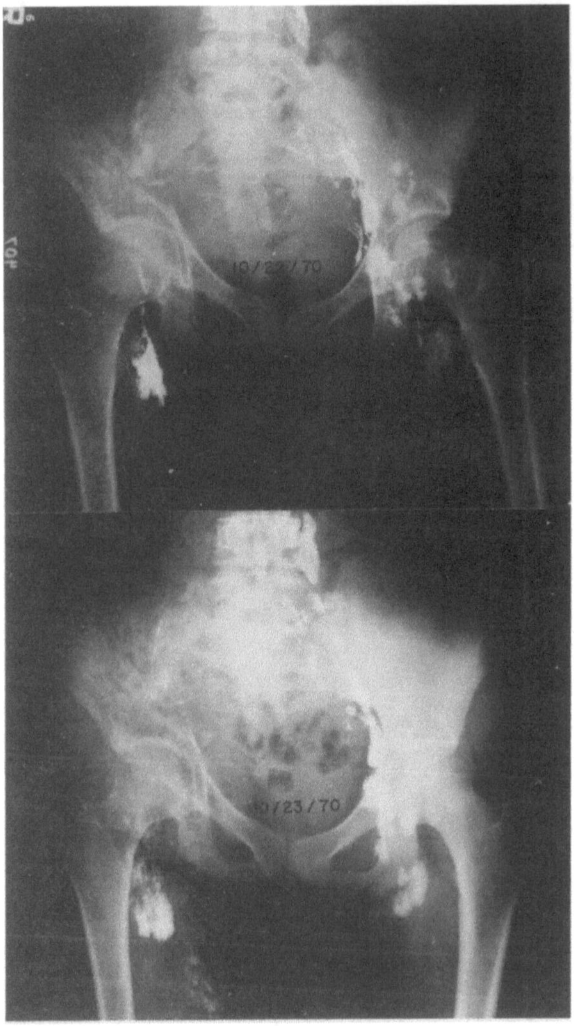

Fig. 2: Vascular phase of lymphogram on a patient with lymphangiomatosis. There is complete obstruction on the right with lymphovenous communications.

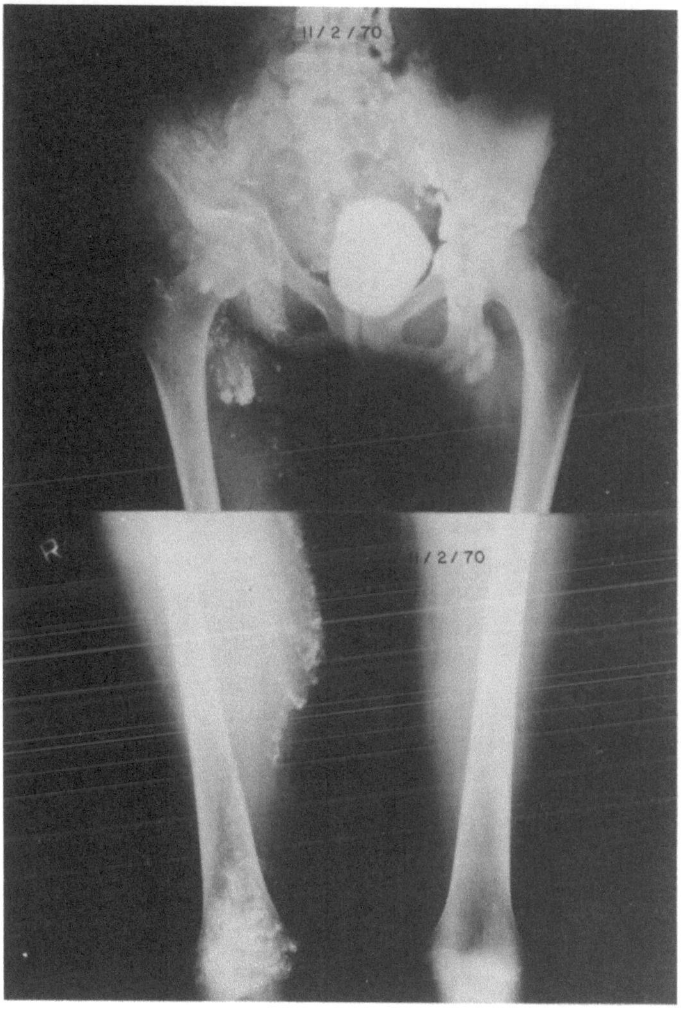


Fig. 3: Lymphadenogram of the patient in Figure 2 demonstrating contrast material within the bone on the right and multiple soft tissue lymphangiomas. The left side is normal.

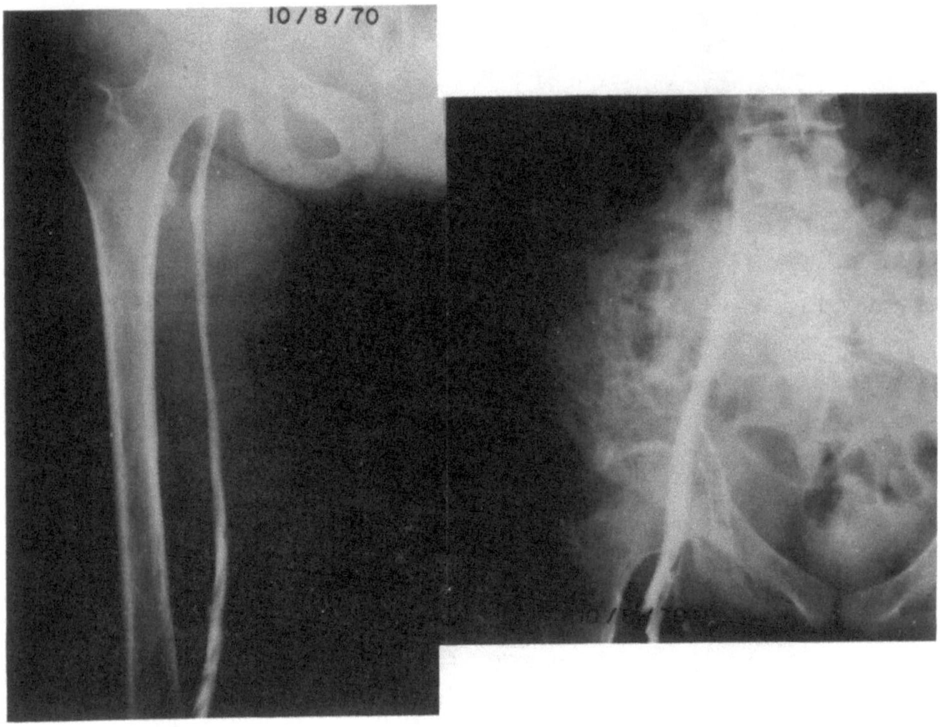


Fig. 4: Venagram on the patient in Figures 2 and 3 demonstrating normal femoral and iliac veins not compressed or obstructed by the disease process.

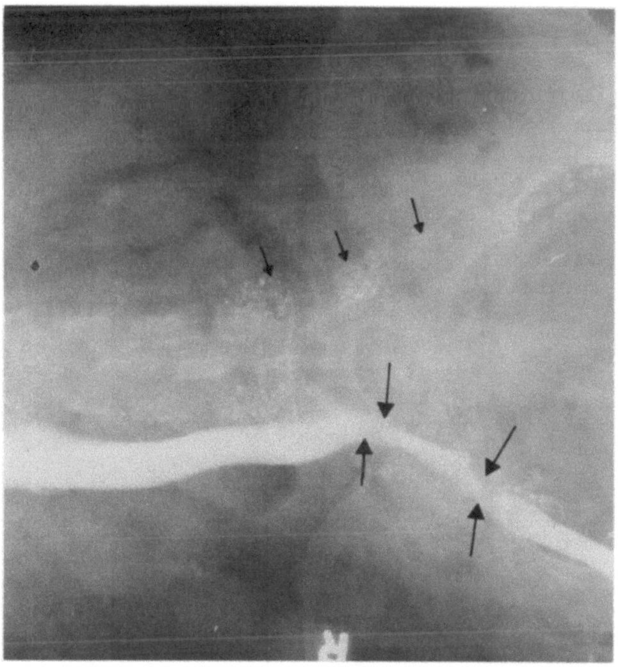


Fig. 5: Inferior venacavagram on a patient with abnormal enlarged lymph nodes (small arrows) demonstrating compression of the pelvic veins by the large nodes (large arrows).

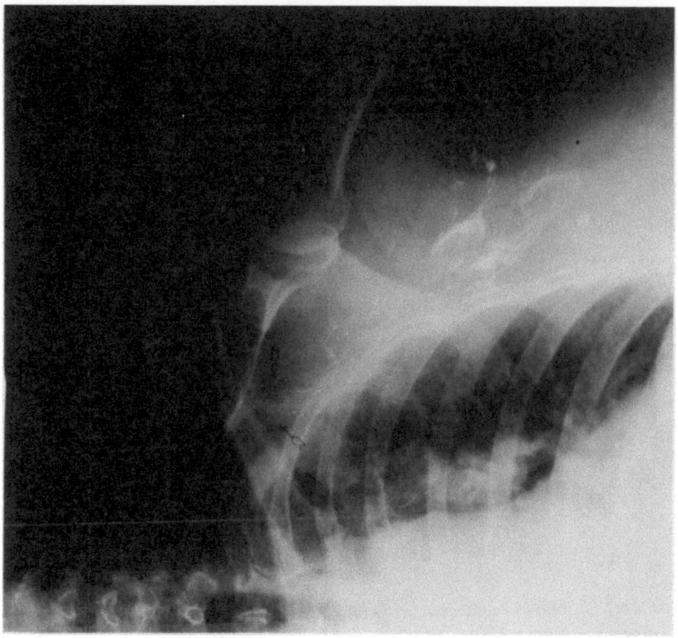

Fig. 6: Left arm lymphogram on a patient with complete lymphatic obstruction in the axilla (arrows).

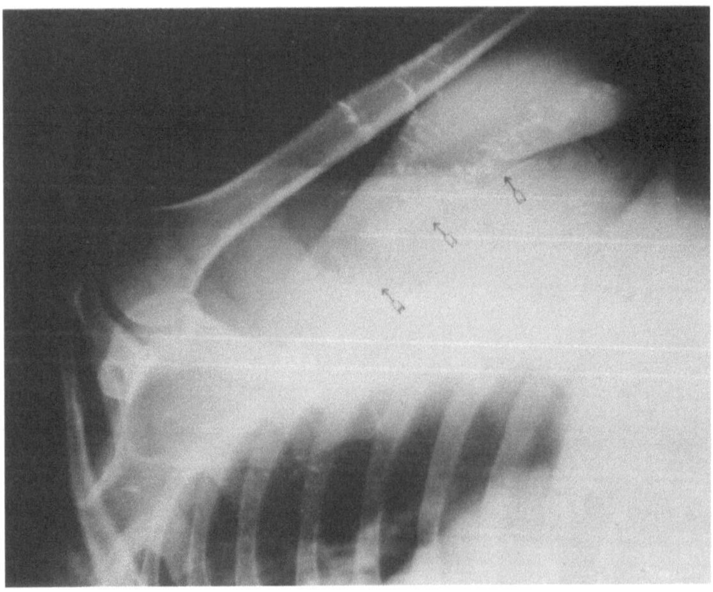

Fig. 7: Lymphadenogram on the patient in Figure 7 demonstrating ectasia and dermal back-flow.

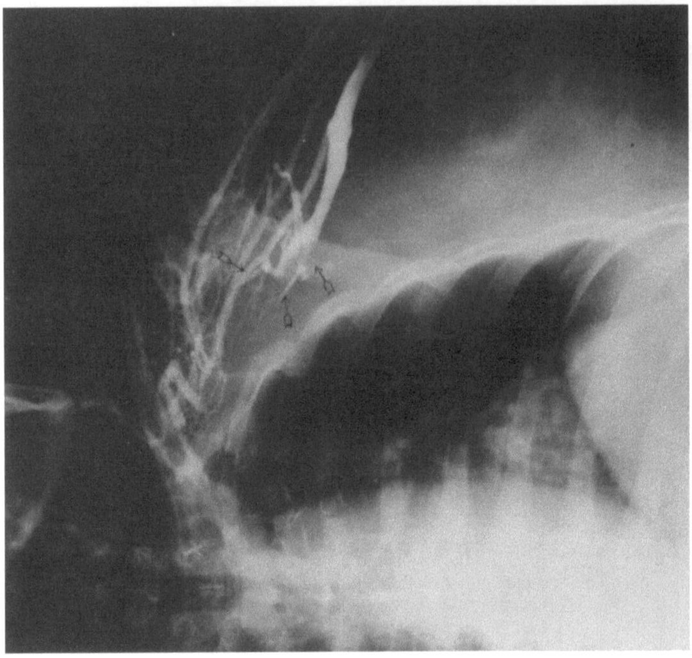

Fig. 8: Venogram on the same patient in Figures 6 and 7 demonstrating occlusion of the axillary vein by the mass (arrows).

trolling the movement of the lymph are muscular activity and the compression of the cysterna chyli by the diaphragm during respiration. The so called "thoracic pump" may also be a factor. It also is well known that venous occlusion increases tissue pressure and therefore lymphatic pressure. Arterial blockade decreases lymphatic pressure. A diagram of Starling's hypothesis demonstrating the interaction between the forces leading to ultra-filtration at the arterial end of the capillary, reabsorption at the venous end, and drainage of the excess interstitial fluid by the lymphatics is shown in Figure 1.

It is difficult to determine the actual cause of the increased lymphatic pressures in our study. In some cases it appears to be due to purely lymphatic involvement alone, one example is illustrated in Figures 2, 3, and 4. In others it appears a combination of lymphatic disease and increased venous pressure due to compression of major veins by pathological lymph nodes is the cause as shown in Figures 5, 6, 7, and 8.

This data suggests that an elevated lymphatic pressure is a non-specific entity, although a reliable indicator of disease. It appears that in lymphatic involvement alone, the opening of lympho-venous anastomoses may occur and the pressure approaches venous pressure. In instances where there is both lymphatic involvement and either venous compression or occlusion, the pressure elevation is of considerably greater magnitude. In patients with elevated pressures a venagram should always be performed.

A pressure of less than 10 cm. of water, when properly performed, appears to be a reliable indication of normal.

The measurement of the intraluminal lymphatic pressure may be of value for patients in which standard lymphography is contra-indicated as in chronic lung disease, irradiated lungs, or sensitivity to iodinated compounds or patent blue dyes.

Summary. The measurement of peripheral lymphatic duct pressure is a technically difficult procedure which can be performed routinely after experience is obtained with the technique. An elevated pressure is a non-specific indication of disease in the lymphatic vessels, lymph nodes, venous circulation, or combinations thereof. A low pressure appears to be a reliable indication of normal. Further correlations will be made relating the magnitude of the lymphatic pressure elevation with venous pressure determinations, venography and lymphography.

References

1. Drinker, C.K. and Field, M.E.: Lymphatics, Lymph and Tissue Fluid. Williams and Wilkins, Baltimore, 1933.

2. Irisawa, A. and Rushmer, R.F.: Relationship between Lymphatic and Venous Pressure in Leg of Dog. Am. J. Physiol. 196: 495-498, 1959.

3. Miller, S., Laine, J.B. and Howard, J.M.: Lymphatic Pressure in Extremities of Dogs. Am. J. Physiol. 206: 63-66, 1963.

4. Szabo, Gy. and Magyar, Zs.: Pressure Measurements in Various Parts of the Lymphatic System. Acta Medica Hungary. 23: 237-241, 1967.

5. Winterberger, A.R.: Radiographic Diagnosis of Lymphangiomatosis of Bone. Radiol. 102: 321-324, 1972.

# CORRELATION OF LYMPHOGRAPHY FINDINGS IN THE ABDOMEN WITH B-SCAN ULTRASONIC LAMINOGRAPHY

Alan R. Winterberger

Roswell Park Memorial Institute

666 Elm Street, Buffalo, New York 14203

Lymphography is presently the most popular method for the evaluation of pelvic and paraaortic lymphatic disease and appears to be the most reliable study short of open surgical inspection and biopsy. It is well known that a negative lymphogram is not conclusive evidence of absence of disease and that a positive lymphogram is a relatively more useful entity in the diagnosis and staging of disease. We have however, as others, been experiencing an increasing number of instances in which the lymphogram was positive radiographically but open surgical lymphoadenectomy results in a histological diagnosis of reactive hyperplasia with no evidence of tumor within the excised lymph nodes. Some of these false positives are due to errors on the part of the surgeon failing to remove the radiographically positive nodes.

Lymphography, although a minor procedure, is an invasive technique and the difficulties associated with the study are well known to all lymphologists.

An attempt has been made to diagnose pelvic and abdominal lymphadenopathy using non-invasive ultrasound. A preliminary evaluation of the method is presented.

Methods. Prior to the usual lymphographic procedure compound B-Mode Ultrasonic Laminography is performed on the patient at two levels, i.e. the anterior-superior-iliac-spines and immediately below the umbilicus. These levels were chosen for the purpose of anatomical reproducibility and standardization.

In the pelvis, the sacrum and recto-sigmoid are identified followed by attempts to localize the pelvic vessels. The patient is allowed to void prior to the scanning so that a distended urinary bladder does not produce confusion or interference.

In the abdomen the lumbar spine is identified followed by localization of the abdominal aorta and vena cava.

After satisfactory scans are obtained, they are recorded on polaroid film from the storage oscilloscope.

The scans are immediately interpreted independently without knowledge of the lymphographic data. The following day after the nodes have collected the contrast material, the scans are compared to the radiographs of the pelvis and abdomen.

Results. Sixty patients were studied in this preliminary series. There were a variety of clinical entities included although the majority of the cases were lymphomas.

The accuracy of diagnosing lymphadenopathy in the pelvis was 70%. The errors were almost always false positives due to artifacts caused by redundant bowel containing fecal matter, enlarged pelvic organs such as the uterus or ovaries, and combinations of both. In the abdomen the accuracy exceeded 90%. The spine, aorta, and vena cava should all be easily identifiable ultrasonographically. If these structures could not be identified, the cause, in this series, was enlarged lymph nodes intimately associated with the ad-venitia of the vessels disturbing the normal acoustic interfaces. The few errors in this series in the abdomen were usually false negatives in which the nodes were diseased without enlargement. Ultrasound has the additional advantage in that it will detect masses non-opacified and only suggested by the lymphogram or nodes not usually visualized by standard lymphography as with hypogastric nodes, or first eschelon testicular nodes. Figures 1 and 2 demonstrate normal scans of the abdomen and pelvis. Figures 3 and 4 depict the lymphogram and ultrasonic scan on a patient with lymphoma prior to radiotherapy. Figures 5 and 6 demonstrate the result of radiation therapy both radiographically and ultrasonographically.

Discussion. A preliminary evaluation of a non-invasive method for the detection of lymphadenopathy in the pelvis and abdomen has been performed. The accuracy of the study in the pelvis is only fair, 70%. In the abdomen the accuracy is good, 90%. The technique is of particular value in the following instances: patients sensitive to iodinated compounds or patient blue dyes, patients with chronic lung disease or radiated lungs, to follow the progress of therapy, and to suggest the timing for repeat lymphography if exacerbation of the disease is suspected clinically and confirmed ultrasonographically.

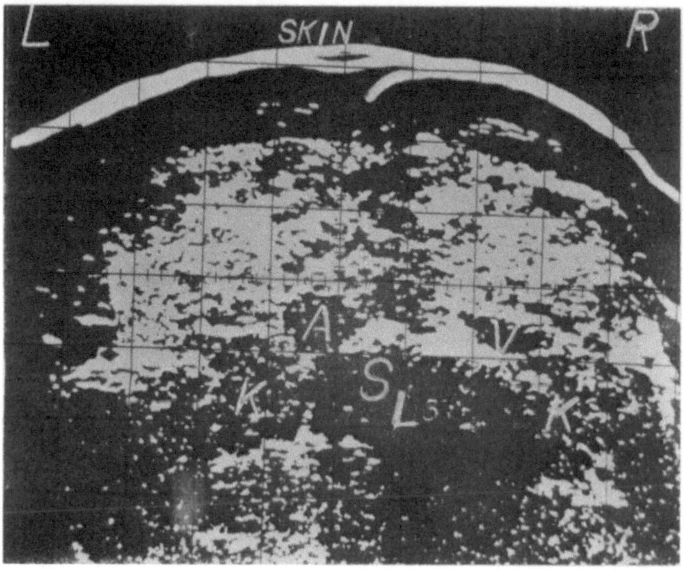


Fig. 1: Ultrasonic scan of a normal abdomen with third lumbar vertebral body, $S_{L3}$; aorta, A; vena cava, V; and the tips of both kidneys, K.

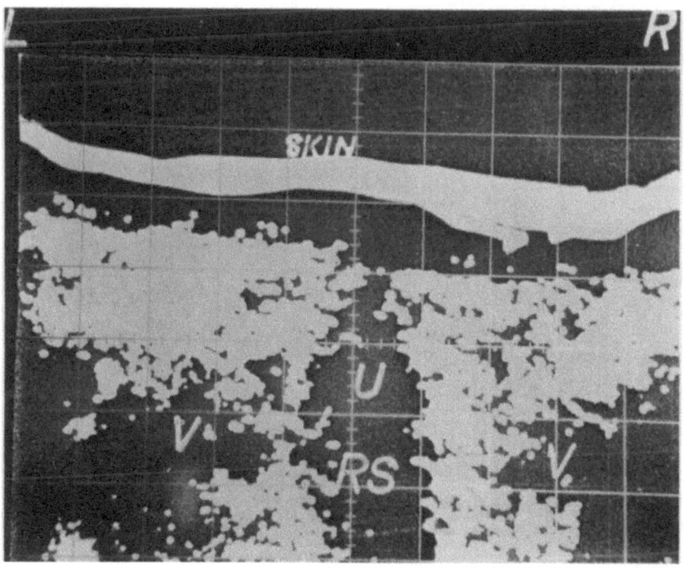


Fig. 2: Ultrasonic scan of pelvis in a normal female with uterus, U; recto-sigmoid, RS; and pelvic vessels, V.

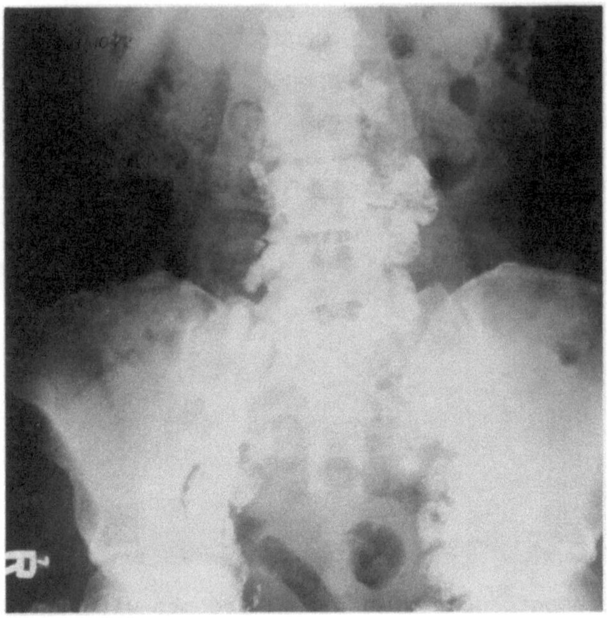

Fig. 3: Lymphogram of a patient with Hodgkin's Disease demonstrating massive lymph node involvement.

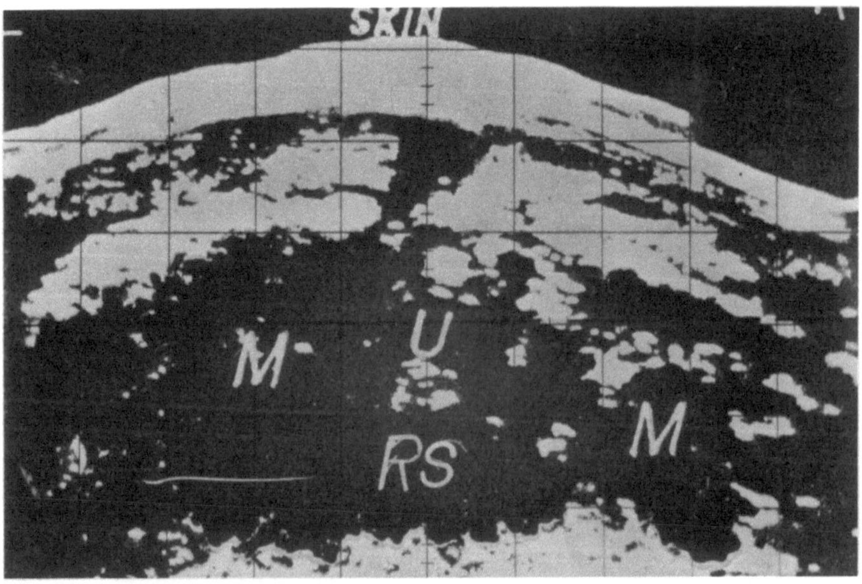


Fig. 4: Ultrasonic scan of the patient in Figure 3 with lymph node masses, M; uterus, U; and rectosigmoid, Rs.

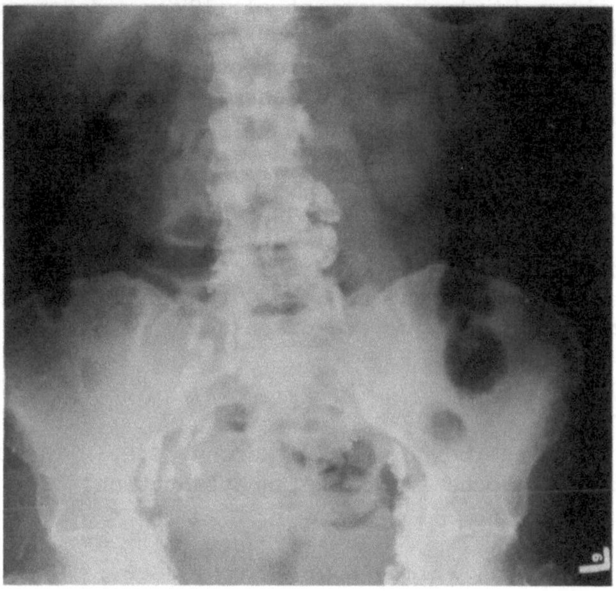

Fig. 5: Repeat abdominal film of patient in Figure 3 after radiation therapy.

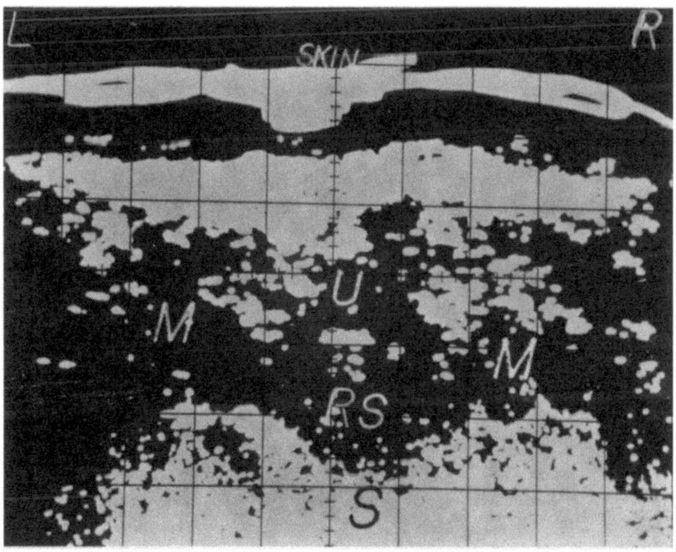


Fig. 6: Repeat ultrasonic scan of patient in Figure 3 demonstrating response to radiation with regression in the size of the masses. Residual lymph node masses, M; uterus, U; and rectosigmoid, S.

We have shown (Winterberger, et al. 1972 and Sampson, et al. 1972) that diagnostic ultrasound is of great value in studying changes in structures known to be present, rather than for "in the blind" searching for suspected masses. It must be emphasized that ultrasonic scanning will detect only enlarged lymph nodes and cannot offer any information about the architecture of these nodes.

Summary. Ultrasonography was compared to Lymphography for the detection of enlarged lymph nodes in the pelvis and abdomen. Preliminary studies indicate the accuracy of ultrasonography is fair in the pelvis and good in the abdomen. The advantages of the non-invasive ultrasonic technique are discussed.

## References

1. Sampson, D., Winterberger, A.R., Murphy, G.P.: The Use of Diagnostic Ultrasound in Renal Transplantation. 29: 77-86, 1972.

2. Winterberger, A.R., Palma, L.D., Murphy, G.P.: Ultrasonic Testing in Human Renal Allografts. 219: 475-479, 1972.

# LYMPHOKINETICS - LYMPHANGIOGRAPHIC DEMONSTRATION OF LYMPHOKINETIC EFFECT OF BENZOPYRONE

R.C. Mayall, A.C.D.G. Mayall, E.T. Mehri,
U.R. Ferretti, and M.V. Villani

Hospital da Gamboa
Rio de Janeiro, Brasil

To study the action of the benzopyrone compounds on the lymph flow we have selected a group of patients with lymphatic diseases of the lower limbs in which there was an indication for lymphangiography.

## Method

The X-ray examination was made with the patient lying down over a sliding table to allow the patient to be monitorized under TV control and to make a serial lymphangiography. On the inner border of the limb there was a radiopaque rule, marking each centimeter on the X-Ray films. The technique of Kinmonth has been used to visualize the lymphatic vessels. The injection of the dye was made under 6 kgrs of pressure and the beginning of the injection was controlled by a chronometer. Under fluoroscopic control using an image amplifier under TV control the progression of the dye was followed and the serial lymphangiography were made, measuring the time to appear the dye on the segment of the limb and the volume of dye injected. The injection was discontinued when the dye arrived on the pelvis and then the needle was cleansed by a saline injection of 10 or 20 mls, up to the complete disappearance of the opacified lymph vessels on the limb. At this moment it was injected 50 or 100 mgrs of benzopyrone compound (Coumarin-rutin) directly within the lymphatic. Immediately after, we injected the dye by the previous technique to make a new lymphangiography, paying the maximum attention to the speed of the flow, the shape of the lymph vessels and the filling of the lymphnodes. The films were taken at the same level, recording the volume of dye injected and the time necessary to reach the same level on the first lymphangiography.

## Radiological Findings

After the injection of benzopyrone compound there was a much better visualization of the lymphatic vessels, with vasodilation, increase in number of visible lymph vessels in a shorter time after the beginning of the injection. As a result of this finding the groin lymph nodes are seen sooner, with better sharpness and higher number, in spite of the smaller volume of dye injected. These effects are very important for the lymphologist's daily life.

## Discussion

The work of Mislin, using a portion of a lymphatic vessel between two valves has demonstrated the myotropic effect of benzopyrones compounds, showing a prolonged regularization of the contractions of the vessel wall with an increase of the lymph volume perfused by minute. Földi, Kovăch, Varga and Zoltan, experimentally have demonstrated the great increase of the lymph flow on the "thoracic ductus", using the same compound,and these findings were confirmed in man, by Bartos and Bazek, on 10 patients with malignant tumors in which there was an indication for the surgical drainage of the "thoracic ductus". The research done by Krajnovic in man and dog, using the intralymphatic injection of this same drug, observed a better result than by intravenous and lesser by intramuscular route. This same author has also observed the shortenning of the time necessary to make the lymphangiography with great advantages for the radiologist and for the comfort of the patient. Sandman has observed better details on the lymphangiographies with great advantage to interpret the plates. More recently, Collard presented a series of papers, about pharmaco-radiology and pharmacotherapy of the lymph vessels in men and experimentally, in which he was able to show an intense lymphokinetic effect of benzopyrones. These experiments were made with an intralymphatic control of the pressure and a selective lymphatic massage was observed. Collard observed also a better and sooner filling with better sharpness of the lymphnodes, resulting of a better regularization of the contractions of the lymphatic walls. Collard recommend systematically the use of these benzopyrone compounds during lymphangiographies and he was able to demonstrate a functional component on lymphedemas that allows to differentiate the fibredemas, in which there is no lymphokinetic effects. With this technique of the intracanalicular low pressure during the injection, the regularization of the contraction reduces the risk of oil embolism and also the metastatic dissemination of malignant cells. During the last Congress of the Union Internationale d'Angéiologie, in 1972, Rio de Janeiro, Scholten has demonstrate that the benzopyrones have a protective effect against the lymphostatic experimental oedema.

| PATIENTS | SEX | DIAGNOSTIC | Dose Coumarin+ Rutin | RESULTS | Radiological Findings after the injection of Benzopyrone |
|---|---|---|---|---|---|
| L.L.G. | F | Left Arm Lymphedema post adenectomy and erysipela | 50 mg | EXCELLENT | Great increase on the number of visible lymph vessels. Slight lymphangiectasy after the injection. Notable increase on the lymph flow. |
| C.J.T. | M | Secondary postphlebitic lymphedema of the legs | 50 mg | EXCELLENT | Better visualization of the lymphnodes. Increase on the number of lymph vessels on the thigh and calf, after the injection, with better shape. |
| J.C.O. | M | Post phlebitic lymphedema on the leg | 50 mg | EXCELLENT | Great vasodilation, with better sharpness and longer distance on the lymph vessel dying after the injection. |
| N.C. | M | Lymphedema of the leg | 50 mg | EXCELLENT | Increase on the number of visible lymph vessels with vasodilation. Much better sharpness. Lymph flow with higher speed. |
| O.R. | M | Iatrogenic and Post phlebitic lymphedema | 50 mg | EXCELLENT | Great increase of the visible lymph vessels with vasodilation. Lymph flow with higher speed. |
| J.S.S. | M | Postphlebitic Lymphedema with fibredema | 50 mg | FAIR | Very little difference on the first plates. Better visualization on the later plates. |
| N.O.R. | F | Lymphedema with fibredema on the leg | 50 mg | FAIR | Better visualization of the lymph vessel. Slight increase of the lymph vessels visualized by the dye. |
| A.P.G. | F | Lymphedema on the leg | 50 mg | EXCELLENT | Faster and better visualization on the knee. |
| I.S.M. | M | Iatrogenic and congenital lymphedema on the right | 50 mg | EXCELLENT | With less 2 ml of the dye and 8 minutes before the text plate of the lymph vessels and lymphnodes. |
| I.S.M. | M | Congenital and iatrogenic lymphedema | 50 mg | EXCELLENT | Seven minutes before the text plate the dye arrived on the pelvis in spite of 1,5 ml short of dye. |

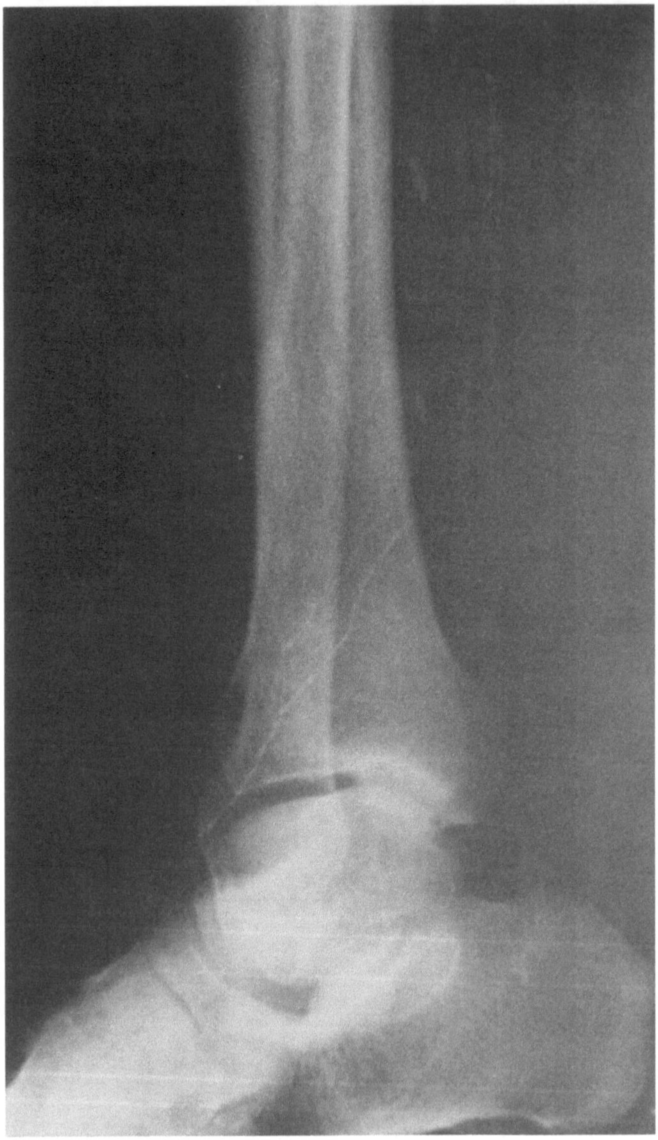

PATIENT N.C. - Before benzopyrone intralymphatic injection

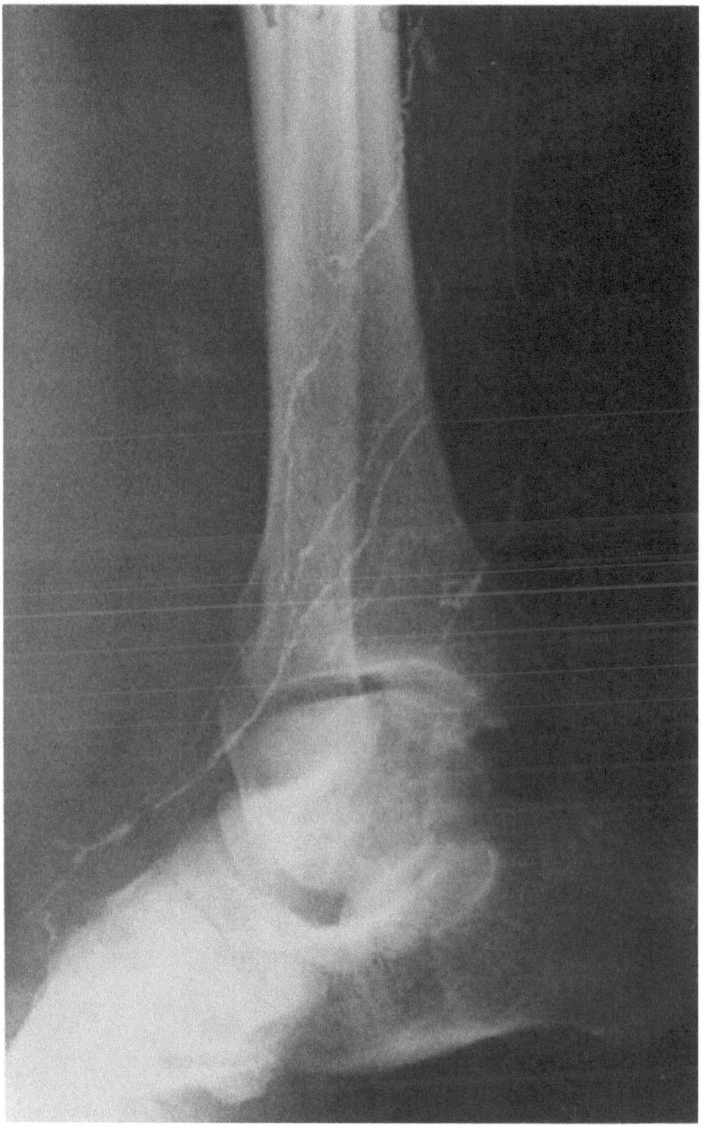

PATIENT N.C. - After benzopyrone intralymphatic injection

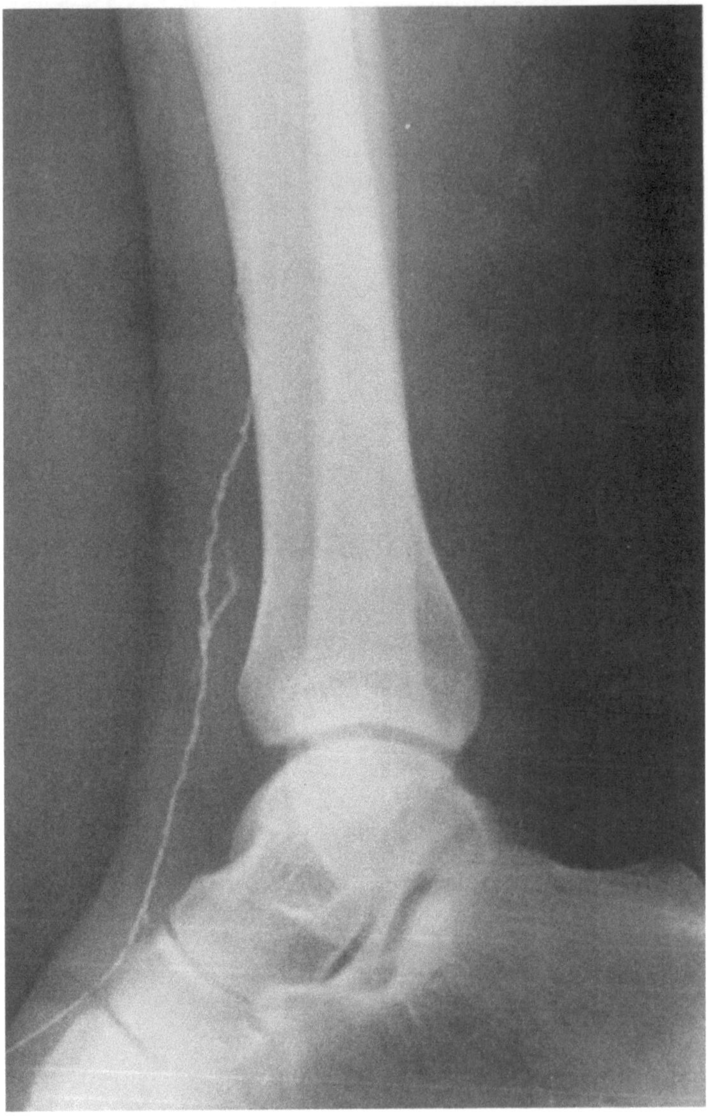

PATIENT J.C.O. - Before benzopyrone intralymphatic injection

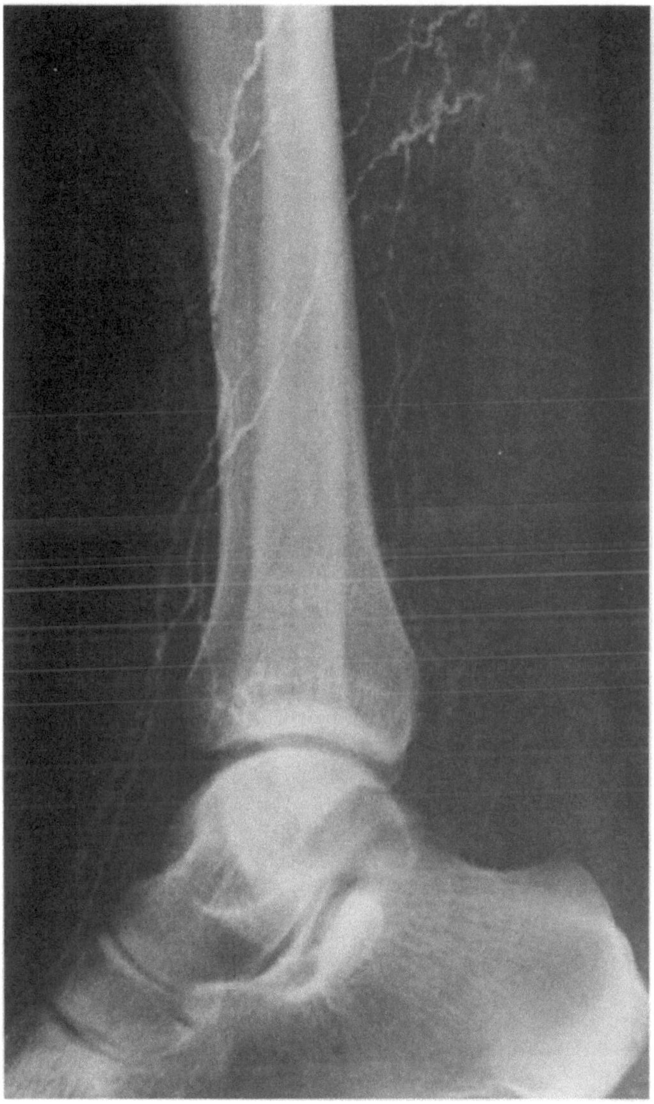

PATIENT J.C.O. - After benzopyrone intralymphatic injection

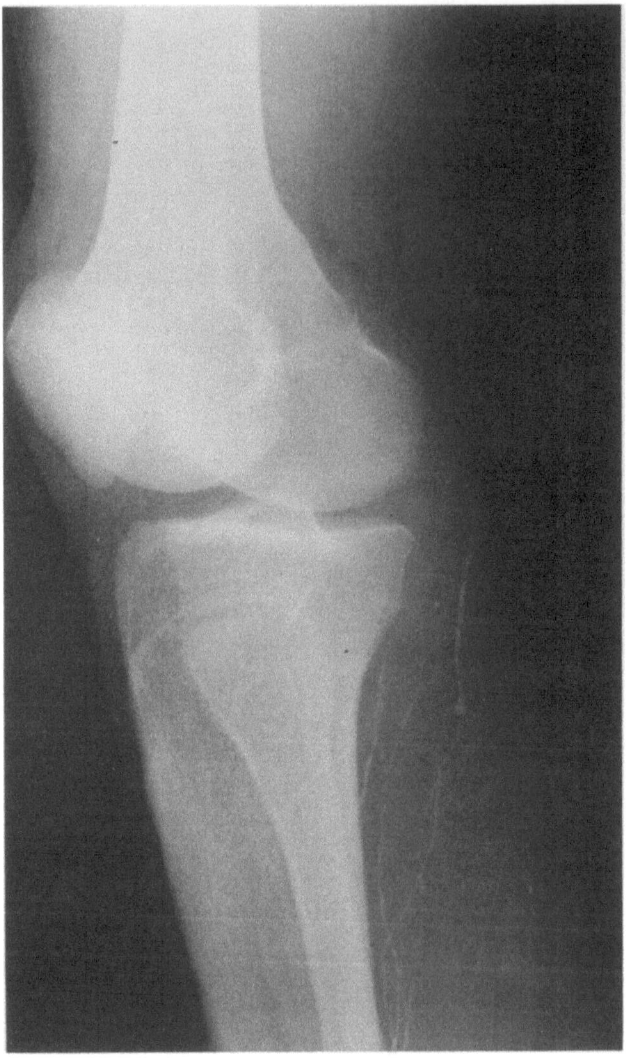

PATIENT A.P.G. - Before benzopyrone intralymphatic injection

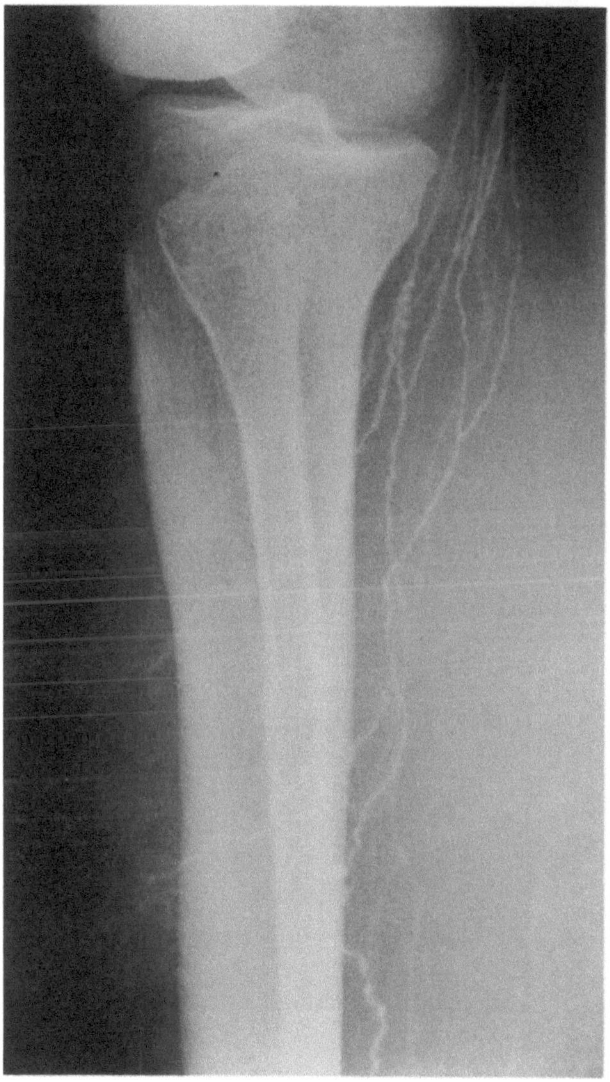

PATIENT A.P.G. - After benzopyrone intralymphatic injection

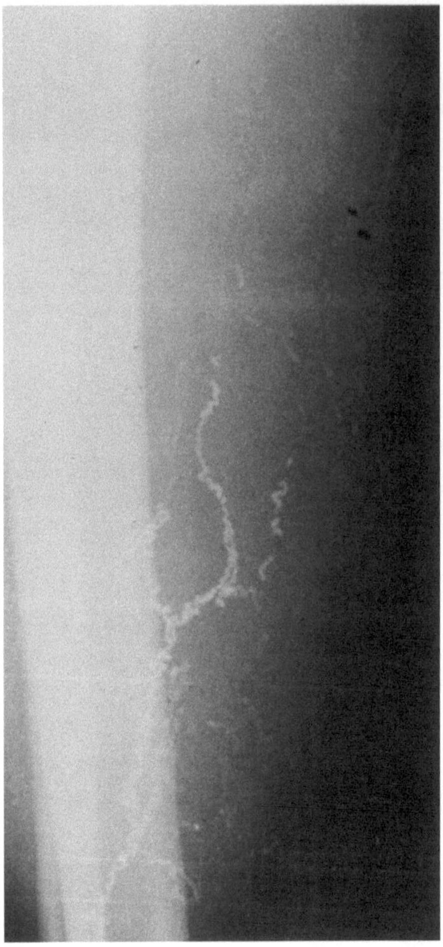

PATIENT O.R. - Before benzopyrone intralymphatic injection

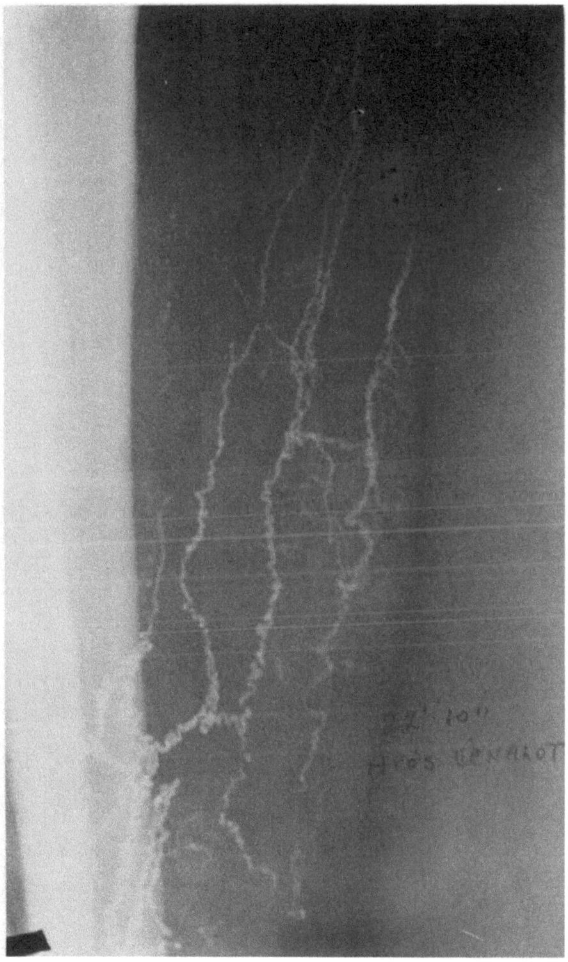

PATIENT O.R. - After benzopyrone intralymphatic injection

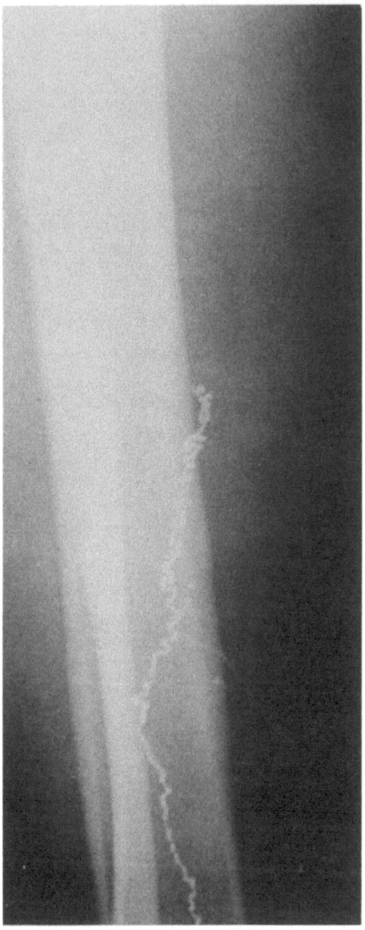

PATIENT J.S.S. - Before benzopyrone intralymphatic injection

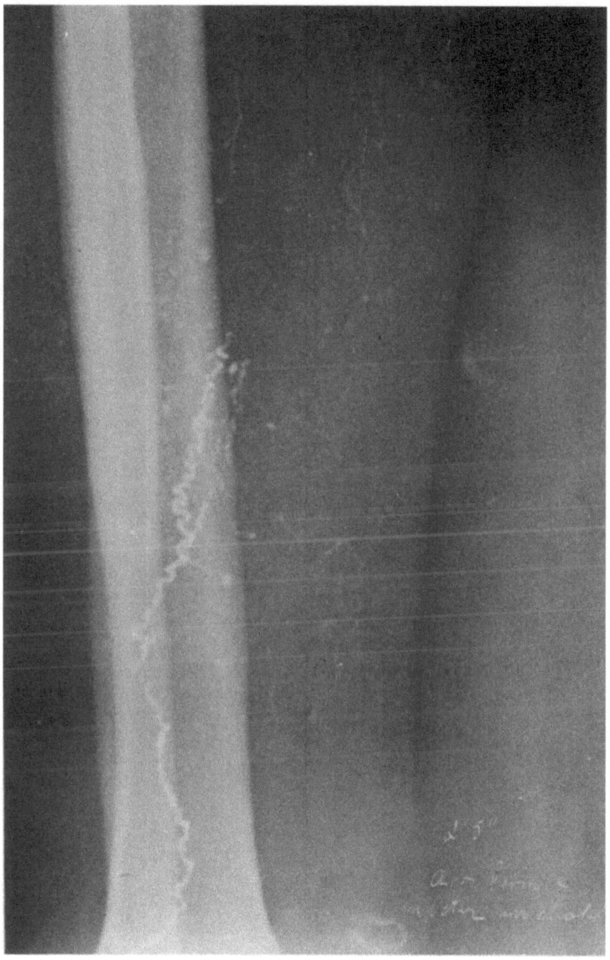

PATIENT J.S.S. - After benzopyrone intralymphatic injection

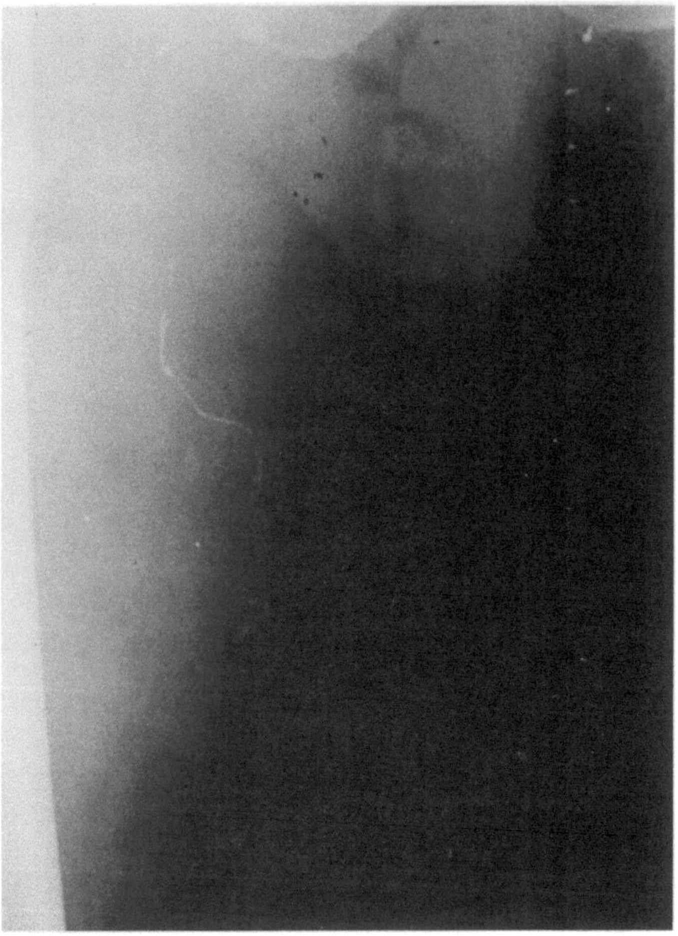

PATIENT I.S.M. - Before benzopyrone intralymphatic injection

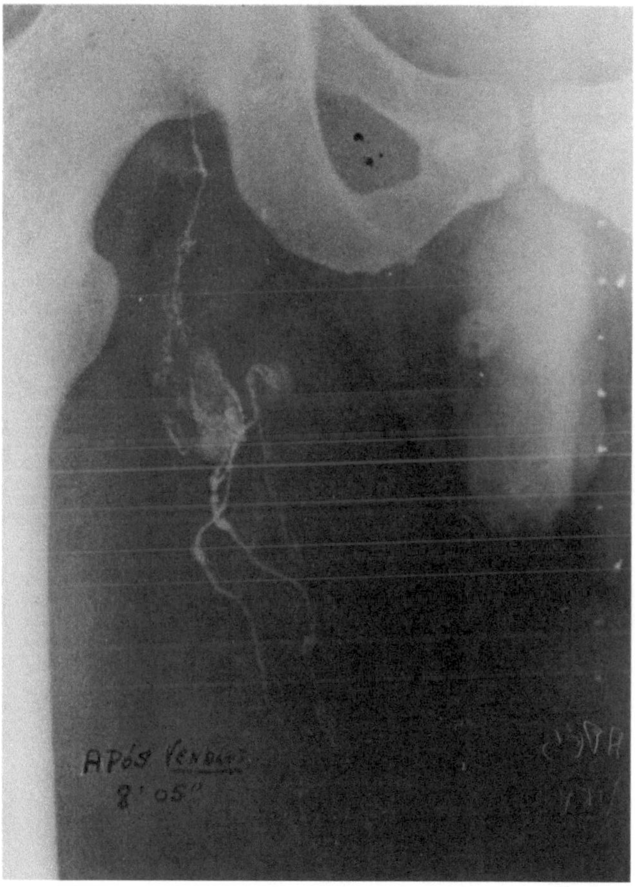

PATIENT I.S.M. - After benzopyrone intralymphatic injection

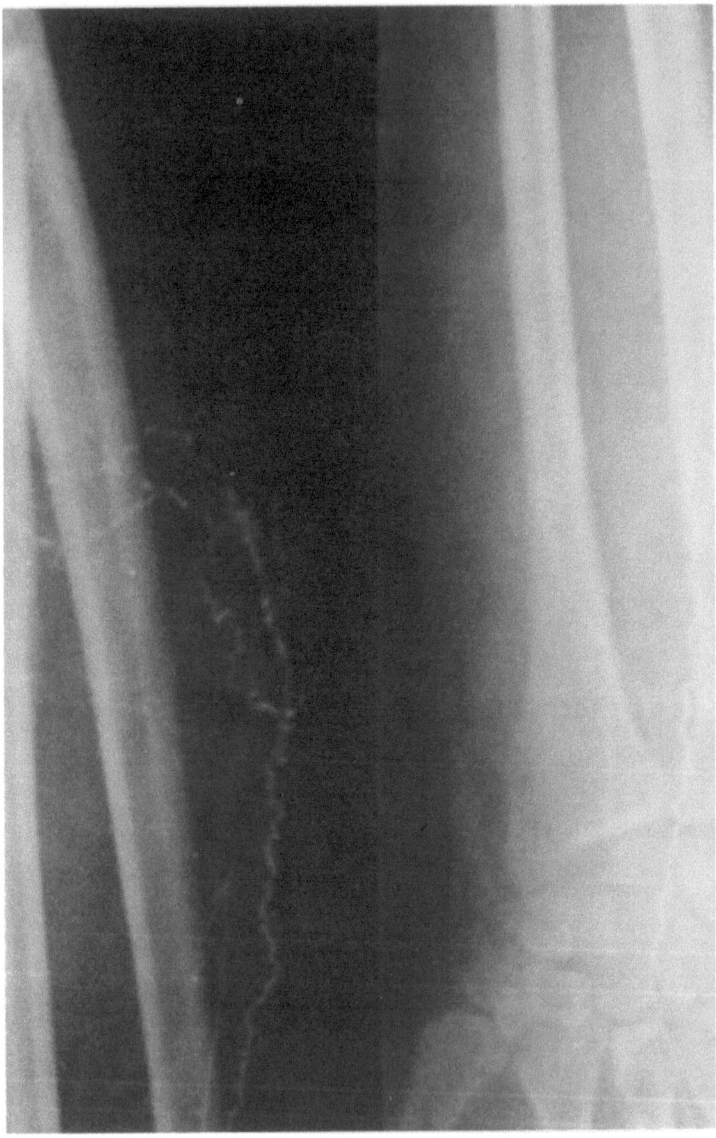

PATIENT L.L.G. - Before benzopyrone intralymphatic injection

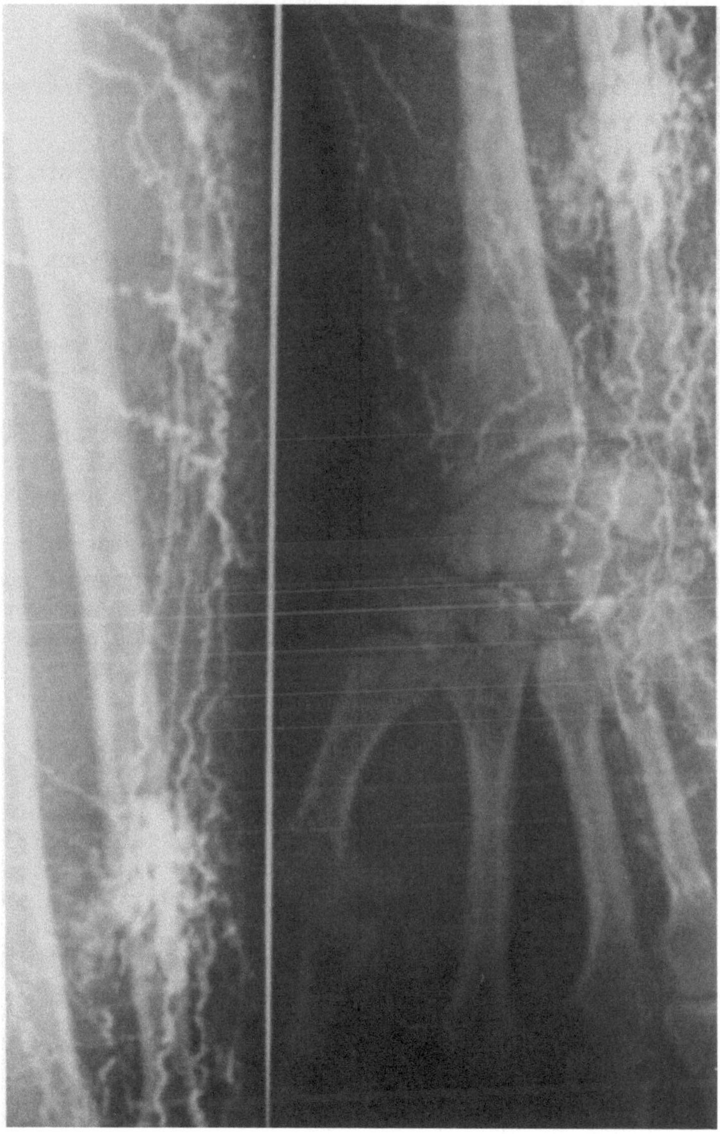

PATIENT L.L.G. - After benzopyrone intralymphatic injection

## Conclusions

Our pharmaco-radiological experiments have fully confirmed the lymphokinetics action of benzopyrones.

When this compound was used by intralymphatic or intravenous route we have observed the following facts:

1. There is a shortening of time necessary to perform the lymphoadenography due to the faster flow of the lymph.

2. In consequence of the regularization of the lymph flow it is necessary to use a smaller volume of dye.

3. Better visualization of the superficial lymph vessels offers big advantages for the clinical differential diagnosis.

4. There is a sharp effect on the speed of the lymph flow, with a vasodilation. These facts show a functional disorder on lymphedema secondary to vasomotor or reabsorption defects of the lymph flow.

We consider the lymphokinetics action of benzopyrone compounds very much useful for the lymphologist's daily activities not only for the medical treatments of lymphostatics edemas but also to shorten the time to observe the lymphadenography.

## BIBLIOGRAPHY

MISLIN, H. Die Wirkung von Cumarin aus Melilotus officinalis auf die Funktion des Lymphangions, Arzneim.Forsch.21:852-853, 1971

FÖLDI, M. KOVACH, A.G.B., VARGA, L., ZOLTAN, OT. Die Wirkung des Melilotus Praeparate Esberiven auf Die Lymphstromung im Ductus Thoracicus des Menschen, Med.Klinik 65; 1701-3, 1970

KRAJNOVIC, P. Lymphographic Investigations concerning the influence of drugs on the lymphatic circulation. XXIII, pg.381-384, Vol.10, Nov.1969.

SANDMANN, W. Lymphographische Befunde bei intraarterielle und intralymphatische applikation eines Coumarin präparates - Herz-Kreislauf- 35 G, N. 2, 4 April 1971, pg. 124-127

COLLARD, M. Etude pharmacoradiologique des effets lymphotropes de la Coumarine (5,6 Benzo-A-Pyrone) Progress on Angiology Vol.2, 1974, pg. 809-812

SCHOLTEN, C.A. L'action Lymphotrope de la Coumarine. Progress on Angiology, Vol. 3, 1974, pg. 813-814

FÖLDI, M. Basic Lymphology - Second Ringelheim Symposium - Folia Angiologica Supplementum, Vol. III, Verlg Haup. & Koska OHG, Berlin, Wien, 1974.

# TECHNIQUE OF FUNICULAR LYMPHOGRAPHY WITHOUT THE USE OF INDICATOR DYES

Hans Kuisk, Clyde E. Blackard, Donald C. Schenk, et al.

Department of Radiology
University of Minnesota
Minneapolis, Minnesota

We have developed a method of doing funicular (testicular) lymphography without injecting indicator dye into the tunica albuginea which carries the potential danger of disseminating tumor cells. Since our preliminary report (4), further experiences have been obtained which are summarized herewith.

We were fortunate to obtain two black American bears (Ursus americanus) for our purpose. To our liking, we found the testicular-lymphatic structures of the bear very similar to that of humans as seen in the accompanying illustrations. Prior to applying our technique on patients, we found human autopsy material very useful for practicing the identification of the lymphatic vessels which sometimes appear quite like the veins of the spermatic cord.

Figures 1 (bear) and 2 (human autopsy material) demonstrate our technique in detail. In this demonstration (Fig. 2), the cord was clamped and saline injected under pressure into the testis. This results in the same effect as when the constricting thread is placed around the cord on an actual patient. The whole procedure is as follows:

The spermatic cord is exposed surgically, the incision being made close to the inguinal ring. The cremasteric fascia is slit longitudinally and pushed away. A heavy, constricting silk thread is placed around the spermatic cord which obstructs and dilates the rich spermatic cord vessels which are seen running in a parallel fashion. The lymphatics can be identified as clear fluid-filled structures while veins appear dark.

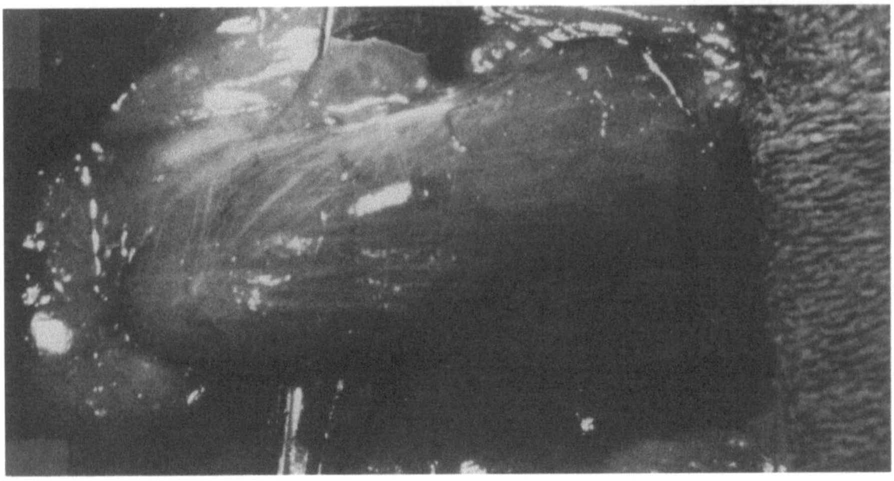

Fig. 1A: Funicular lymphography on an American black bear (Ursus americanus) Exposed funicular cord of the bear, the inguinal ring lies at the viewer's left.

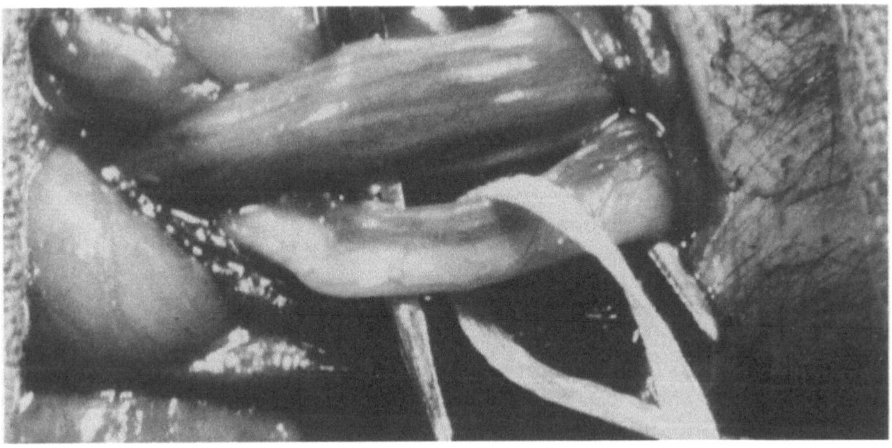

Fig. 1B: The cremasteric fascia has been split longitudinally and pushed away. The pulled down structure is the ductus deferens.

A 27 gauge lymphography needle is used for which an improvised handle is made making use of a sterile adhesive bandage (Fig. 2A). One end of the adhesive portion of the bandage is cut short and the distal portion of the tubing is pressed against it. A vertical split is now made just below the proximal part of the needle. The lower flap, thus formed, is folded around the tubing and pressed

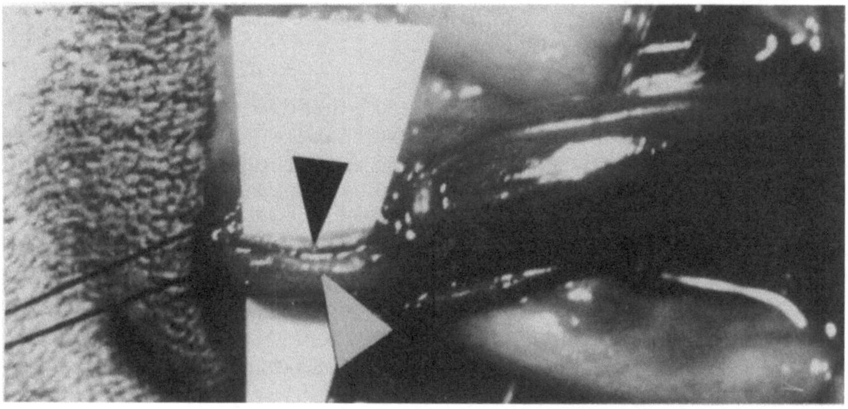

Fig. 1C: A constricting silk thread has been placed around the cord close to the inguinal ring to obstruct and dilate the parallel running vessels. The upper arrow points to a vein while the lower arrow shows a lymphatic trunk recognizable by its content of clear colorless lymph.

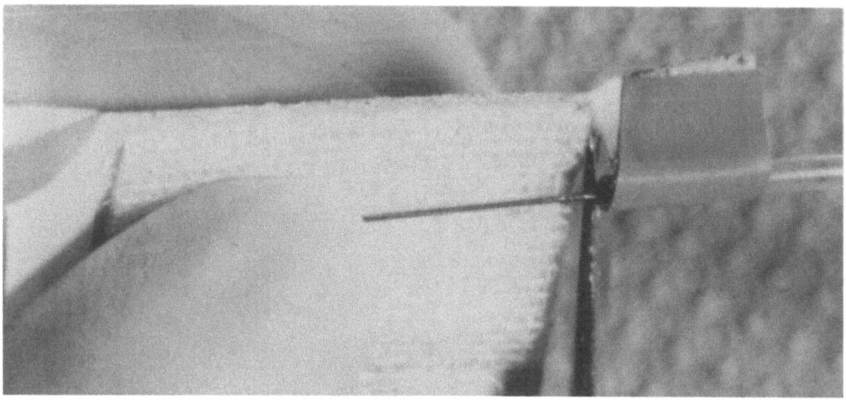

Fig. 2A: Demonstration of the described technique on autopsy material. Making an improvised handle for the lymphograph needle. The end of a sterile adhesive bandage (at viewer's right) has been cut short; the distal end of the tubing is pressed against the midportion of the exposed adhesive surface, and a vertical cut made just below the proximal free part of the needle. The lower flap produced this way is folded around the tubing to form a handle. The bare residual adhesive surfaces must be cut off to avoid the needle sticking to the gloved fingers after its insertion.

against the upper portion of the adhesive surface. This forms a useful handle to manipulate the needle. The remaining bare adhesive parts are cut off carefully in order to avoid the sticking of the needle to the gloved fingers.

Next, the sharp cutting edges of the needle are semi-dulled by simply rubbing it against the corrugated handle of the scalpel. This prevents the sharp needle tip from cutting through the delicate wall of the lymphatic vessel after it has been successfully inserted.

Prior to the cannulation, the proximal part of the needle is immobilized by piercing the needle through an avascular portion of the cord (Fig. 2B) and after the insertion (Fig. 2C), the distal part of the needle is secured in place by a 6-0 silk suture which also seals the vessel around the needle. Occasionally, in order to better identify the cannulable vessel a white plastic wedge can be slipped beneath it which facilitates markedly the inspection of the vessel through the magnifying glasses (Beebe' binoculars) which we always carry when doing any type of lymphography.

The "white background" and the improvised handle are routinely used in our pedal lymphographic technique (3,5). The material from which the "white background" is cut comes from the water repellent portion of sterile adhesive bandages or any other commercially available 0.1 mm thick, white opaque plastic sheet which can be gas sterilized.

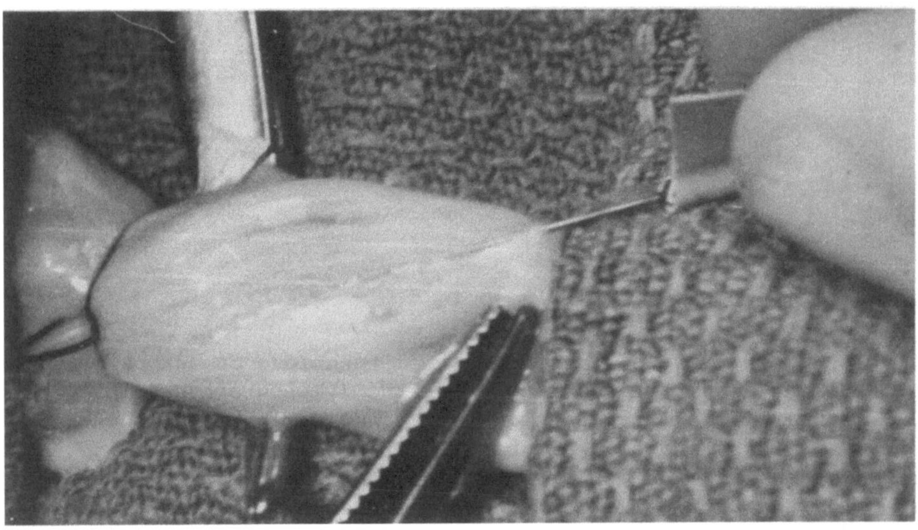

Fig. 2B: After the sharp cutting edges of the needle have been semidulled, it is pierced through an avascular part of the cord for immobilization.

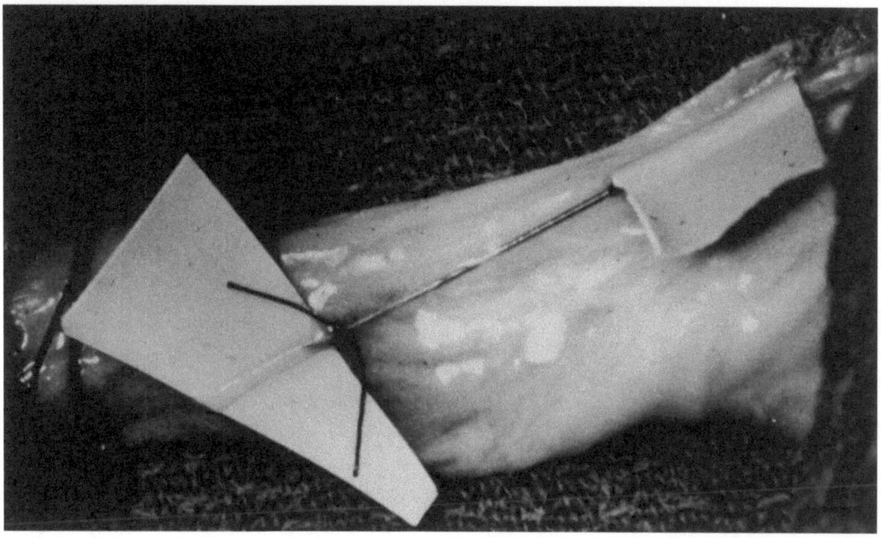

Fig. 2C: Sometimes a white plastic wedge can be placed beneath the lymphatic for better visualization. After insertion the distal end of the needle is immobilized with 6-0 silk suture which also seals the lymphatic around the needle.

After a trial injection of saline, about 3 ml of Ethiodol is injected under low pressure. We are using an improvised gravity type of injector made of a heavy wire on which a 5 cc Luer lock syringe is suspended under a 450 grams lead weight.

Several scout-roentgenograms are taken during the injection (Fig. 3C) and the follow-up films after 48 hours allowing the patient more rest.

One of our patients on whom we did funicular lymphography gave a lymphangiographic picture much different (Fig. 4) from the usual testicular pathway seen in Fig. 3C. The spermatic lymphatic trunk, instead of crossing cranially to end in the para-aortic nodes as usual (1,2,3), turned medially, instead, toward the lower level of the sacro-iliac joint and opacified the external and common iliac chains. One can interpret this occurrence in two ways: 1. that we have injected one of the trunks which drains the epididymis or 2. that this is the more rare type of pathway which drains the testis proper described already before the turn of the century and verified later by others (7). This also appears to be the same pathway described recently by McBrien, Edwards, and Kinmonth (6) who found this channel essential for drainage of the tunica vaginalis. In none of their 18 idiopathic hydrocele patients did this pathway

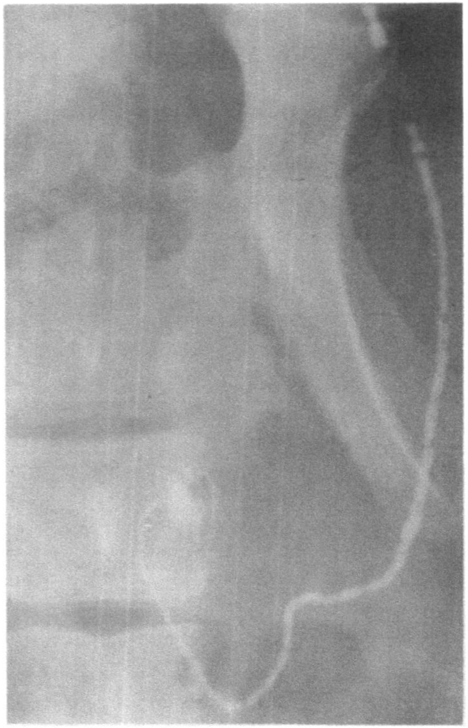

Fig. 3A: Right-sided funicular lymphangiogram of our first bear showing the similarity with the human structures. The ascending testicular lymphatic trunk is seen curving down to the primary drainage node from where a lumbar trunk is seen emerging. It runs cranially later to form the thoracic duct.

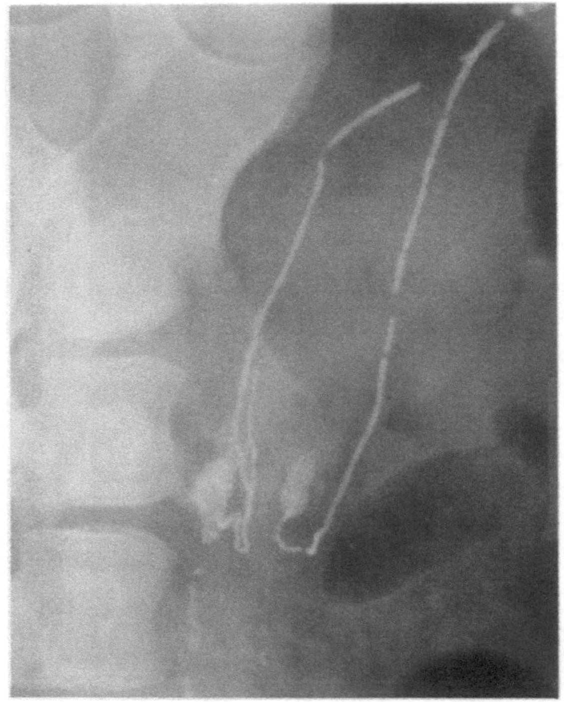

Fig. 3B: The oblique view of the funicular lymphangiogram of our second bear. It shows the same cranial arching of the testicular lymphatic trunks, large efferent lumbar trunks which start the formation of the thoracic trunk at the upper portion of this picture.

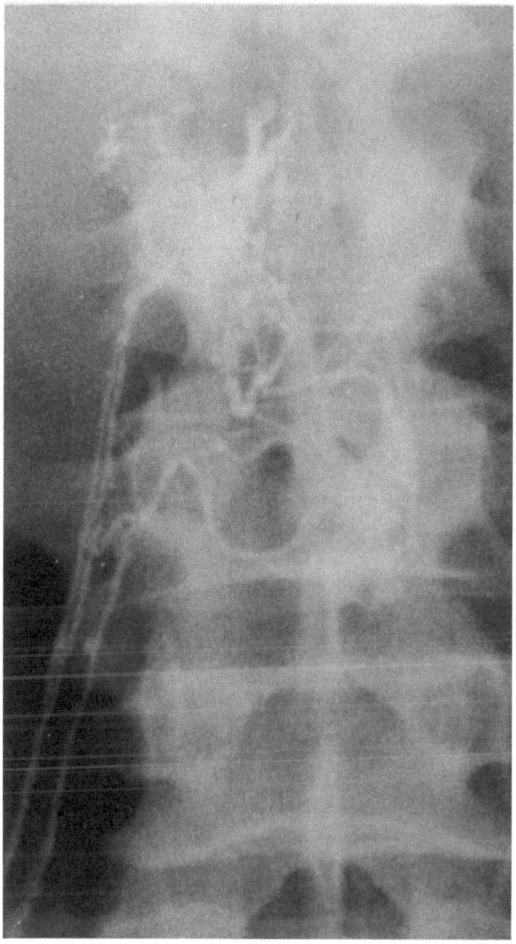

Fig. 3C: A close up view of a right-sided normal funicular lymphangiogram on human showing the preaortic cross-over of the lymphatics.

opacify through testicular lymphography.

Another interesting finding is noticed in the present study. The funicular lymphography showed profusion of Ethiodol only through the medial part of a common iliac node located at the S-1 level leaving a ragged lateral border. Pedal lymphography, however, which is always done as a supplement to a testicular study, demonstrates afferent vessels which entered the lateral portion of this node as well, and produced full opacification of this node as seen on the

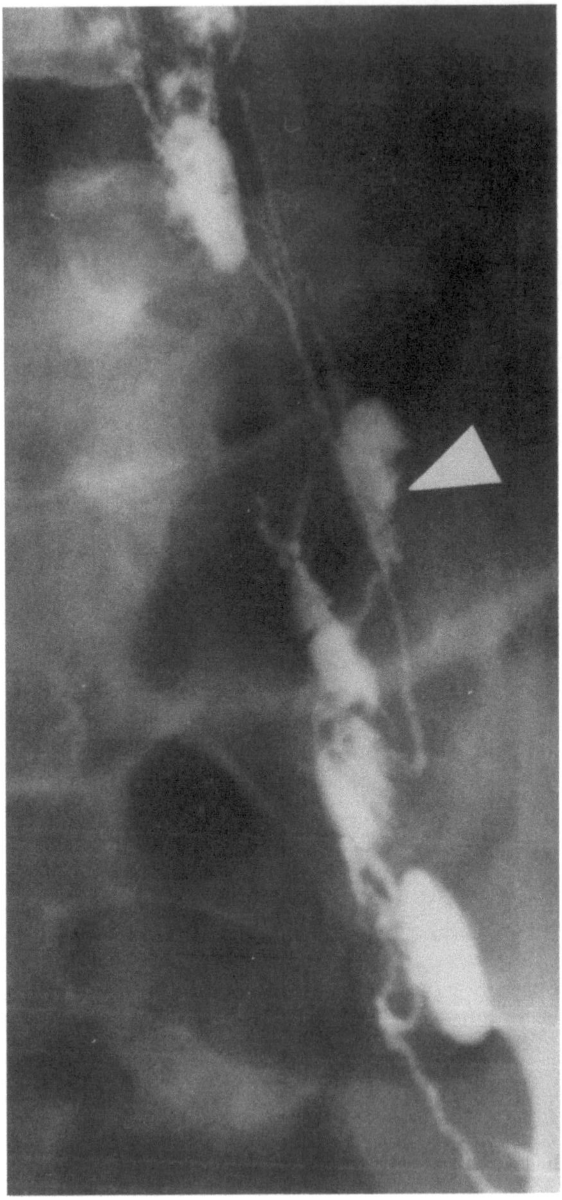

Fig. 4A: The external and common iliac lymphatic chains have become opacified during funicular lymphography. This presents either a rarer type of testicular drainage proper, or a pathway from the tunica vaginalis, or one of the pathways of the epididymis. Notice the perfusion of the medial portion of a common iliac node only (arrow), leaving a rugged lateral border.

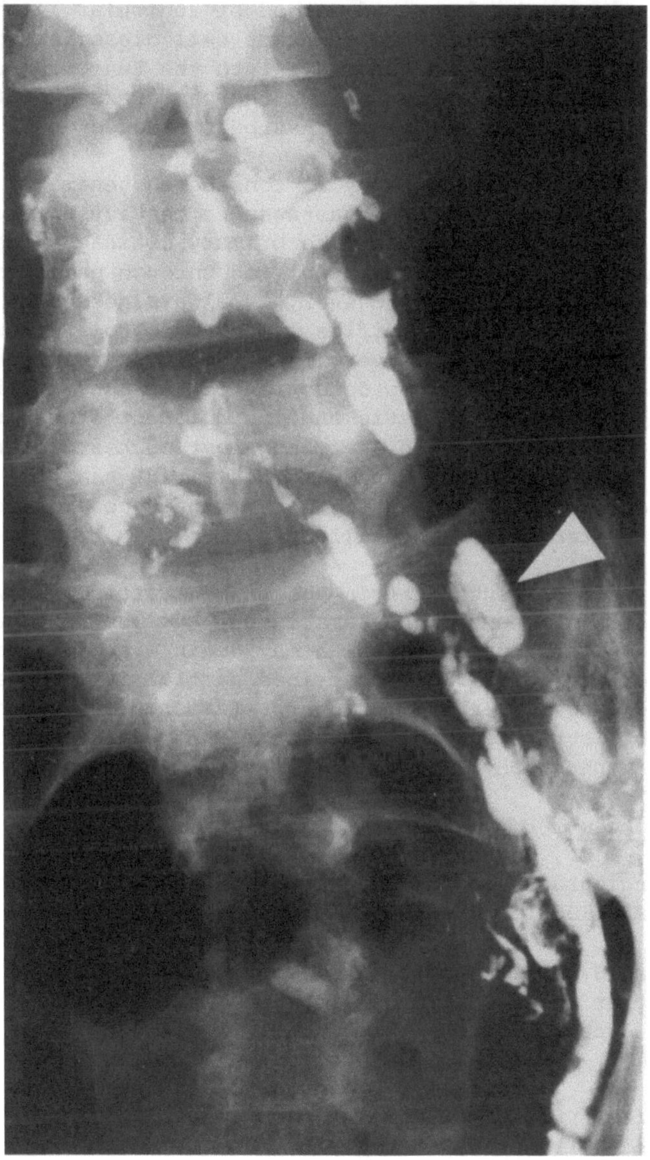

Fig. 4B: Pedal lymphograph, which is always done as a supplement to testicular studies shows, in this case that afferent vessels from a different pathway have entered the lateral part of the same node opacifying it fully.

lymphadenographic phase (Fig. 4B).

Conclusion. The described method of funicular lymphography removes the concomitant hazard of tumor cell dissemination because the need for injecting indicator dye into the tunica albuginea has been eliminated. This method allows the performance of funicular lymphography even when the testis has been removed.

Although pedal lymphography is considered generally sufficient for evaluation of lymph node metastases in testicular tumors, Chiappa, et. al. (2) have shown that the primary drainage nodes of the testicle may not always become opacified through pedal routes. Bilateral pedal lymphography, however, is always needed to supplement a testicular study as it opacifies lymph nodes to a wider extent. Testicular lymphography, however, does remain an important investigative procedure which allows detection of the many possible variations in the drainage of testis and its adjacent structures, carrying a high significance in the management of testicular tumors. The interesting finding by Wahlqvist, et al (8) that the thoracic duct may connect a primary testicular drainage node directly with the venous system is worth recalling.

The findings illustrated in the present article show that afferent vessels of one and the same lymph node may originate from different lymphatic pathways which may drain even different anatomical parts of the body. Such described partial lymph node filling may cause diagnostic errors in interpretation. The purpose of this presentation is to widen the interest for further research in funicular lymphography.

References

1. Busch, F. M., Sayegh, E.S., Chenault, O.W., Jr.: Some uses of lymphangiography in the management of testicular tumors. J. Urol. 93 (1965): 490-495.

2. Chiappa, S., Uslenghi, C., Bonadonna, G., et al.: Combined testicular and foot lymphangiography in testicular carcinomas. Surg., Gynec., Obstet. 123 (1966): 10-14.

3. Kuisk, H.: Technique of lymphography and principles of interpretation. Series of Modern Concepts of Radiology, Nuclear Med. and Ultrasound, ed. by L.E. Etter. Warren H. Green, St. Louis, 1971.

4. Kuisk, H., Blackard, C.E., Schenk, D.C., Panning, W.P.: A method of funicular (testicular) lymphography by eliminating indicator dye. Radiology 96 (1970): 198-201.

5. Kuisk, H., Panning, W.P.: A simple, practical technique of lymphangiography, Radiology 88 (1967): 576-583.

6. McBrien, P.M., Edwards, J.M., Kinmonth, J.B.: Lymphography of the testis and its adnexa in the normal and in idiopathic hydrocele. Arch. Surg. 104 (1972): 820-25.

7. Rouviere, H.: Anatomie des lymphatiques de l'homme. Masson et Cie, Paris, 1932.

8. Wahlqvist, L., Hulten, L., Rosencrantz, M: Normal lymphatic drainage of the testis studied by funicular lymphography. Acta. Chir. Scand. 132 (1966): 454-465.

# COMPLICATIONS OF LYMPHOGRAPHY

P. Ruben Koehler, M.D.

Department of Radiology
University of Utah Medical Center
Salt Lake City, Utah

The following report, summarizing the more serious complications associated with lymphography, is based on a survey taken from 1966 to 1968 by the International Congress of Lymphology. Although the number of lymphograms performed over the last 7 or 8 years has increased greatly, it is believed that the relative distribution of complications is the same.

## MATERIAL

Some 326 questionnaires were mailed to members of the International Society of Lymphology and to authors of publications dealing with lymphography. Eighty-three investigators returned these questionnaires.

It is obvious that this type of survey is open to much criticism. Since the term "complications" has not yet been thoroughly defined, many interpretations must be expected. Consequently, each person answering the questionnaires uses his own criteria as to what he considers a complication. The duration of time between the procedure and the onset of complication has also not been defined. As a result, some incidents occurring as late as 21 days after lymphography have been associated with the procedure. Frequently, clinical follow-up of patients who underwent lymphography was less than ideal, perhaps minimizing the number of reported complications. In most instances, however, information on serious complications is relayed to the physician who performed the examination so that these complications are most likely reported here.

Despite these reservations, the value of this survey is

that it reflects the experience of investigators who performed over 32,000 lymphograms. Because of the large number of examinations done, it is felt that a general statement covering the incidence of serious complications associated with lymphography is justified.

In the hope of receiving maximum cooperation the questionnaire was made as simple as possible. The person receiving the questionnaire was requested to estimate as accurately as possible, the total number of lymphograms done in his institution and to report only the more serious complications. Detailed clinical data of serious complications was requested, but frequently not supplied.

## RESULTS

The complications were divided into the following groups:

1. Fatalities attributed to the procedure of lymphography
2. Pulmonary complications, including pulmonary infarction, pulmonary edema and other severe pulmonary reactions
3. Cardiovascular incidents, including hypo- or hypertensive crises
4. Hypersensitive reactions to:
    a. Radiopaque contrast media
    b. Vital blue dye
5. Neurologic disorders
6. Other complications

The total number of lymphograms performed exceeded 32,000. In the vast majority the lymph vessels of the feet were cannulated. In over 99% the radiographic contrast media used were Lipiodol UF, Ethiodol and Myodil.

## FATALITIES

The total number of fatalities reported was 18. This is an incidence of 1:1,800. The following causes of death were reported:

| | |
|---|---|
| 1. Cardiac failure | 2 |
| 2. Respiratory death | 7 |
| 3. Cerebral death | 3 |
| 4. Not stated | 6 |

The time between lymphography and the onset of symptoms ranged from two hours to five days. The time between the onset of symptoms and death ranged from three hours to 21 days.

Since in many instances the clinical data returned with the questionnaires was insufficient, it was chosen not to describe any of the cases in detail.

PULMONARY COMPLICATIONS

1. Pulmonary infarcts - 81 - incidence 1:400. It was hoped that pulmonary oil embolization was not included in this category and that the cases reported would have the classical clinical and radiological signs of pulmonary infarction. It is the author's impression that the reported incidence is much too high and in all likelihood many cases of pulmonary oil embolization have been included* (the presence of oil in the lung a short time after lymphography is very common, and is usually without clinical manifestion or significance).

2. Pulmonary edema - 10 - incidence 1:3,200.

3. Pneumonia - 13 - incidence 1:2,500 (with radiographic evidence of pulmonary infiltrates and elevation of temperature lasting more than 24 hours).

4. Hemoptysis - 10 - incidence 1:3,200 (since pneumonia and hemoptysis are not considered serious, it is believed that the true incidence of such complications is much higher than this material reflects).

CARDIOVASCULAR COMPLICATIONS

A surprisingly small number of pure cardiovascular complications were reported. Only six instances of hypotensive crisis were listed. This is an incidence of 1:5,000. One patient required digitalization because of acute cardiac failure.

---

* A detailed description and hypothesis of the pathophysiology of the interaction of the oil with the lungs can be found in: Koehler, P.R.: Lymphography. Complications and accidents. Proceedings of Lymphology, ed. A. Rüttimann, George Thieme, Stuttgart, 1966, p. 306-307.

## HYPERTENSIVE REACTIONS

A total of 40 patients developed hypersensitive reactions to the oily contrast medium. In 57 instances allergic reactions to the vital blue dye occurred. Hypersensitive reactions to the different vital blue dyes are shown in Table 1.

Table 1. Hypersensitive Reactions

| | Number of Cases |
|---|---|
| Ethiodol, Lipiodol or Myodil | 40 |
| Vital Blue Dye (Total) | 57 |
| Patent Blue Violet | 47 |
| Alphazurine 2G | 3 |
| Brilliant Green | 1 |
| Sky Blue | 1 |
| Not Specified | 5 |

Hypersensitive reactions ranged from hives, to angioneurotic edema with or without laryngospasm, to vasomotor collapse. In many instances a local anesthetic was mixed with the vital blue dye, but since hypersensitivity occurred in patients who had negative skin reactions to the local anesthetic, it is suggested that the vital blue dye may be the allergic component.

## GENERAL DISORDERS

Severe cerebral disorders were reported in 9 cases. This is an incidence of 1:3,500 lymphograms. In all 9 patients definite neurological signs developed; motor disfunctions, paraplegia and deep coma lasting for weeks were reported. Six of the 9 recovered within two to three weeks without permanent impairment. In three instances death occurred. In most patients the neurological signs appeared within the first 48 hours after the procedure, developed gradually, reaching a peak in 4 to 7 days, and then slowly subsided. Unfortunately, here too the clinical information available does not permit any detailed discussion.

## OTHER COMPLICATIONS

Other complications reported were:

| | |
|---|---|
| Prolonged fever (more than 24 hours) | 24 |
| Lymphatic fistulae | 4 |
| Lymphatic stasis of leg | 2 |

## CONCLUSIONS

This relatively simple and somewhat incomplete questionnaire represents the experience of about 70 investigators who performed more than 32,000 lymphograms. Because of the large number of examinations involved it is believed that the survey reflects the approximate incidence of the more serious complications in lymphography. The number and incidence of complications is tabulated in Table 2. The results showed that the rate of serious complications is relatively low and that in regard to complications this type of radiographic examination compares favorably with other radiodiagnostic procedures.

Table 2. Number of Cases & Incicence of Complications

| | Number of Cases | Incidence |
|---|---|---|
| Death | 18 | 1:1,800 |
| Pulmonary infarcts | 81 | 1:400 |
| Pulmonary Edema | 10 | 1:3,200 |
| Pneumonia | 13 | 1:2,500 |
| Hypotensive Crisis | 6 | 1:5,000 |
| Hypersensitivity Reaction | | |
| Oily Contrast Medium | 40 | 1:800 |
| Vital Blue Dye | 57 | 1:600 |
| Cerebral Disorders | 9 | 1:3,500 |

## References

1. Koehler, P.R.: Lymphography. Complications and Accidents. Proceedings of Lymphology, ed. A. Rüttimann, Georg Thieme, Stuttgart, 1966, p. 306-307.

2. Koehler, P.R.: Typical Fatal Reactions After Lymphography. Cancer Chemotherapy Reports, Vol. 52, No. 1, January 1968, p. 113-118.

3. Koehler, P.R.: Complications of Lymphography. Lymphology, Vol. 1, No. 4, December, 1968, p. 116-120.

# Malignant Diseases

# SUPRACLAVICULAR LYMPH VESSEL LIGATION IN MALIGNANT TUMORS OF THE PARANASAL SINUS, ORAL CAVITY, AND HYPOPHARYNX

H.-J. Nickol

Ear, Nose, and Throat Clinic of the General Hospital
Hamburg-Altona, West Germany

Lymphatic vessels and nodes of the neck do not exhibit the specific and constant drainage patterns characteristic of the blood vessels and nerves in this area. The pathways of one side cross often making it difficult to identify the appropriate lymph nodes. Rouviere and Taillens established a generally accepted scheme which has been confirmed by Walter, Fisch, and Becker. In a film in 1965, we were able to demonstrate cranially directed lymphatic pathways showing physiologic spontaneous movement of the middle and greater lymphatic vessels. Thus, primary metastasis of the larynx behind the insertion of the sternocleideomastoid muscle in the nuchal area can occur (Nickol). Tumor metastases can be found in all lymph nodes of the neck.

We believe that while lymphovenous anastomoses are of importance in transporting tissue fluid, they play only a minor role in transport of tumor cells, especially in the neck area. Distant metastases of head and neck tumors of any kind have been demonstrated in only 3 to 5% of the cases. Moreover, the vertial lymphatic system terminates at the level of the clavicle and represents the major inflow of lymph into veins. Only very few cranially running lymphatic vessels have been identified below this line. Also, caudal diseased lymph nodes are rarely described above the clavicle except for the lymphatic vessels which pass from the thorax underneath the subclavian vein and enter this vein rather than the jugular vein. Thus we find an important barrier of the lymph system in the head and neck between the caudal and cranial parts of the body. Only the paratracheal lymph pathways cross this border in both directions.

In my opinion, the lymph system of the neck should be viewed as a closed unit and treated as such. In therapeutic approaches one should consider not only the lymph vessels and lymphatic nodes along the internal jugular vein or along the phrenic nerve, but, as in X-ray therapy, the surgeon should try to eliminate the whole system. If tumor exists at one margin of the lymphatic unit, the whole block of the suspected side has to be extracted -- total en bloc neck dissection -- except for biopsy excisions of single preserved nodes. No clear results can be obtained with partial resections and, therefore, these have to be rejected (Bocca).

A malignant lymph system disease evolves by spreading and advancing of malignant tumors but may also arise as a systemic disease such as Hodgkin's disease. One can count 10,000 cancer cells per square millimeter of tumor tissue. Most likely the outflow of tumor cells begins at a very early point. One has to consider that with each careful and restricted lymph node dissection some unknown colonies in the fringe areas are likely to be overlooked and thus escape treatment (Fisch, Wustrow).

Microscopic examination has clearly shown that it is impossible to abolish tumor spread by X-ray or by cytostatic drugs. After treatment with 6000-7000 rDD, lymph vessels remain patent for particles including tumor cells. The physiological spontaneous movement of the vessels may be impaired as well as their elasticity, but tissue pressure propels lymph and its contents onward, often bypassing X-ray-destroyed lymph nodes. If the metastatic nodes become smaller or even disappear, drainage into the veins remains open (Kley, Nickol, Jung).

In the search for a new surgical method to obtain better results, we took advantage of the anatomic structure of the neck.

## Methods

Above and parallel to the subclavian vein, there are no vital nerves and vessels. Here, however, one finds the most intensive concentration of caudally running vessels. To display the subcutaneous fat and lymphatic tissue, it is necessary to perform a skin-platysma incision of 10 cm under local anesthesia. After isolating the internal jugular vein, a lateral silk ligature should be pulled from the jugular vein above the scalenus muscles laterally under the anterior rim of the trapezius. Here the thread is placed outside and knotted. Then all lymph vessels are tied and allowed to dam up slowly. The lymphatic congestion can be visualized up to the lower edge of the larynx (Figs. 1 and 2).

Right after lymphatic ligation, irradiation of the whole lymph unit with telecobalt is begun. The primary tumor should be

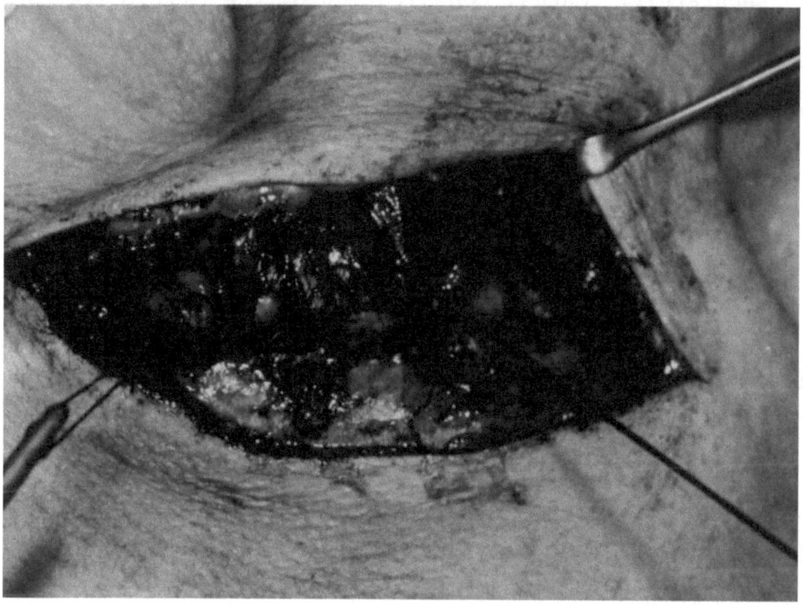

Fig. 1

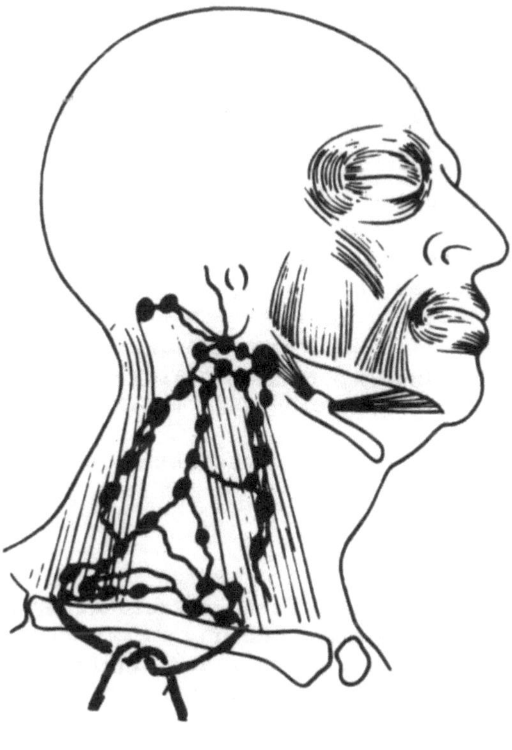

Fig. 2

X-rayed separately. Mutual consultation by the radiologist and otolaryngologist determines continuation of treatment after half of the tumor dose, or 3000 rDD.

The following points are important for the first method, the "sandwich method":

1. Has the primary tumor been largely eliminated?
2. Are the palpable lymph nodes still evident?
3. Does a strong X-ray reaction of the mucosa exist in the region of the primary tumor?

If question 1 is answered positively and questions 2 and 3 negatively, then the operation performed is a total en bloc neck dissection. At the same time, the primary tumor is extensively removed. An average interval of 18 days between the last X-ray and the operation is allowed to elapse.

If question 1 is answered negatively and questions 2 and 3 positively, the patient is X-rayed with 6000 rDD, and the total en bloc neck dissection follows. The interval between completed irradiation with 6000 rDD and the operation should be at least 6 and if possible 10 weeks.

The surgical procedure should be undertaken to control the primary tumor (Böhme, Miehlcke, Fletscher, Monnier-Kuhn, Wullstein, Spitalier, Nickol). According to the classification of the ICPR and the UICC, only tumors of stages $T_1$ and $T_2$ and metastases $N_0$, $N_1$, $N_2$, and rarely $N_3$ are considered. Wider tumor invasion cannot be controlled even by our method.

The en bloc neck dissection is performed by the method of Dietzel (Fig. 3). The incision can be extended further. Tissue components such as fat, lymph vessels, lymph nodes, and nerves, including the accessory nerve, are removed caudally above and parallel to the subclavian vein as far as the base of the skull on the neck muscles with removal of the sternocleidomastoid muscle and the omohyoid muscle. The jugular vein is totally isolated and all inflow tied off. The wall of the vein must remain intact.

If lymph tissue is adherent, then this vessel may also be resected.

## Histology

If the "sandwich method" is applied, then the histology after 3000 rDD is as follows. There are small, medium, and moderately dilated lymph vessels, which contain a transparent liquid and only scattered leukocytes in lumen. Complete obliteration of the pathways of the lymph nodes has not developed (Fig. 4).

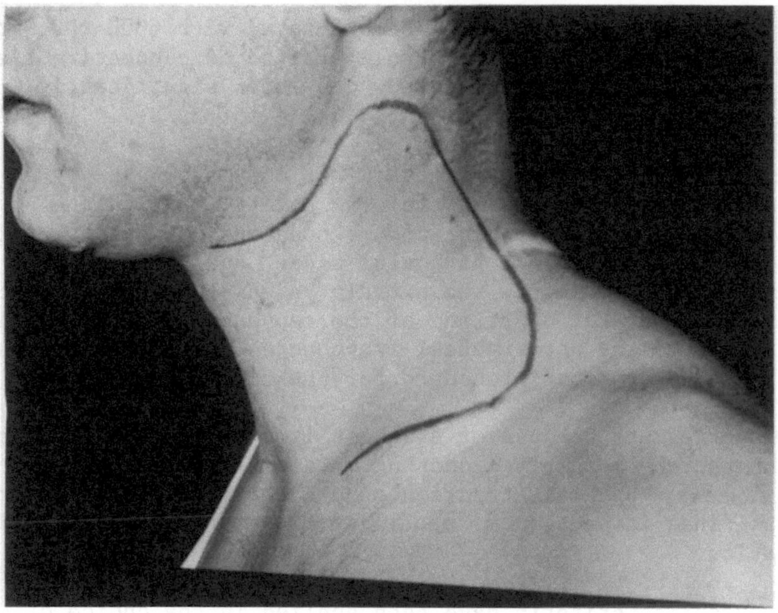

Fig. 3

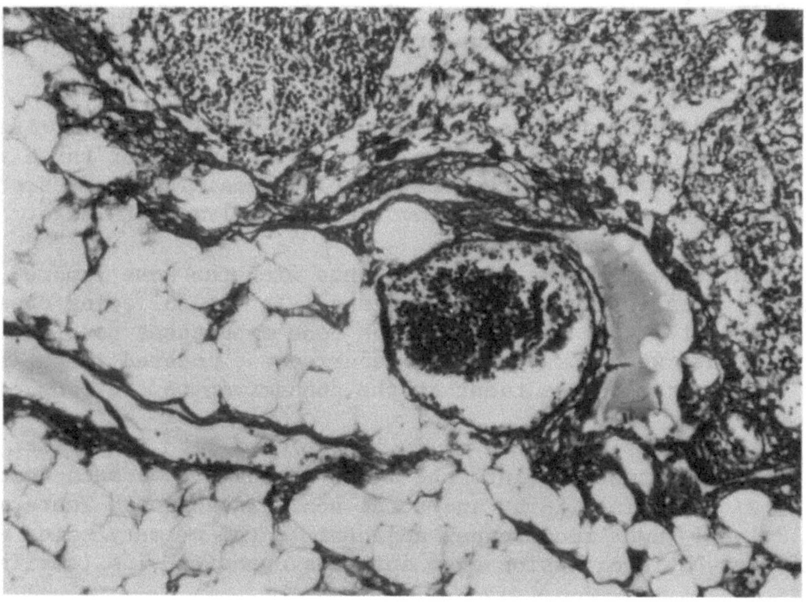

Fig. 4

If the neck lymph unit has been X-rayed with 6000 rDD, then the vessel system is altered. Proliferation of connective tissue and edema of the endothelium narrow the lumen significantly. Total obstruction is not present (Fig. 5).

Initial treatment by the method has only been used by us for strictly unilateral tumors of the oral cavity, soft palate, uvula, tonsils, fringe of the tongue, and mesopharynx, as well as for tumors of the nasopharynx, paranasal sinus, and hypopharynx. According to our experience, the extralaryngeal tumors, tumors of the larynx and of the upper end of the esophagus metastasize in 25% of cases to the paratracheal lymph nodes. These tumors have to be excluded from our procedure for the time being.

Danger exists because of stagnant lymph flow from lymphatic ligation thereby possibly promoting metastasis to the paratracheal lymph vessels. Special attention should be directed to the fringe areas at final inspection as each ligature opens up collateral circulation.

Very strict criteria have been applied in the choice of cases. We believe, however, that our success so far should extend the applicability of this method.

During a period of 5 years, 159 patients have been operated on by us for malignant tumors in the head and hypopharynx (stages $T_1$, $T_2$, $N_2$, and eventually also $N_3$). In 25 of these cases, we performed lymphatic ligation. The primary tumor in those 25 cases was predominantly in the oral cavity, where we had the most concrete and visible control.

Of the 25 patients who underwent ligation, 10 have survived over a period of ten years, 4 for four years, and 2 for three years. No patient had lymph node recurrence. The remaining 9 cases showed local tumor recurrence without involvement of lymph drainage.

In our second series of 41 patients with the same tumors, we utilized lymphatic ligation in 26 cases. In the following observation period of 2 to 5 years, no lymph node metastases have occurred. However, there were three primary recurrences, located in the tonsilar fringe area of the tumor at the connection to the tongue.

Thus, success was achieved in 51 patients with lymphatic ligation. No metastases into the lymph drainage have been demonstrated with combined X-ray and total neck dissection. There were only 12 local tumor recurrences adjacent to the primary tumor without new lymphatic extension even into the opposite side (see Table 1).

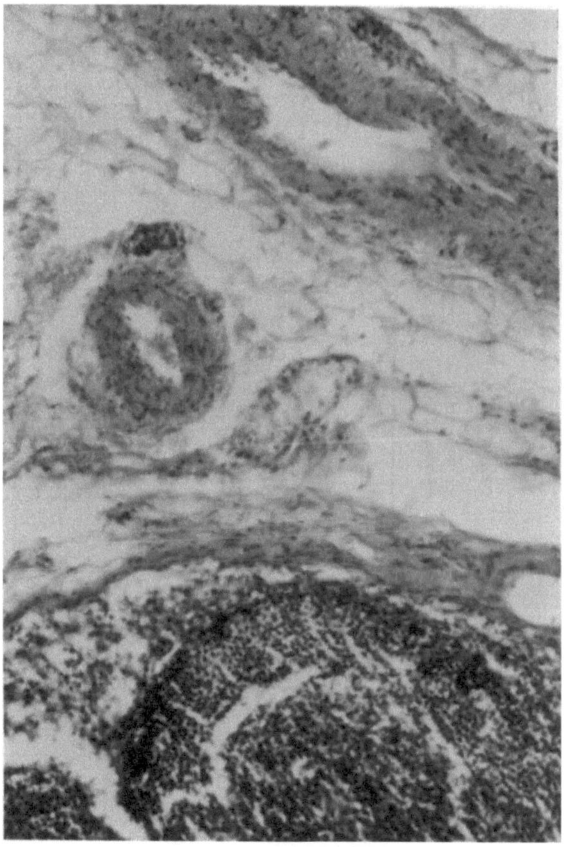

Fig. 5

TABLE 1. Tumor Localization and TNM System

(a) usual therapy (operation and X-ray)
(b) lymph ligation with X-ray and operation

51 lymph ligations on 200 tumor patients in 10 years

| | | $T_1$ | | | | $T_2$ | | | | $T_3$ | | | | $T_4$ | | | | Recurrence | | |
|---|---|---|---|---|---|---|---|---|---|---|---|---|---|---|---|---|---|---|---|---|
| | | $N_0$ | $N_1$ | $N_2$ | $N_3$ | $N_0$ | $N_1$ | $N_2$ | $N_3$ | $N_0$ | $N_1$ | $N_2$ | $N_3$ | $N_0$ | $N_1$ | $N_2$ | $N_3$ | Local | Lymph nodes | Free |
| Paranasal sinus | a | | | | | 3 | 4 | | | 2 | 3 | 5 | | 2 | 1 | 1 | | 9 | 8 | 4 |
| | b | | 1 | | | 2 | 1 | 1 | | 1 | | 1 | | | | | | 1 | | 5 |
| Tonsils | a | | 1 | 5 | 2 | | 9 | 5 | 3 | | 4 | 4 | | | 2 | | | 11 | 12 | 12 |
| | b | | 1 | 1 | | | 2 | 2 | | | 5 | 9 | 1 | | 1 | | | 4 | 1 | 17 |
| Oropharinx | a | | 1 | | | | | | | | 2 | 3 | | | 1 | | | 2 | 4 | 1 |
| | b | | | 1 | 1 | 1 | 1 | | | | 2 | 1 | 1 | | | | | | | 8 |
| Tongue | a | | 2 | 3 | | | 2 | 1 | | | 9 | 1 | 1 | | 1 | | | 8 | 11 | 1 |
| | b | | 1 | 1 | | 1 | 2 | | | | 1 | 3 | 3 | | 1 | | | 2 | | 11 |
| Hypopharynx | a | 1 | | | | 2 | 18 | 9 | | 2 | 18 | 7 | 3 | 3 | 3 | | | 21 | 38 | 7 |
| | b | | | | | | | | | | 1 | | | | | | | | | 1 |
| Total | a | 1 | 4 | 8 | 2 | 5 | 33 | 15 | 3 | 4 | 36 | 20 | 4 | 5 | 8 | 1 | | 51 | 73 | 25 |
| | b | | 3 | 3 | 1 | 4 | 6 | 3 | | 1 | 9 | 14 | 5 | | 2 | | | 7 | 1 | 43 |

I wish to propose that in other regions of the body with dense lymphatic drainage, tumor treatment can be improved by ligation of the respective lymph system and prompt X-ray treatment following radical surgery.

In summary, malignant tumors of groups $T_1$ through $T_3$ and $N_0$ through $N_3$ can be controlled with best results by complete elimination of the primary lymph unit. The lymphatics at their entrance into the venous systems should be

(a) ligated first,
(b) X-rayed,
(c) finally, operated on as radically as possible.

The results are excellent, with no further metastases into the regional drainage and collateral pathways.

## References

Becker, W. (1963), Arch. Ohren, Nasen, Kehlkopfheilkd., 182:126.

Bocca, E. (1972), in: Kopf- und Hals-Chirurgie (H. H. Naumann), George Thieme, Stuttgart.

Böhme, P. E. (1963), Chirurgie, 34:97.

Dietzel, K. (1960), Arch. Ohren, Nasen, Kehlkopfheilkd., 176:801.

Fletcher (1963), Amer. J. Roentgenol. 90:990.

Fisch (1966), Fortschr. Hals, Nasen, Ohrenheilkd., 14.

Jung, H. (1974), Z. Laryngol. Rhinol. 53:769.

Kley (1963), Arch. Ohren, Nasen, Kehlkopfeilkd., 182:399.

Monnier-Kuhn (1959), J. Fr. Oto-Rhino-Laryngol., 8:887.

Miehlke, A. (1959), Z. Laryngol. Rhinol. 38:524.

Nickol, H. J. (1965), Habilitationsschrift, Hamburg.

Nickol, H. J. (1966), HNO (BLU) 14:105.

Nickol, H. J. (1970), Proc. 2nd Int. Laryngol. Lymphol. 1968, George Thieme, Stuttgart, p. 227.

Nickol, H. J. (1967), Arch. Ohren, Nasen, Kehlkopfeilkd., 188:562.

Rouviere, P. (1932), Anatomie des lymphatiques de l'homme, Masson & Cie, Paris.

Spitallier, J. M., et al. (1961), Press. Med., 69:2549.

Taillens, J. P. (1967), Progress in Lymphology, Georg Thieme, Stuttgart, p. 275.

Walter, H. E. (1948), Krebsmetastasen, Schwabe, Basel.

Wullstein, H. L. (1968), Fortschritte der Kiefer- und Gesichts-Chirurgie, Vol. 3, Georg Thieme, Stuttgart.

Wullstein, H. L. (1941), Arch. Ohren, Nasen, Kehlkopfheilkd., 149:517.

Wustrow, F. (1965), Urban und Schwarzenberg, München.

# EXPLORATION OF THE HEAD AND NECK LYMPHATIC SYSTEM USING COLLOIDAL GOLD-198

Dr. Federico J. Gruart

Calle Austria 2626

Buenos Aires, Argentina

Taking advantage of the lymphophilic quality of colloidal gold-198, we used this radioisotope to study the head and neck lymphatic system.

Hultborn in 1955 utilized colloidal gold for the first time to explore the lymphatic drainage of the breast in cancer involvement of this system. Later Leborgne used the same procedure to check whether axillary lymphatic dissection had really been radical. Other authors performed similar investigations in the same and other regions, reaching similar conclusions.

The method demonstrated

(a) the lymphophilic property of colloidal gold;
(b) the presence of lymphatic spread of cancer.

Based on these findings, we applied the technique of scintigraphy to visualize the head and neck lymphatic system. This paper includes the study of 50 cases of whom 25 were patients free of head and neck pathology, and the other 25 had different types of tumors located in this area.

## Technique

Using the perlingual route as in lymphadenography, topical anesthesia of the tongue edge was carried out and colloidal gold injected in varying quantities (200 to 400 microcuries) unilaterally or bilaterally according to the study plan.

The injection was made in the submucous level or intramuscularly (to spread the radioactivity to the opposite side). The dose of Au-198 was given in divided doses, one-third to the anterior half of the tongue and two-thirds in the posterior half of the tongue. Following the radioisotope injection, the tongue was gently massaged and scintigrams taken one and 24 hours later. These times were the most important and illustrative, but we have also prolonged the studies for days with interesting observations.

The results of this technique confirmed that the anterior third of the tongue drains through the lymphatic capillaries to the submental lymphatic nodes and the posterior half drains to the subdigastric nodes first and from there to the jugulocarotid lymphatic group. The colloidal gold spreads later from the submental nodes to the submaxillary group and from there to the jugulocarotid groups. Still later, the radioisotope is visualized along the entire jugulocarotid lymphatic chain.

The reticular system of the lymph nodes is the one that fixes the radioisotope, and the density of the images varies with isotope concentration, which in turn is related to the degree of cancer invasion of these nodes.

Neoplastic tissue does not fix the colloidal gold, so that cancer invasion shows as an area of poor or absent uptake of radioisotope. The scintigrams that furnished the above information were those taken one and 24 hours after the injection in frontal and profile positions right, left, or bilaterally according to the study planned.

## Summary and Conclusion

It is evident that scintigraphy obtained after injection of colloidal gold-198 is a practical method to investigate the condition of the major head and neck lymphatic groups (the ones most frequently invaded by cancer metastases).

The reduction in radioisotope uptake, which may be partial or total depending upon the stage of the cancer, can predict preoperatively the likelihood of lymph node metastasis. Scintigraphy is also of value as a postoperative test of the thoroughness of the resection. We therefore recommend that this technique be utilized in other centers.

# EXAMINATION OF THE THORACIC DUCT LYMPH IN MALIGNANT ABDOMINAL DISEASES (with special reference to the pulmonary metastases)

F. Lukic, J. Skrk, N. Poniz, M. Us-Krasovec,
L. Sebek, G. Klanjscek, and M. Bohinc
The Institute of Oncology and
The Institute of Transfusion
Ljubljana, Yugoslavia

## Introduction

Metastatic tumors sometimes appear in unexpected locations. As summarized by many authors there exist classically (WALTER and BATSON) five types of tumor cells spread in the venous circuit to and from the lung. Another type of tumor spread to the lung is possible by distribution of the cancer cells along the lymphatic ways and the thoracic duct, before it drains into venous system. To this type of the malignant cell distribution our study is dedicated. We are dealing with the following aspects of thoraic duct lymph:

- x ray presentation of the thoracic duct,
- flow and pressure measurement of the thoracic duct lymph the operation and in the early postoperative period,
- appearance of the malignant cells in the thoracic duct,
- total number of the white blood cells in the thoracic lymph,
- some biochemical examination of the thoracic duct lymph,
- lymphocyte blast transformation index and HLA antigen identification of the thoracic duct lymphocytes.

## Method

Eleven patients ranging from 35 to 70 years were explored for cannulation of the thoracic duct lymph. The thoracic duct lymph for examination was gained by the cannulation in the neck region. To reach agreement on the extent of the malignant abdominal diseases of our patients the TNM classification was used (except liver). Four cases of stomach cancers were explored, 3 cases of rectum cancers, 3 cases of ovary cancers and 1 case of liver cancer in advanced stage of the primary tumors T - 3 or T - 4. In all patients there were distant metastases of various locations present.

Flexible Silastic tubes for the cannulation were used. For one day cannulation also polyethylene tubes were successful. The operative treatment was the standard one. Valves in the duct often preclude introducing the cannula for more than 1 or 2 centimeters. The thoracic duct cannula was connected to a sterile glass collection flask which was washed with heparin solution (1:500). The thoracic duct samples were collected for examination eight times in time intervals of two hours. The drained lymph wasn't replaced. At the end of the lymph collection the tube was ligated with silk for 12 hours and then slipped out.

Retrogradeductography was performed with Lipiodol UF. Lipiodol was injected by Rüttimann apparatus (1 ml/1 Min.). For lymphocytes separation of thoracic duct lymph the same method was used as for lymphocytes separation in the blood. Standard procedures were used for other examinations. Lymphocytes blast transformation was examined morphologically after PHA stimulation.

## Results

Eleven patients were explored for cannulation of the thoracic duct lymph. The following results were obtained:

- x ray presentation of the thoracic duct:

the upper part of the thoracic duct was demonstrated in all cases. The diameter of the thoracic duct varied from 3 - 8 mm. There was observed dilatation of the thoracic duct till 20 mm. If still more contrast was injected there exist retrosternal pain.

- flow rate and pressure of the thoracic duct lymph: lymph flow ranged from 0,2 to 3,7 ml/min (normal 0,5 to 1,5), lymph pressure ranged from 2,0 to 40 cm $H_2O$ (normal 5,0 to 12,0) during the operation and in the early postoperative period. The flow and pressure were enhanced after fatty diet, deep breathing, coughing or manual pressure on the upper abdomen. The values varied quickly and frequently.

- appearance of the malignant cells in the thoracic duct: single tumor cells and/or tumor cells clusters were identified in the thoracic duct in 3 cases: in two cases of stomach cancer and 1 case of the rectum cancer.

- total number of the white cells in the thoracic duct lymph:

total white blood cells varied in the thoracic duct during the day, nutrition, and work (from 300 to 3400). Differentiation of cell population revealed 90% lymphocyte purity.

- some biochemical examinations of the thoracic duct lymph value of the glucosa varied from 93 to 118 mg%, value of cholinesterase varied from 220 to 700 mE/ml, value of the alkaline phosphatase varied from 5 to 18 IU. The study of alkaline phosphatase isoenzymes revealed high values of the intestinal isoenzymes alpha - 1 and alpha - 2 fractions.

The protein content of the thoracic duct lymph was 3,2 (1,7) to 5,1 gr%, 1,9 (0,9) to 3,1 gr% on account of the albumin.

Biochemical values varied as all values of the thoracic duct lymph in connection and dependancy with blood values. All blood values were at the time of examination in normal range.

- lymphocytes blast transformation index and HLA antigen identification of the thoracic duct lymphocytes.

Our series of lymphocytes blast transformation index and HLA antigens examinations is too small to find out the definitive results. In some examinations (2 of them) the values were as follows:

Lymphocytes blast transformation index of the thoracic duct lymphocytes was 63,4%, for peripheral blood lymphocytes however 41,6%.

In the peripheral blood there were revealed predominantly HLA - 2 and - 3 antigens, but in the thoracic duct lymph lymphocytes only HLA - 2 antigens.

## Discussion

X - ray presentation of the thoracic duct demonstrated the topographical, anatomical and pathological (occlusion, fistulation) state of the duct in the upper mediastinum. The examination will probably find the diagnostic value in the clinical medicine.

The flow rate and pressure, total white cells number, biochemical values of the thoracic duct lymph varied quickly and frequently. There exists some evidence which indicates that the immunological properties of blood and lymph are different.

Malignant cells in the thoracic duct lymph were found only in three patients (28%). We have inspected the appearance of the malignant cells in more cases and predominantly in the cases of liver and ovary cancer, because of their close connection to the thoracic duct (via liver lymph or diaphragm and mediastinal lymphatic vessels in cases of ovary cancer with ascites). In our cases the malignant cells in the thoracic duct lymph were positive in cases with stomach and rectum cancer.

About factors, which may influence the occurence of tumor cells in the thoracic duct (grade of malignancy, stage of cancer, surgical or diagnostic manipulation) we didn't find any criteria. Our opinion is that surgical and manual manipulation of the tumor mass may influence the appearance of the malignant cells in the thoracic duct.

The unsolved question is if the malignant cells in the thoracic duct lymph represent circulating cells which are unable to implant and will eventually be killed or produce metastases. 21 years after radical mastectomy lymph node metastases were found in outer axillary region without other signs of cancer recurrence. There is a possibility that the malignant cells were dormant in the lymph node all the years and the lymph didn't influence or harm the malignant cells.

How the tumor cells enter the thoracic duct deserves consideration. The malignant cell gains the thoracic duct presumably through the lymphatic node by known routes or directly, without transpassing the lymphatic node. In the thoracic duct there exist many ways, how the malignant cell attacks the pulmonary lymphatic system, via reversal flow:

- by detached emboli from metastatic mediastinal lymph node,

- if the hilar nodes are blocked there exists a reverse pulmonary lymphatic flow in the centripetal direction,

- direct reversal flow from the thoracic duct to pulmonary lymphatic vessels, via bronchomediastinal trunks, paratracheal lymphatic vessels, bronchopulmonary lymphatics, interlobular lymphatics, peribronchial, perivenous lymphatics to visceral pleural lymphatic vessels.

The sluggish lymph stream, trapping of the lymph, pressure changes (e.g. caused by work, intrathoracical pressure) appear frequently through the day in the thoracic duct and may perhaps influence the adhesion of malignant cells to lymphatic vascular endothelium. During enhanced lymphatic pressure, the thoracic duct is extended and so the valve system may become incompetent. In such a way reverse lymphatic flow is possible and malignant cell may contact the lung on lymphatic way without entering the blood circulation. Tumor cells may stick to the endothelium or roll away along the vessel wall. Intralymphatic adhesion is a reaction between malignant cells and environment - the lymph stream. The possible list of factors which may affect his process is long, but there were discussed only some of them.

## Conclusion

Tumor spread to the lung by distribution of the cancer cells along the lymphatic ways and the thoracic duct is possible before it drains into venous system. In the thoracic duct there exist many ways, how the malignant cell attacks the pulmonary lymphatic system. But there rise a number of questions without answer:

- are cancer cells found in the lymph viable?
- what role does the host resistence play?
- are circulating malignant cells in the lymph a bad thing?
- how to obviate the lymphatic route of cancer dissemination during the surgery?

ENDOLYMPHATIC THERAPY OF LYMPH NODE METASTASES USING $^{32}P$ AND $^{131}I$ LIPIODOL UF

H. Weissleder

Deutsche Klinik für Diagnostik, Department of Radiology,

6200 Wiesbaden - Germany F.R.

Lymphography can be used for therapeutic purposes by giving an intralymphatic injection of a contrast medium, which contains radioactive material. The method enables an internal irradiation of the inguinal, iliac and lumbar and axillar lymph nodes. The doses are approximately 100,000 rads. The immediately neighbouring and blood forming organs remain to a great extent unharmed.

According to the literature, by the middle of 1973, 1500 patients in all had been treated endolymphatically in greatly differing centres throughout the world. The total number of treated patients is estimated to lie between 2000 and 2500 by the end of 1974. Although this is a relatively small amount, a number of clinics have records of long term observations of up to 10 years.

In Germany in 1972, members of the ISL established a working team with the aim to standardise endolymphatic radionuclide therapy, including the dosimetry and follow-up examinations. Examination and treatment data are noted centrally. The computer centre also controls those follow-up examinations which are to be carried out regularly. By 31st December 1974, 260 patients were registered, chiefly with malignant melanoma.

At an international workshop in December 1973 we discussed our results with colleagues from Austria, England, Canada, Italy and Switzerland, and arranged to work co-operatively.

INDICATIONS

In principle all primary and secondary malignant lymph node diseases are suitable for endolymphatic radionuclide therapy; that is so far as local radiation therapy is indicated, and the affected lymph nodes are situated in the drainage area of lymphatic vessels which can be punctured. However, it must be guaranteed that the dosage reaching the malignant tissue is sufficient to exterminate it. Lymph node metastases from solid tumours of the lower extremities, with their well-known resistance to percutaneous radiation therapy, should be regarded as cases strongly indicated for endolymphatic therapy. However, if the treatment is to be successful, only those lymph node metastases which have not exceeded a certain size, can be considered. As the maximum range of beta rays from $^{32}P$ is 8 mms, with an average of 2.8 mms, the greatest therapeutic effect is to be expected with micro and the smaller metastases with a cross-section below 5 mms. However, the primary requirement is an even distribution of the radioactive contrast medium mixture throughout the affected lymph nodes.

EDWARDS (1972), JANTET (1969), and we too, use the method almost exclusively for the treatment of lymph node metastases in malignant melanoma of the lower extremities. With this tumour, metastases in the regional lymph nodes can be proved early and relatively frequently with the aid of bioptic examinations. Comparative examinations showed that histologically metastases occur in up to 50% in inguinal lymph nodes of normal size.

Malignant tumours of the testis and the penis are limited in their suitability for endolymphatic therapy. The treatment of lymph node metastases from gynaecological carcinomas presents problems, as it is not possible to include the regional lymph nodes completely. In addition, advanced carcinoma metastatic spread can cause a block in the lymph flow, and thus hinder an accumulation of the injected radionuclide in the metastatic lymph nodes.

The indications for endolymphatic radionuclide therapy in lymphatic systemic diseases are considerably more difficult to define than in lymph node metastases of solid tumours, as here we already have tested and successful treatment methods. In these cases endolymphatic therapy is only important as additional treatment in order to keep down the dosage volume of the percutaneous irradiation. However, successful treatment can only be expected when the distribution of radioactivity in the lymph nodes allows for even and sufficient irradiation. This cannot be guaranteed in Hodgkin's disease, chronic lymphatic leukemia, lympho- and reticulo sarcomatosis, as usually the affected lymph nodes demonstrate larger storage free zones.

## CONTRAINDICATIONS

Endolymphatic radionuclide therapy should not be carried out when the expected therapeutic result is out of proportion to the possible side effects and the effort involved for this treatment.

In detail the following contraindications arise:

1. Therapy resistant respiratory and/or cardiac insufficiency because of the possible radiation load from overspill of the radioactive contrast medium into the lungs.
   Following percutaneous radiation therapy of the mediastinum and/or lungs endolymphatic radionuclide therapy should only be carried out if the results of the lung function examinations are satisfactory.

2. Previous percutaneous irradiation of the infradiaphragmal lymph nodes.
   The storage capacity of the lymph nodes is considerably reduced, due to radiation fibrosis. A sufficient concentration of radioactive material contrast medium mixture can then no longer be guaranteed. In addition, there is a strong likelihood of an increased spillover of radioactive substance into the lungs.

3. Lymph blocks and/or lymphovenous shunts, due to operation or extensive retroperitoneal lymph node metastases, so as to avoid radiation damage in the affected areas, as well as in the lungs and portal venous system.
   In addition those lymph nodes situated behind others, in relation to the point of injection, receive only an insufficient amount of radioactive material, thus the desired therapeutic effect is no longer certain.

4. Generalised metastatic spread.

5. Chylous ascites, chyluria and chylothorax.

In animal experimental examinations KOEHLER et al. (1968) found that previous diagnostic lymphography does not have any significant influence on the storage capacity of the lymph nodes for radioactive material, even if the interval is as short as 3 to 5 days. This view is in fact disputed; however exact examination results proving otherwise are lacking. Our own observations of two patients with malignant melanoma, who had undergone diagnostic lymphography 4 weeks previous to endolymphatic radionuclide therapy, support KOEHLER's results. In spite of this it is to be recommended that the next proceedings following lymphography should depend on the individual case, and the length of the interval.

PRELIMINARY EXAMINATION OF THE PATIENT

As a rule, the patient is admitted to the clinic the day before the proposed endolymphatic radionuclide therapy, so that the following examinations can be carried out:

- Admission examination
- Laboratory examination (eg. blood count, sedimentation rate, serum electrophoresis, transaminasis)
- Lung function examination (CO diffusion, $0_2$ load)
- Chest X-ray in 2 planes
- Pregnancy test for women of child-bearing age

With regard to the thyroid gland block the opinions are somewhat divided. When applying higher dose of $^{131}I$-marked Lipiodol UF a block in the thyroidal iodine absorption with Lugol's solution or sodium perchlorate is inevitable. When using the now usual standard dosage of $^{32}P$, $^{131}I$ Lipiodol such a procedure is, in the opinion of PFANNENSTIEL (1972), no longer necessary, as less than 2% of the added $^{131}I$ with 0.5 - 1.0 mCi, appears in the form of iodide.

EXAMINATION TECHNIQUE AND MEASUREMENTS FOR RADIATION PROTECTION

The radioactive triolein contrast medium mixture is delivered by the manufacturer in ready-for-use leadlined injection syringes. The following dosage is used by the German working group "ENDO-LYMPHATIC RADIONUCLIDE THERAPY":

- 2 mCi $^{32}P$ and 0.5 mCi $^{131}I$ in 3.5 cc. Lipiodol UF (for each side of the lower extremities).
- 5 mCi $^{32}P$ and 0.5 mCi $^{131}I$ in 3.5 cc. Lipiodol UF (for injection on one side only).

For application to the upper extremities the dosage volume is merely reduced.

The therapeutic effect emanates from the $^{32}P$ (Tri-N-octyl-phosphate). $^{131}I$ is added in the form of iodine triolein merely because of the dosimetry.

The radioactivity in the whole body and lungs as well as in the pelvic and lumbar lymph nodes is measured by a profile scanner at definite time intervals following $^{32}P$, $^{131}I$ administration. The next slide shows an example of this with high uptake of radioactivity in the retroperitoneal lymph nodes and only small amounts of radioactivity over the thoracic region.

The examination table is covered with plastic sheets as protection against contamination. Disposable gloves are used in the usual way for all manipulations on the syringes and connecting tubes. Instruments which come into contact with the radioactive substance, as well as the operation clothes and swabs, are packed into small plastic bags at the end of the injection, and then brought to the Nuclear Medical Department for measurement of radioactivity. There the contaminated parts are destroyed in the correct way or, if appropriate, left until their radioactivity has worn off.

## CONCLUSION

On the average, 12.5% of the total injected radioactivity, 4 mCi $^{32}P$ 1 mCi $^{131}I$ Lipidol UF (R), remains in the injecting system. With a number of patients the total amount available was further reduced due to contamination of operation sheets, swabs and instruments. In spite of this, sufficient radioactivity still remains to irradiate the lymph nodes. The larger portion of the radioactivity actually injected (approximately 2/3 of the total amount) is stored in the lymph nodes. The average irradiation dose to the lymph nodes is 94000 rads. A detectable concentration of radioactivity in the lungs was registered in 80% of the treated patients. The radiation dose to the lungs is dependent on the technical procedure. With bilateral injection it was found to be approximately 233 rads. Radiation damage has not yet been observed.

The amount of radiation reaching the examiner and the medical assistants is extremely low when using the standard dosage of $^{32}P$ and $^{131}I$. The total energy of the $^{32}P$ and the $^{131}I$ energy is given off in the form of beta rays. The gamma part of the $^{131}I$ is so small that if attention is paid to the distance no radiation dosage worth mentioning is to be expected.

For the pre-operative examination, that is before the removal of the primary tumour, the injection at the usual point on the dorsum of the foot is, as a rule, sufficient.

With the post-operative treatment, which means after removal of the primary tumour, the situation is more difficult, particularly if the efferent lymphatic vessels have to be servered. The most certain and sensible method of post-operative endolymphatic therapy is the direct puncture of the lymphatic vessels proximal to the operation area.

Should the endolymphatic therapy have taken place preoperatively, then the operation can be made 10 to 14 days later. The dose on the surface of a lymph node is at this time about 2 to 3 rads/hr.

SIDE EFFECTS

The side effects will remain within justifiable limits if the technical procedure is correct and the indications are strictly observed.

Blood count and serum-protein alterations are observed over a period of 2 to 4 weeks if $^{131}I$ is used on its own. Leuko-and lymphopenia is involved here, as well as slight reticulo-and thrombocytosis. Such marked blood cell count alterations have no longer been observed since the use of $^{32}P$ in combination with 0.5 to 1.0 mCi $^{131}I$.

In animal experimental examinations (KLOSS et al., 1970) the radiation load to the bone marrow was found to be minimal. After 2 mCi of $^{32}P$ tri-n-octyl-phosphate marked Lipiodol UF had been injected into dogs weighing 20-40 pounds a maximum of 3-5 rads was measured. On 5$^{th}$ day the activity concentration in the blood reached a peak of 0.00052% of the dosage per cubic of whole blood. The concentration in bone lay well below 0.001% of the dosage per gram bone. According to examination carried out by CROIZAT et al. (1969) the total radiation dosage in man lies between 6 and 12 rads. The amount depends on the dosage of the injected radioactivity.

The temporary rise in the acute phase proteins alpha$_1$-glycoprotein, alpha$_1$-antitrypsin, alpha$_2$-macroglobulin and haptoglobulin is interpreted as a result of necrotic softening, due to the intensive radiation therapy (KLEMM et al., 1968/69).

Irregularities in menstruation have been reported particularly by CHIAPP et al. (1971). Amenorrhoea occured in 12.7% of 110 treated women. In the majority of cases the amenorrhoea was only temporary, and from these, 1/3 later became pregnant. The children did not demonstrate any abnormalities during the observation period.

In endolymphatic therapy, just as in the diagnostic lymphography, a portion of the applied substance flows via the thoracic duct into the lungs. The amount is directly dependent on the volume injected, as well as the number and storage capacity of the lymph nodes passed through.

According to the results of ZUM WINKEL (1967) the radiation load on the lungs, using an injection of 20 mCi $^{131}I$, lies between 120 and 920 rads. Using the same radionuclide, PFANNENSTIEL et al. (1970) registered radiation loads between 100 and 3100 rads maximum. The latter is however an exception.

In the early days of endolymphatic therapy a total of four deaths was observed. These can be regarded to be results of the raised radiation load on the lungs. Those patients of ours all suffered, without exception, from generalised Hodgkin's disease with lung attack and previous percutaneous radiation therapy to the lungs, mediastinum and abdominal region with a dosage of at least 4000 rads. The combined effect of percutaneous irradiation and endolymphatic radionuclide therapy in these lungs from the basic disease, was fatal.

The following consequences can be drawn from the observations:

1. The indication for endolymphatic therapy is fundamentally dependent on the results of the lung function tests. All patients with a respiratory insufficiency resistant to therapy should be excluded from endolymphatic treatment.

2. The volume of the radioactive contrast medium mixture was reduced by about half.

When applying the present standard doois of 2 mCi $^{32}P$ and 0.5 mCi $^{131}I$ to each side, the load on the lungs lies between 0 and 1000 rads. This is based on the results to date from 102 patients. Aproximately 80% of them had a radiation load of less than 400 rads. If, for any reason, the whole of the injected standard dosage should reach the lungs, then a radiation load of 2500 rads is to be expected.

From our observations, it can be said that when there is no previous damage to the lungs or other restrictions in the respiratory functioning, then radiation loads on the lungs of up to 1400 rads do not cause radiation fibrosis, either clinically or radiologically.

Concentrations of radioactivity in the liver and spleen are only slight, so long as the lymph flow is not interrupted. The total loads registered were in the liver 30 to 60 rads, in the spleen 50 to 175 rads and in the kidneys 50 to 115 rads. (CHIAPP et al., 1966; FAVA and RONVORONI, 1965; LORD and KINMONTH, 1969). CHIAPPA et al. (1971) observed in 2 patients with Stage IV Hodgkin's disease a liver insufficiency accompanied by jaundice, and a rise in the direct and indirect serum bilirubin an the transaminasis.

These patients died within a few days with very extensive liver necrosis. Follow-up examinations over a period of 2 years were carried out on a patient with a measurable radiation load on the spleen, and did not show any alterations which could be proved clinically, haematologically or biochemically.

Up till now local radiation damage has been observed at the puncture and around the lymph nodes. In the main this can be attributed to extravasation (JANTET, 1966; EDWARDS and KINMONTH, 1968).

Altogether 6.3% of the patients treated by CHIAPPA et al. (1971) suffered from side effects and complications, half of which could be put down to amenorrhoea. From a total of 426 treated patients, 3 showed necrosis after extravasation, and another 3 patients lymphangitis.

RESULTS

Long term results are only available from a few centres at present. KENDA et al. reported at a meeting in Wiesbaden in 1973 about the treatment of 426 patients suffering from malignant lymphoma. They found a marked reduction in the rate of relapse in patients with primary negative lymphography reports (8%) as compared with a group of untreated patients (23%).

Encouraging results are reported by EDWARDS (1972). He found that a 5 year survival rate for malignant melanoma was the case in 80% of Stage I and 21.4% of Stage II.

In all cases the endolymphatic therapy immediately followed an extensive excision of the primary tumour. One or several efferent lymphatic vessels of the operation area were catheterised under anaesthetic. This is followed by the infusion of the radioactive substance. From a comparable group in the same hospital, who were only treated surgically, 58.9% of Stage I and 12.5% of Stage II, reached a 5 year survival rate.

At present a comparable study is running in Great Britain on the value of endolymphatic therapy in malignant melanoma of the lower extremities. The results till now show a marked lower rate of relapse in the lymph nodes, (2.3% of the radioactively treated patients, as compared with 19% of those receiving conventional treatment).

In the same group skin metastases were observed more often following endolymphatic therapy (16%) as in those not treated (6%).

Unfortunately, however, some of the institutes taking part have only little experience in endolymphatic therapy.

## CONCLUSION

Endolymphatic radionuclide therapy is absolutely indicated in the treatment of Stage I malignant melanoma of the lower extremities. The therapeutic procedure with other localisation, or Stage II of the disease, must be individually decided on, according to the situation in each case as it arises.
In diseases of the lymphatic system endolymphatic therapy can only be regarded as additional treatment.

In the hand of the experienced person, endolymphatic radionuclide therapy involves only a slight risk for the patient, providing the following points are strictly observed: through consideration of the indications and contra-indications, observation of the recommendations concerning the volume and radiation dosage of the radionuclide applied, and careful technical procedure during the treatment. According to the present stand, endolymphatic therapy is to be regarded as a valuable supplementary treatment, which enables an improvement in the survival rate.

# THE CELLULARITY OF PERIPHERAL LYMPH IN LYMPHOMAS

A. Engeset, K. Bremer, and S.S. Froland

The Norwegian Radium Hospital

Montebello, Oslo 3, Norway

A large quantity of the lymphocytes migrate from the blood into the tissue and back to the blood again. This recirculation takes place largely within the lymph nodes, but on a smaller scale also in other tissues.

There are at least two types of lymphocytes; the T-lymphocytes derived from the thymus and the B-lymphocytes which are from other sources and which are plasma cell precursors. It is impossible by light microscopy to distinguish B- and T-cells. They can, however, be classified by some other methods. We have employed the ability of the T-lymphocytes to form rosettes with sheep erythrocytes under special conditions (E-rosettes). The B-lymphocytes contain immunoglobulin on the membrane which can be demonstrated by immunoflourescence. In our laboratory about 40 per cent of mononuclear cells in the blood of healthy people are T-cells by these techniques and 10-20 per cent are B-cells. Some of the other cells are probably monocytes.

The malignant lymphomas have for many years been studied mainly by morphological parameters. Recently we have employed a functional test, a study of the lymphocyte circulation kinetics in non-lymphoid tissue and the participation of B- and T-cells in this traffic. Lymphocyte circulation to and from non-lymphoid tissue can be followed by study of the cells in peripheral lymph as demonstrated in animals by Hall and Morris (2). Applying this method in man we have collected peripheral lymph for days and weeks in about 80 patients with malignancies, most of which were lymphomas. The patients under study walk around, the glass vials taped to the leg, connected to a polyethylene tube inserted into a lymphatic (1). Two to twenty ml lymph is collected daily, containing about 200 cells per microliter of which 80-90 per cent are lymphocytes. The material is still too small for definite conclusions, but there are some trends which might be of interest.

Four groups have been studied. They are patients with small superficial carcinomas, untreated and irradiated Hodgkin's disease and chronic lymphocytic leukemia. Figure 1 gives the mean cell number per microliter lymph in the individual patients. There is a wide range of values in each group and all are overlapping. However, the mean value is lower in the Hodgkin patients especially those who have been irradiated. Irradiation had been done 5-35 months before the study.

Figure 2 shows that there is a correlation between the lymphocyte number in blood and lymph in patients with untreated Hodgkin's disease. There was no such correlation in patients who had been irradiated or in those with chronic lymphocytic leukemia.

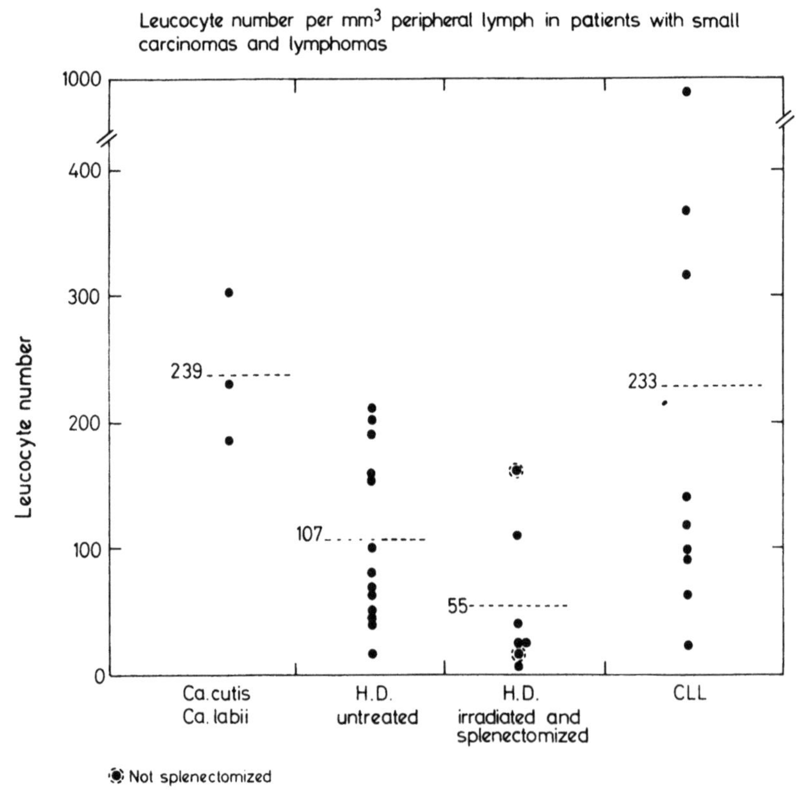


Fig. 1: The mean cell number per microliter lymph in the individual patients.

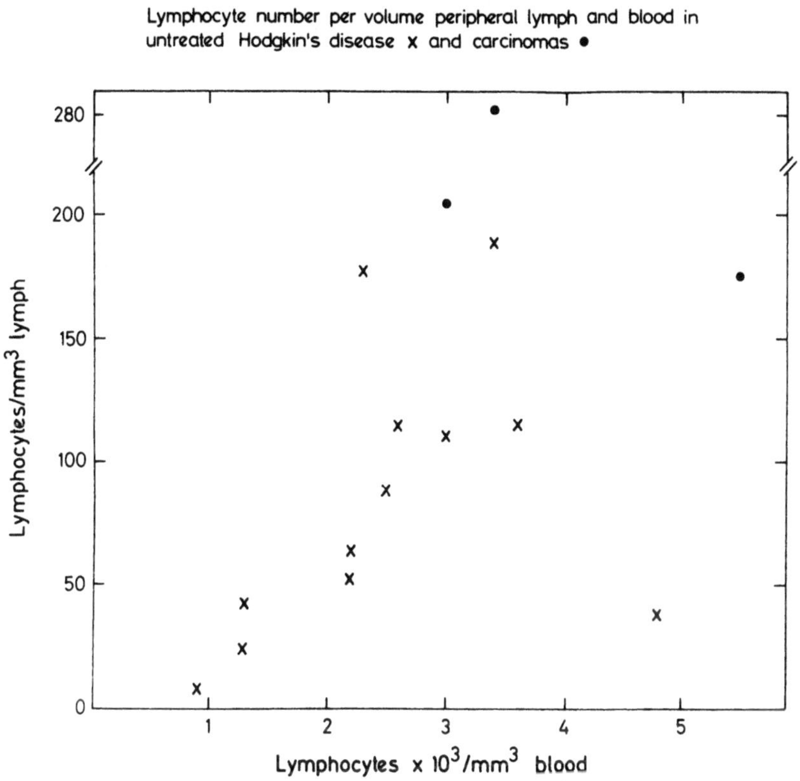


Fig. 2: The correlation between the lymphocyte number in blood and lymph in patients with untreated Hodgkin's disease.

Figure 3 gives the ratio between lymphocytes in lymph and blood. The carcinoma patients had about 20 times as many lymphocytes per volume blood as per volume lymph. This group is used as an index representing 100 per cent and to which the other groups are related. Figure 3 shows that the other patients have relatively fewer cells in the lymph compared to the blood values. This is most pronounced for the treated Hodgkin patients and for the fraction of patients with chronic lymphocytic leukemia with more than 5000 lymphocytes per microliter of blood. In these two groups a higher percentage of the blood lymphocytes were B-cells than in the untreated Hodgkin patients and the controls (Fig. 4). None or very few B-cells were found in the lymph. In a small group of patients investigated, the E-rosette forming cells - the T-cells - however, were about twice as numerous in the lymph as in the blood, comprising about 60-80 per cent of the lymph leukocytes.

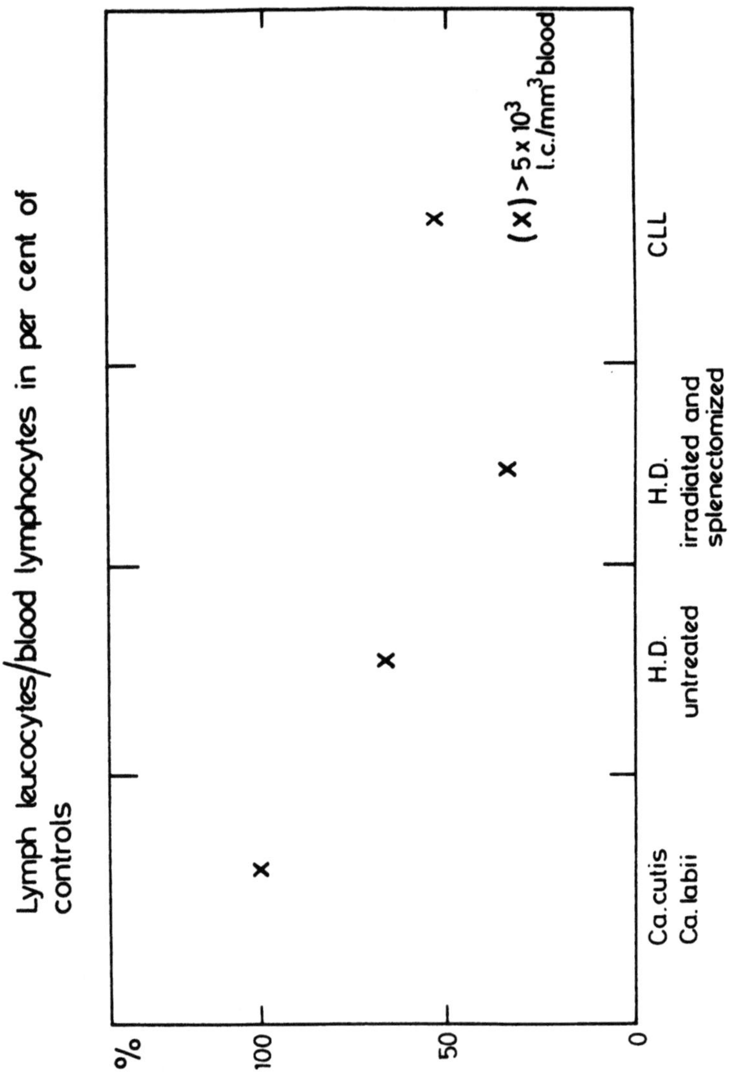


Fig. 3: The ratio between lymphocytes in lymph and blood.

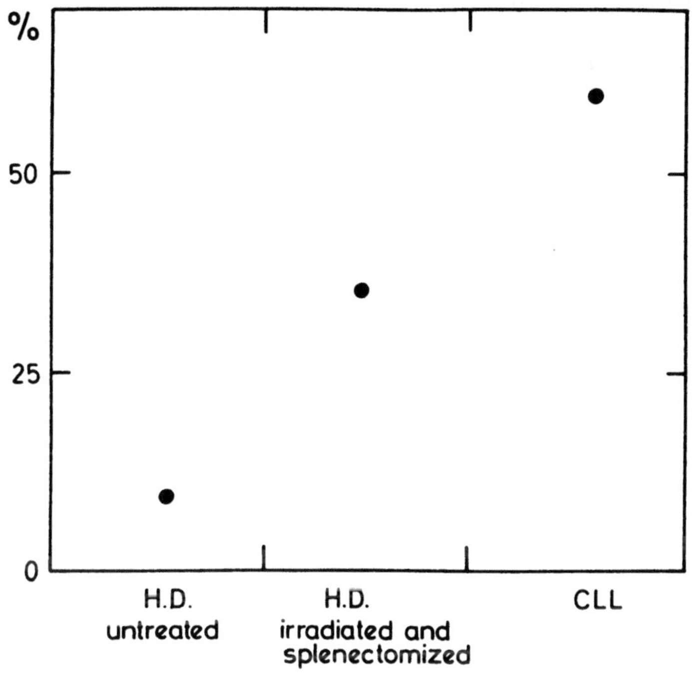


Fig. 4: Percentage of blood lymphocytes (B-cells) in untreated Hodgkin patients and controls.

In conclusion. There is correlation between lymphocyte number in blood and lymph in patients with untreated Hodgkin's disease. These patients have a normal ratio between B- and T-cells in the blood. In patients treated for Hodgkin's disease and in untreated lymphocytic leukemia, the lymphocyte number in the lymph is lower than would be expected from the lymphocyte number in the blood. These patients have a high percentage of B-lymphocytes in the blood and low or very few B-cells in peripheral lymph. These observations show that the B-cells do not migrate into the lymph to the same extent as the T-cells, either because they do not migrate into the tissue from the blood vessels or they do not return to the lymphatics.

The low lymphocyte number in peripheral lymph probably reflects that the tissue contains few T-cells which might explain the reduced cellular immune response so often observed in these groups of patients.

References

1. Engeset, A., Hager, B., Nesheim, A.: Studies on human peripheral lymph. Lymphology 1973, 6, 6-12.

2. Hall, J.G., Morris, B.: The lymph-borne cells of the immune response. Quart. J. exp. Physiol. 1963, 48, 235-247.

# THE PEDICLED GREATER OMENTUM IN RECONSTRUCTIVE SURGERY FOLLOWING TREATMENT OF CERTAIN CANCERS

M. Abbes

Department of Surgery
Cancer Center Antoine Lacassagne
Nice, France

Since 1963 after Kiricuta, the use of the greater omentum (G.O.) has taken a large place in repair following surgery of cancer, essentially for defects in irradiated areas but also for fistulae closure, amputated breasts reconstruction and as a cover of large non-irradiated tumoral resection areas.

Although some authors now develop techniques of free grafting of GO by microvascular anatomoses, we prefer the security given by a pedicled omental flap.

We present our experience of 14 cases after a short study of the reasons for its choice and of our procedure.

## THE REASONS OF A CHOICE

Many studies have proved the value of G.O. as a nutritive graft.

a) Its vascular richness is due to the epiploic arteries network which stems from the gastroepiploic arch, mainly coming from the right gastroepiploic artery, a branch of the gastroduodenal artery. The left gastro-epiploic artery, in a more posterior plane, anastomoses with the vertical epiploic vessels and with the left extremity of the gastro-epiploic arch.

b) The physiological activity has been studied by Kraft, Langhamer, Ax, Fischer, Krusman, Krisek
Capacity of resorption: it allows the absorption of liquids and cell destruction products, by the "windows"

in the initial lymphatic ducts of the G.O.
Capacity of inflammation with immunitary reaction which causes the efficient reaction of adhesion in peritonitis. These properties explain its trophic activity on atonic, necrotic or infected tissues. It allows the closure of Fistuale, the protection of exposed bones and vessels while it stops the necrotic or infectious process, so frequent after intensive radiotherapy. This explains the ability of G.O. to bud and receive semi-thick skin grafts.

## TECHNIQUE

Use of the G.O. out of the abdominal cavity requires lenthening by vascular sections, preferably based on the right pedicle. The gastro-epiploic arch is separated from the stomach and the left pedicle ligated after a "colo-epiploic detachment." Sometimes a transversal, horizontal approach can be used with a better aesthetic result than a vertical midline laparatomy. We did not try Adley's procedures, but only Kiricuta's meche and flag techniques.

Exteriorization of the G.O. must avoid any striction and the incision of the skin will be preferred to the subcutaneous tunnel.

Fixation of G.O. causes no problem, and, if covered by a skin graft, the peripheral sutures are usually sufficient. No drains are used.

## INDICATIONS OF G.O. IN CANCEROLOGY

In a first step, we have used G.O. after surgery in irradiated areas, where classical techniques had failed. We now use it immediately with success.

A. INTRA-ABDOMINAL USE = 2 cases

1) Case Nº 1

A 25 year old male presented a reticulosarcoma of the left hemi-pelvis treated by cobalt therapy (5000 R) and chemotherapy.

April 74: colo-vesical fistula

May 74: excision and closure of the fistula; suture of the bladder and colic resection with interposition of the G.O. Good result.

2) Case Nº 2

A 12 year old girl, treated by cobalt (8000 R) in 1973 for an osteosarcoma of the left ilio-pubic branch.

April 74: occlusion by stenosis of the sigmoid colon with inguinal fistula and a risk of vascular ulceration (the left iliac vein presented a stenosis)

Oct 74: colic resection with curettage of iliac bone and of the fistula up to the vessels. Interposition of the G.O. on the surface of the pelvis and exteriorization by the inguinal fistula.

Good results.

B. <u>EXTRA ABDOMINAL USE</u>: 12 cases

1) <u>Radionecrosis</u>: 8 cases in the E.N.T., thoracic, breast and inguinal areas.

a) E.N.T.:

3 males, 66-68 and 69 years old, underwent major surgery:

pharyngolaryngectomy for recurrence after irradiation (7000 R) of E.N.T. cancers (1 piriform sinus, 1 larynx, 1 retromolar triangle).

Lesions were 2 pharyngostomas and 1 oropharyngostoma; wide resection of the irradiatied tissues, pharynx closure, transposition of the G.O. to cover the exposed vessels, and rotation of a deltopectoral flap were performed with good results except for 1 case; necrosis by striction in the subcutaneous tunnel, though the pharyngeal suture remained closed.

b) Inguinal radionecrosis: 1 case.

70 year old woman, inguinal lymphatic metastases of anal cancer treated by irradiation.

Necrosis and recurrence occurred 3 years after irradiation (7000 R).

In Sept. 73: right inguino-crural dissection with large skin resection, transposition of the G.O. and local skin flap were performed.

Good result in spite of the recurrence 1 year later.

c) Mammary cancerology (4 cases)

-Axillary sclerosis (1 case): 72 year old woman who underwent Halsted + coblat (6000 R) for cancer of the right breast.

Progressive development of swollen arm + axillary sclerosis + fistula. Axillary liberation, skin and fat resection, transposition of the G.O. and skin grafting were performed on Sept. 73.

Good results on pain and mobility, less satisfactory on the swollen arm.

-Thoracic wall radio-necrosis (3 cases)

3 women: 63, 65, and 70 years old

Breast cancer treated by cobalt + surgery, followed by thoracic wall radionecrosis in the 12 months following operation.

Skin and wall resection was performed in all cases with transplantation of the G.O., once on a Marlex mesh prosthesis.

Cover was once a local flap and twice a skin graft. Good results.

2) The G.O. out of irradiation: 4 cases

a) 1 pharyngostoma after pharyngolaryngectomy + neck dissection without irradiation.

Closure by transposition of the G.O. + rotation of a Bakamjian flap

b) 1 presternal skin cancer

Wide skin and sternal resection, repaired by Marlex mesh prosthesis, transposition of the G.O. and skin graft.

Good result in spite of a nylon allergy.

STEWART-TREVES SYNDROME - REPORT OF 3 CASES

A. K. Cordeiro, F. F. Baracat, A. Carrasco, and
A. J. Brandi

Instituto Arnaldo Vieira de Carvalho and
Faculdade de Medicina de Valença
São Paulo, Brazil

Swelling of the upper limb after radiacal mastectomy is a common and distressing problem for internists, gynecologists, and surgeons who care for patients with cancer of the breast. This complication can arise both in the presence and absence of recurrent tumor. When associated with recurrence, palliation can be undertaken until the spread of cancer interferes with vital functions. On the other hand, when the cancer has not recurred, treatment of the lymphedema may take a very protracted course, and a variety of modalities have been recommended but often with questionable success.

The present study describes an unusual complication of development of a new specific tumor--the so called Stewart-Treves syndrome--in the lymphedematous upper limb after radical mastectomy for breast cancer.

## Materials

CASE I: M.J.R., a 62-year-old white Brazilian female presented with numerous cutaneous lesions disseminated in the right lymphedematous upper limb and in anterior, lateral, and posterior regions of the right hemithorax. A right radical mastectomy for adenocarcinoma had been performed 8 months earlier. Lymphedema of the right upper limb developed promptly postoperatively. Physical examination revealed cutaneous lesions presenting a variable color from red to purple with occasional ulcerations. The mastectomy scar showed an intense ulcerated lesion of red-purple color. The patient's general condition was debilitated.

The diagnosis of lymphangiosarcoma was made. The patient was treated with chemotherapy following refusal of an interscapulothoracic

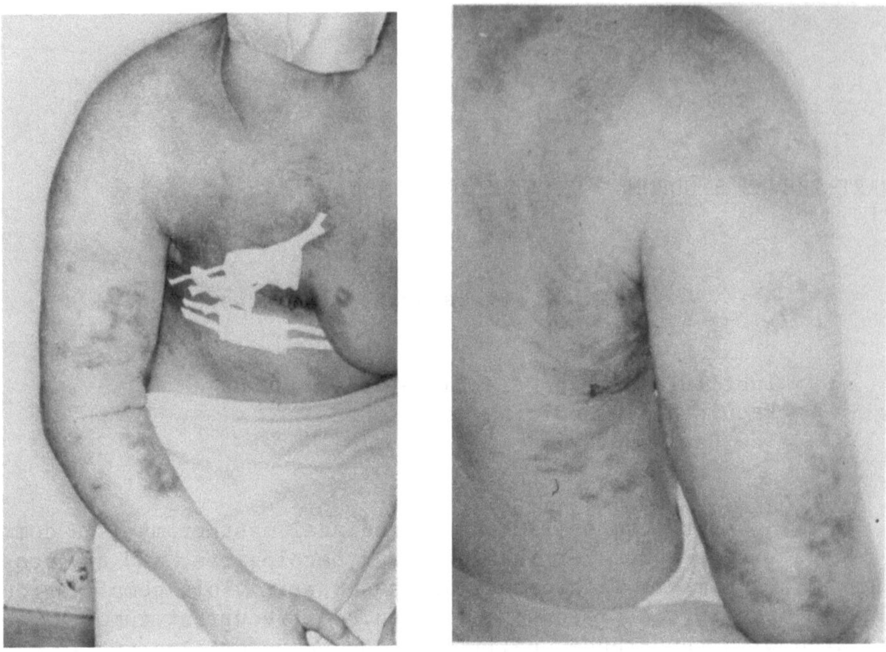

Fig. 1. Case I (M.J.R.) Cutaneous lesions of tumor dissemination in lymphedematous right upper limb and right hemithorax.

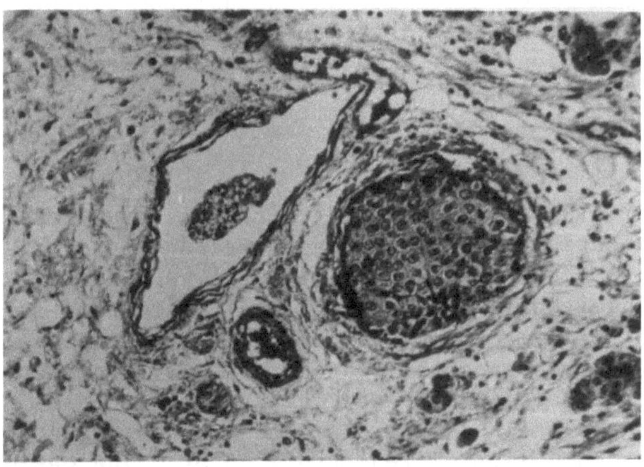

Fig. 2. Case I (M.J.R.) Histopathological examination showing presence of neoplastic emboli in vessels (artery, vein, and lymphatic trunk).

amputation. She died 10 days later (Fig. 1). Permission was obtained for a biopsy (7 cm x 4 cm x 4 cm) of the medial surface of the right arm from skin to periosteum. Macroscopic examination revealed whitish confluent tumor nodules with ulcerated granulations. Microscopic examination revealed undifferentiated carcinoma in cutaneous, subcutaneous, and muscular layers. Tumor emboli were noted in arterial, venous, and lymphatic trunks (Fig. 2).

CASE II: I.C.C., a 53-year-old white Brazilian female, had a right radical mastectomy in April, 1970, with histopathological diagnosis of adenocarcinoma. Lymphedema of the right upper limb developed 2 months after surgery. In November, 1970 the patient presented with cutaneous lesions in the surgical scar, anterior, lateral, and posterior regions of the right hemithorax, as well as in the lymphedematous upper limb. These cutaneous lesions resembled "hemangioma" with purple color, irregularity, and occasional ulceration. Skin biopsy revealed undifferentiated carcinoma and lymph node biopsy revealed solid undifferentiated carcinoma. The diagnosis of postmastectomy lymphedema with Stewart-Treves syndrome was made and an interscapulothoracic amputation recommended to but refused by the patient. Systemic and sternal chemotherapy was carried out without improvement, and the patient expired in January, 1971. Autopsy was refused (Fig. 3).

CASE III: A.G.A.R., a 57-year-old white Brazilian female, had a radical mastectomy performed for adenocarcinoma of the left breast, and radiotherapy was carried out postoperatively. Ten months after operation a local recurrence appeared and was treated by radiotherapy, oophorectomy, chemotherapy, and hormone therapy. Following this second course of treatment, her left upper limb became lymphedematous. About 1 month later, the patient observed numerous cutaneous lesions disseminated throughout the edematous left upper limb and the anterior, lateral, and posterior regions of the thorax. These cutaneous lesions were irregular, sometimes confluent, and ulcerated with a color varying from whitish to purple. Skin biopsies of arm, forearm, and thorax revealed lymphangiosarcoma. The patient refused an interscapulothoracic amputation as well as continued chemotherapy. Three days later she left the hospital and was lost to follow-up (Figs. 4,5,6).

## Comments and Conclusions

The clinical development of Stewart-Treves syndrome includes a three-stage sequence:

(1) Breast cancer + radical mastectomy;
(2) Postmastectomy lymphedema of upper limb;
(3) Appearance of cutaneous lesions in lymphedematous upper limb.

This sequence was observed in our three cases.

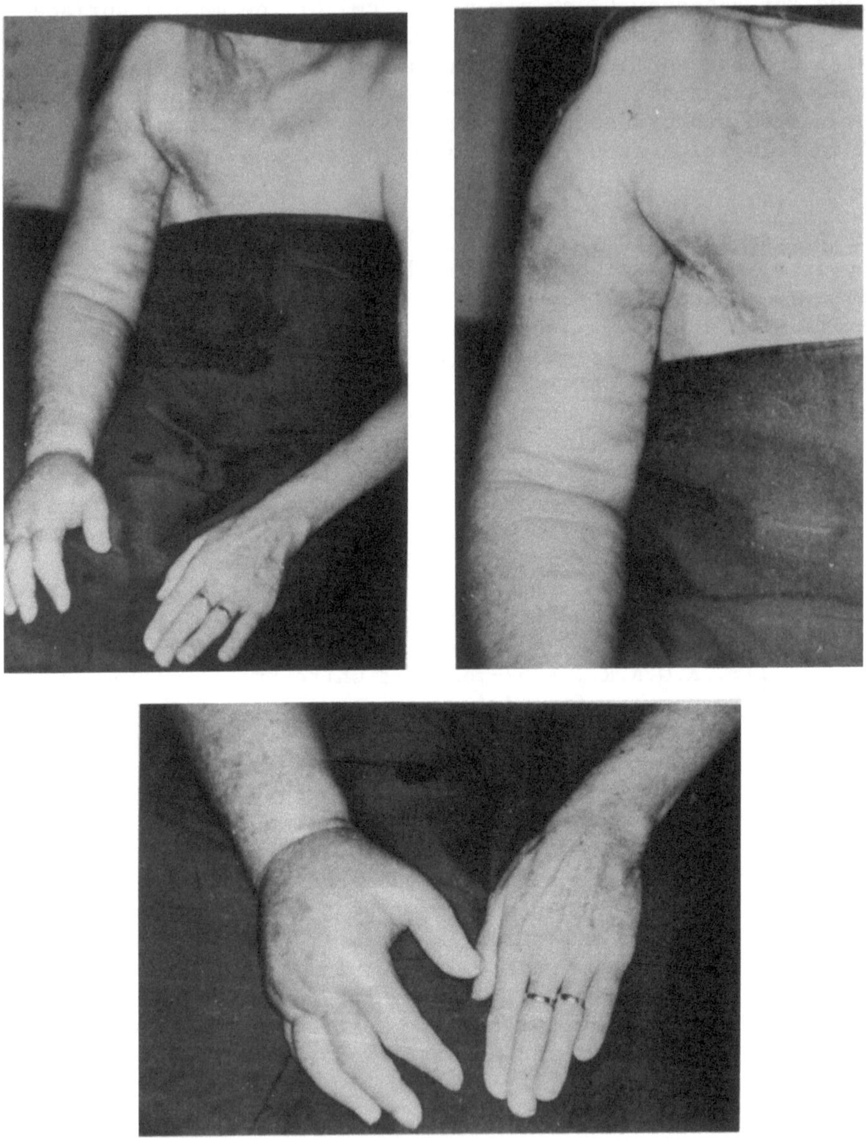

Fig. 3. Case II (I.C.C.) Cutaneous lesions (some ulcerated) of disseminated tumor in intermammary region, mastectomy scar, right hemithorax and lymphedematous right upper limb with red wine color of hemangioma.

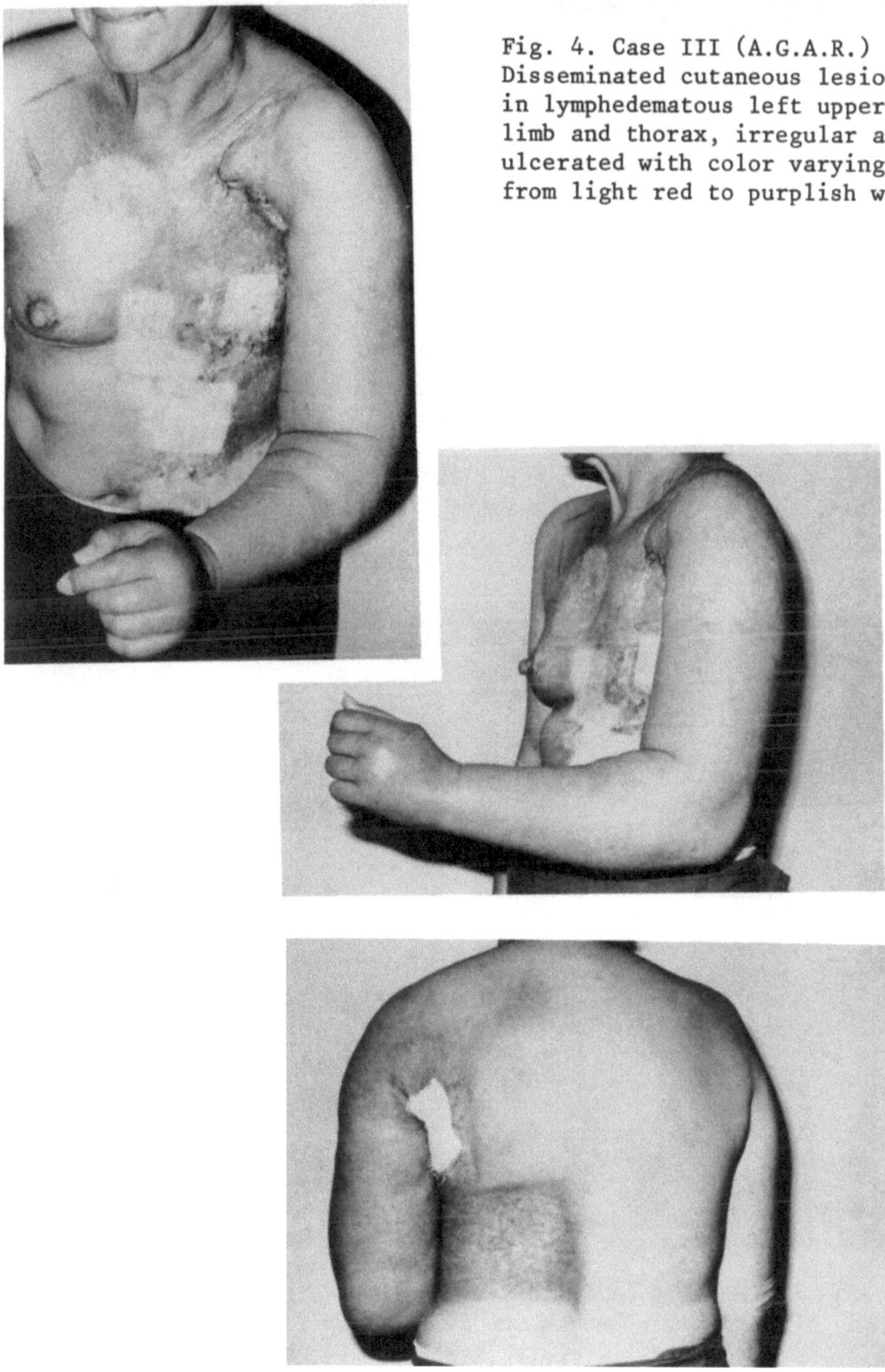

Fig. 4. Case III (A.G.A.R.) Disseminated cutaneous lesions in lymphedematous left upper limb and thorax, irregular and ulcerated with color varying from light red to purplish wine.

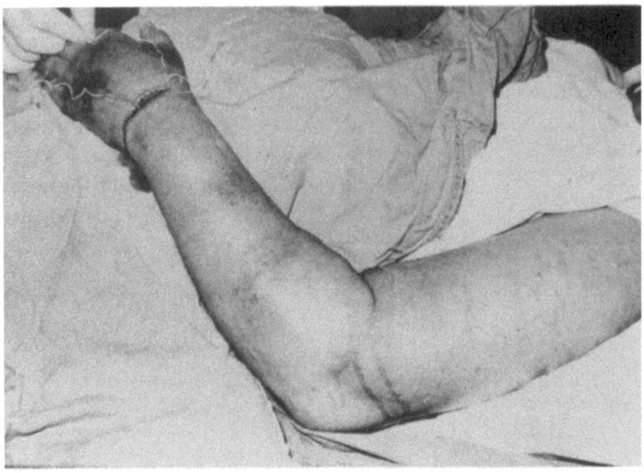

Fig. 5. Case III (A.G.A.R.) Visual lymphangiogram. Small nodular lesions are noted in the left arm and forearm.

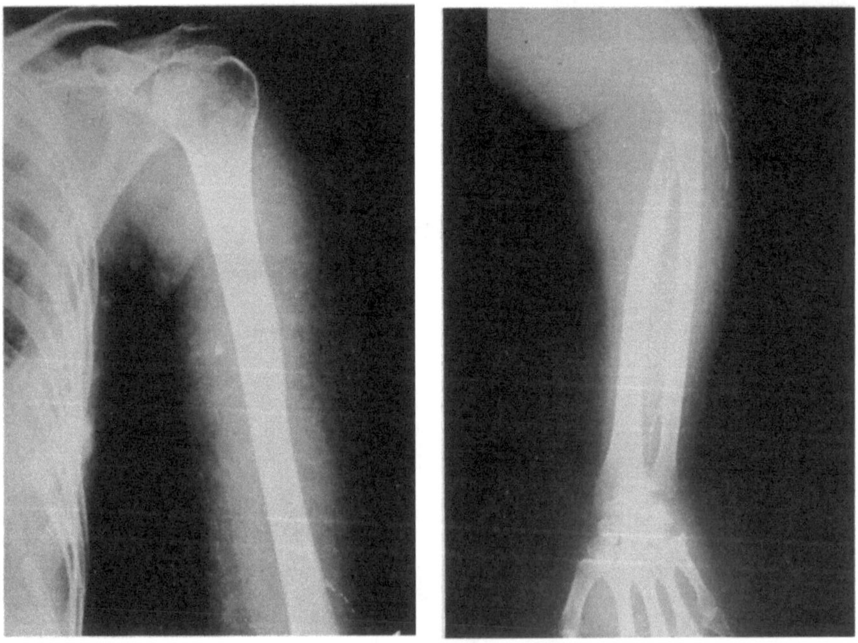

Fig. 6. Case III (A.G.A.R.) Lymphography. Left forearm: lymphatic trunks are dilated and irregular; Left arm: irregular lymphatic trunks showing deposition of contrast in small rounded lesions. Dermal backflow of contrast is noted.

The malignant cutaneous lesions occur at a frequency that is fortunately very low (0.5% of patients with postmastectomy lymphedema of upper limb) and the mean age is 64 years (62 years in our case I, 53 years in case II, and 57 years in case III). The relation between mastectomy and appearance of cutaneous lesions in the lymphedematous limb is on the average 10 years, but there are cases with earlier and later appearance. In the great majority of cases, the first cutaneous lesion appears in advanced lymphedema. The lesions sometimes resemble an ecchymosis of purple color (case II), a red or brown nodule, or, in rapidly developing cases, new clear or reddish plaques, mammiform and hemorrhagic (cases I and III). The tumor spreads rapidly to adjacent tissues of the upper limb and thorax (cases I, II, and III). Radiotherapy can retard the growth only temporarily (case III), but radical surgery can produce marked improvement when the tumor is localized to the lymphedematous upper limb.

The patient usually dies rapidly of metastasis, generally to the lungs and pleura (cases I and II). Relatively few patients die of intercurrent disease. Survival is usually measured in months (the great majority of patients die within one year), but occasionally patients have survived for five years.

Pathologic anatomy reveals macroscopically thickened superficial cutaneous coats with frank thickening of the dermis reflecting the degree of lymphedema. Different levels present numerous hemorrhagic nodules, irregular margins, confluence (cases I, II, and III) that seems to stop at the adjacent tissues but occasionally invades these tissues even deeply into the muscles, aponeurosis, and great vessels which may become thrombosed (cases I and III).

Histologically, certain features recur so that four pathologic groups can be distinguished:

Type 1 - Angiosarcomatous tumors represent the great majority of cases (9,15,20) (case III).

Type 2 - Tumors presenting as epithelial metastases have been described by Laffargue and other authors (4,9,10,19).

Type 3 - Mixed tumors (angiosarcomatous and epithelial) are more frequently observed than pure epithelial tumors. Both features coexist in the same nodule, which makes it impossible to identify with certainty one or the other tumor (1,9).

Type 4 - Undifferentiated cell tumors have been described by Ferraro and other authors (2,7,9) (cases I and II).

## Differential Diagnosis

Even though the diagnosis may be evident from the history, other clinical and histologic entities may present in a similar fashion. Two particular diseases must be differentiated: breast cancer metastasis and Kaposi's disease.

Cutaneous breast cancer metastases are very frequent and late centrifugal metastases are not at all rare. However, in certain cases, the distinction between late cutaneous breast cancer metastases and Stewart-Treves syndrome can be artificial.

Kaposi's disease affects certain specific populations, is more frequent in the lower limbs, is rarely preceded by lymphedema, and does not give rise to true metastases. However, some authors do not see a fundamental difference between Stewart-Treves syndrome and Kaposi's disease (13).

## Pathogenesis

For Stewart-Treves (20), appearance of a second tumor in patients operated upon previously for breast cancer suggested the presence of a circulating carcinogenic factor. This theory is not well-accepted. For Laffargue (11), cutaneous propagation of breast cancer seemed more reasonable.

Actually, two main theories have been advanced to explain Stewart-Treves syndrome:

1. Metastatic recidivation of breast cancer theory. This theory is defended in large part by French and Italian authors (9) and by Salm (19) on the basis of clinical and histologic arguments.

2. Malignant vascular origin theory. This theory is defended by the majority of Anglo-Saxon authors (9,13) also on clinical and histologic grounds.

Neither theory can explain all the features of the Stewart-Treves syndrome.

## Treatment

Treatment modalities proposed to prevent the spread of the cutaneous lesions of Stewart-Treves syndrome are many, attesting to the inadequacy of any individual approach. These treatments may be combined in the same patient (case III). Three different approaches --radiotherapy, cytostatics (cases I and II), and surgery (local excision, amputation, or interscapulothoracic disarticulation)-- may be distinguished.

Peterson and Servelle (9) believe that the appearance of the Stewart-Treves syndrome in lymphedema can be prevented. While lymphedema itself is usually impossible to prevent during breast cancer surgery, once it appears it can be minimized by appropriate management.

Servelle (9) proposes a radical cure of lymphedema by superficial lymphangiectomy in different stages. Pataro (9), however, has shown the appearance of cutaneous tumor even after healing of lymphedema. We propose that postmastectomy lymphedema of the upper limb be treated by lymphovenous anastomosis between the superficial lymphatic trunks and humeral vein.

## Conclusions

Stewart-Treves syndrome is a specific clinical entity of unclear etology and pathogenesis.

Lymphedema is an essential element of the syndrome, but other variables determine the appearance and morphology of the lesions.

## References

1. B. L. Bachulis, W. Jacob, and G. J. Arthur - Postmastectomy lymphangiosarcoma in a patient with carcinoma of the rectum, Amer. J. Surg., 113:289, 1967.

2. R. Cruse, W. C. Fischer, and F. C. Usher - Lymphangiosarcoma in postmastectomy lymphedema, a case report, Surgery, 30:565, 1951.

3. C. A. Danese, E. Grishman, C. Oh, and D. A. Dreilling - Malignant vascular tumors of the lymphedematous extremity, Ann. Surgery, 166:245, 1967.

4. J. Delarue - Les récidives métastases brachiales des cancers du sein (et les pretendues lymphangiosarcomes des bras lymphoedémateux après mammectomie), Mim. Acad. Chir., 88:98, 1962.

5. R. N. Disimone, A. M. El-Mahdi, T. Hazra, and S. Lott - The response of Stewart-Treves syndrome to radiotherapy, Radiology, 97:121, 1970.

6. B. Duperrat, J. Jourdain, G. Noury, and J. L. Lainé - Syndrome de Stewart-Treves, Soc. Franc. Dermat. et Syphil., Reunion Dec. 1971, 650.

7. L. R. Ferraro - Lymphangiosarcoma in postmastectomy lymphedema: a case report, Cancer, 3:511, 1950.

8. L. R. Finlay-Jones - Lymphangiosarcoma of the thigh, Cancer, 26:722, 1970.

9. B. Hery, R. Masse, and J. M. Le-Fur - Le syndrome de Stewart-Treves. Un nouveau cas rapporté. Revue de la literature, Bull. du Cancer, 59(3):269, 1972.

10. G. Kitchen - Lymphangiographic studies in a case of postmastectomy lymphangiosarcoma, Brit. J. Radiology, 45:388, 1972.

11. M. M. Laffargue, F. Pinet, and R. Le Go - Syndrome de Stewart-Treves (métastases épithéliomateuses ou angiosarcome dans le gros bras compliquant la mammectomie), La presse Medicale, 41 (6):1506, 1960.

12. S. Liszaver and R. C. Ross - Lymphangiosarcoma secondary to chronic lymphedema, Canad. Med. Ass. J., 76:475, 1957.

13. W. D. McCarthy and G. T. Pack - Malignant blood vessel tumors, Surg. Gyn. & Obst., 91:464, 1950.

14. D. H. Mackenzie - Lymphangiosarcoma arising in chronic congenital and idiopathic lymphoedema, J. Clin. Path., 24:524, 1971.

15. B. McSwain and S. Stephenson - Lymphangiosarcoma of the edematous extremity, Ann. Surgery, 151:649, 1960.

16. F. Martorell - Tumorigenic lymphedema, Angiology, 2:386, 1951.

17. T. A. Marrick, R. A. Erlandson, and S. I. Hajdu - Lymphangiosarcoma of a congenitally lymphedematous arm, Arch. Path., 91:365, 1971.

18. J. M. Ryan, P. Lober, and B. J. Kennedy - Lymphangiosarcoma in chronic postmastectomy lymphedema, Minnesota Med., 57:538, 1974.

19. R. Salm - The nature of the so-called postmastectomy lymphangiosarcoma, J. Path. Bact., 85:445, 1963.

20. F. W. Stewart and N. Treves - Lymphangiosarcoma in postmastectomy lymphedema. A report of six cases in elephantiasis chirurgica, Cancer, 1:64, 1948.

21. A. H. Woodward, J. C. Ivins, and E. H. Soule - Lymphangiosarcoma arising in chronic lymphedematous extremities, Cancer, 30:562, 1972.

# Lymphedema

# LYMPHEDEMA: STUDY OF COLLAGEN METABOLISM

A. K. Cordeiro, F. F. Baracat, E. Bolanho, and A. J. Brandi

Instituto Arnaldo Vieira de Carvalho, São Paulo, Brazil
Faculdade de Medicina de Valença, Rio De Janeiro, Brazil

The fibroblast is the commonest cell of connective tissue and the one principally responsible for the formation of collagen fibers and the amorphous intercellular matter, the "ground substance."

The amorphous ground substance of the connective tissue is colorless, transparent, and optically homogeneous, and is formed principally of mucopolysaccharides and proteins.

The degree of polymerization of these mucopolysaccharides is very variable and is directly related to the viscosity of the amorphous ground substance.

Through its hydrophilia each molecule of glycoprotein joins up with a large number of water molecules; the total amount of water present in the amorphous substance of connective tissue is found in the solvation layer of glycoproteins.

Adjacent to the amorphous substance may be observed a minimal quantity of a fluid, the interstitial plasma or liquid, the composition of which is similar to blood plasma in regard to ions and diffusible substances. The interstitial plasma contains small quantities of plasma proteins of low molecular weight which pass through the walls of capillaries.

Under normal conditions, the quantity of interstitial liquid is insignificant.

## Materials and Methods

Our material consisted of 30 cases of lymphedema of the lower limbs, of varied clinical etiology.

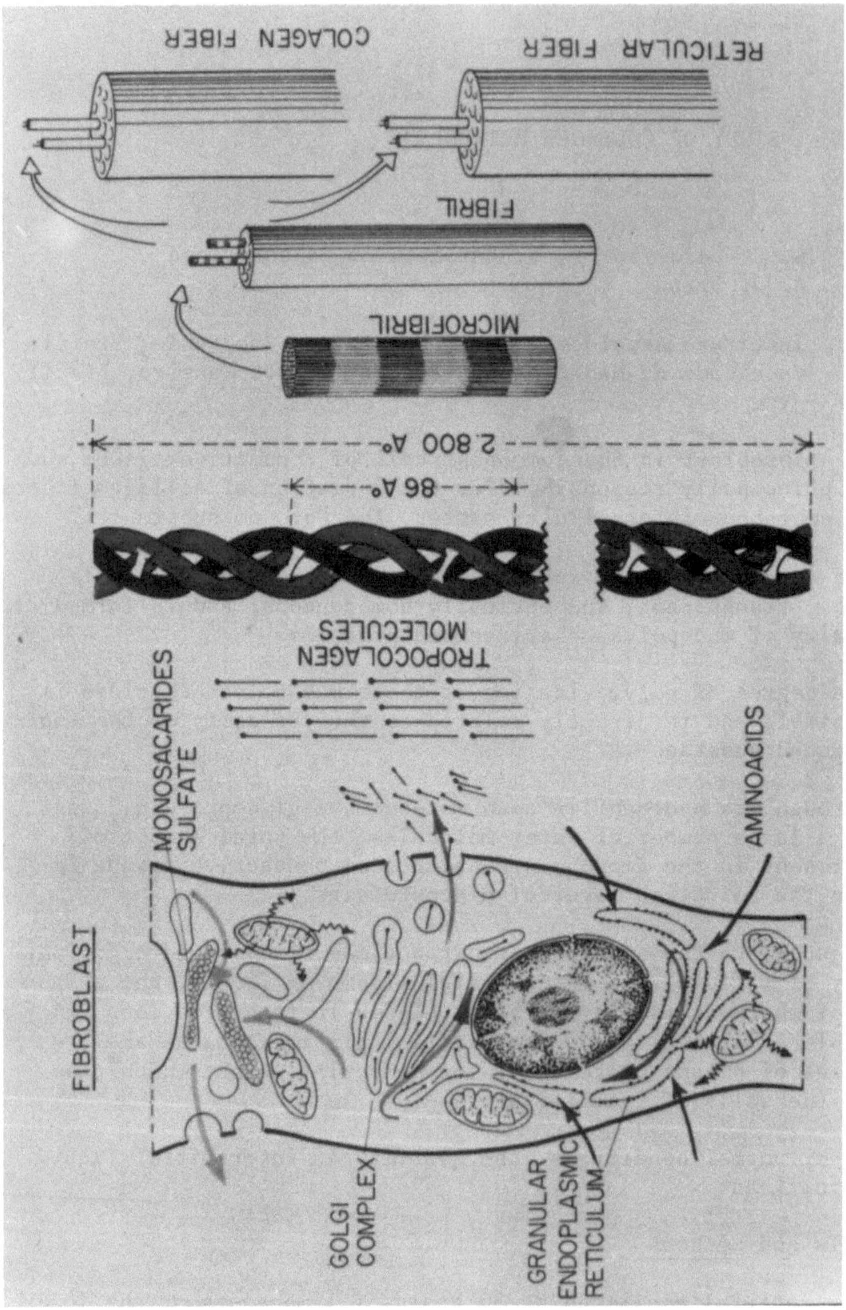


Fig. 1. Fibroblast: collagen metabolism.

Our method of study was the following:

1. Clinical examinations: normal and specialized.

2. Genetic studies: sex chromatin and karyogram, sometimes of parents of patients.

3. Laboratory examinations: hemogram; sedimentation rate; hematocrit; total and fractionated serum proteins; urea; blood sugar; lipid electrophoresis; electrophoresis of proteins; K, Na, and Cl serum values. Special study was made of prolinemia and prolinuria, hydroxyprolinemia and hydroxyprolinuria. In these studies we followed the techniques described by Troll and Cannan (8) for proline and by Stegeman (6) for hydroxyproline.

4. Histopathological and histochemical examination of material extracted during operations. This material was studied with the following stains: H.E., PAS, Masson trichrome, Gomori trichrome, and Alcyan Blue.

5. Lymphography: by Kinmonth's technique (4) for superficial lymphatic system; Tosati's technique (7) for deep lymphatic system; and Romero Marques' technique (5) for deep lymphatic system.

6. Therapeutic studies with N-acetyl hydroxyproline with a daily dose of 3 capsules of 200 mg orally.

## Discussion

Lymphedema was studied in relation to alterations in collagen and cell function.

Földi (3), in studying the function of mesenchymal cells in lymphedema, came to believe that there exists an important "biochemical factor" in lymphedema. The cells of interstitial tissue suffer disturbances of both oxygenation and exchange of several substances which are necessary to their normal function, and lymphedema is, to a certain extent, brought about by a serious lesion of mesenchymal cells produced by lymphatic stasis; later on, these same cells are responsible for development of fibrosis.

De Bruz (1) and Duran-Reynolds (2) maintain that alterations in glycoprotein polymerization depend on enzymatic alterations. Thus the mucinases, just as hyaluronidases, condroitinase, and mucoidinase, can alter the biology of connective tissue, changing the degree of viscosity of the interstitial space and further influencing the hydrodynamics of interstitial-capillary exchange.

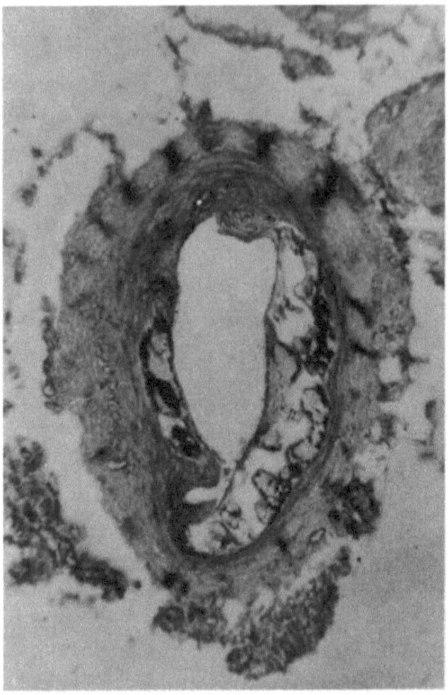

Fig. 2. Fibrosis of perivascular lymphatic tissue. Chronic inflammatory process with degeneration of lymphatic vascular wall (X 100, stain: Gomori)

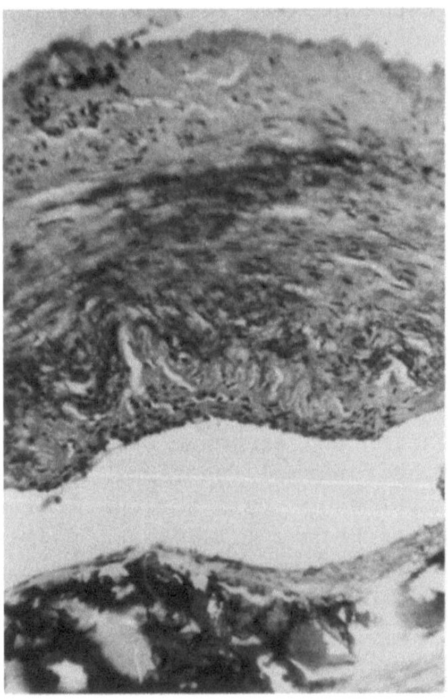

Fig. 3. Fibrosis of perivascular lymphatic tissue. Chronic inflammatory process with degeneration of lymphatic vascular wall (X 100, stain: Gomori)

Thus, alterations in the hormonal secretions, either of depolymerizing hormones (ACTH, cortisone, aldosterone, folliculin), or polymerizing hormones (progesterone, testosterone), or even lack of vitamin E can interfere with the depolymerizing processes of hyaluronic acid and consequently disturb the processes of exchange between capillaries and the interstitial space.

It seems clear that the common denominator of all types of lymphatic stasis brought about by different mechanisms and cellular alterations is accumulation of proteins in the interstitial space. Lymphatic stasis, with increase of interstitial proteins, would stimulate a proliferation of fibroblasts with consequent deposition of connective tissue.

This fibrosis of lymphatic perivascular connective tissue, increasing progressively in association with a chronic inflammatory process, leads to a progressive thickening of the region: elephantiasis. The lymphatic collector ducts involved by sclerosis of these tissues are first progressively blocked and later on completely blocked, causing the delay in lymphatic circulation and consequent worsening of the edematous condition (Figs. 2,3).

Therefore, in all processes of insufficiency of lymphatic circulation in which there is interstitial edema, in time there may be observed the evolution of connective tissue to a fibrosclerotic form.

## Conclusions

We may conclude that in lymphedema there is actually a factor, either genetic, chemical, or enzymatic, which, acting on RNA, leads to alterations in connective tissue through modifications in collagen metabolism with consequent formation of irregular fibrous tissue which may be observed in long-standing lymphedemas.

It appears to us that one of the important alterations in collagen metabolism is related to the metabolism of proline and hydroxyproline.

In congenital lymphedemas this is easily explained by genetic abnormalities.

In primary lymphedemas of praecox or tarda type, in our opinion genetic alterations are also involved.

In secondary lymphedemas, in a general way, these are related to chemical alterations of proteins in interstitial space due to edema of extended duration.

References

1. De Bruz, in: M. Battezzati and I. Donini, Il sistema linfatico nella pretica clinica, Piccin Editores, Padova, 1967, p. 180.

2. F. Duran-Reynolds, La substance fondamentale du mesenchyme et les facteurs de diffusion dans l'infection, Sem. Hôp. Paris, 28:1047, 1952.

3. M. Földi, Diseases of lymphatics and lymph circulation, Akademiai Kiadó, Budapest, 1969.

4. J. B. Kinmonth, G. W. Taylor, and R. A. Harper, Lymphangiography, Brit. Med. J., 1:840, 1955.

5. Romero Marques and L. Ferreira, Linfografia de linfaticos profundos e de la pierna y muslo, Angiologia, 13:51-55, 1961.

6. H. Z. Stegeman, Z. Physiol. Chem., 311:41, 1958.

7. E. Tosati, La linfoangiografia per lo studio dei linfatici ed dei linfedemi dell'arto inferiore, Rass. Clin., Scient., 33:161, 1958.

8. W. Troll and R. K. Cannan, J. Biol. Chem., 200:803, 1953.

# PROLINE AND HYDROXYPROLINE IN LYMPHEDEMA

A. K. Cordeiro and F. F. Baracat

Instituto Arnaldo Vieira de Carvalho

São Paulo, Brazil

The fundamental component of collagen is the triple chain of tropocollagen which is changed into components of connective tissue:

(1) microfibrils
(2) fibrils
(3) insoluble fibers: reticular and collagen
(4) membranes
(5) aponeurosis

The peptide chain renders the characteristic helix sensitive to temperature modifications. Denaturation occurs at temperatures slightly higher than normal body temperature and collagen becomes susceptible to the action of some proteolytic enzymes.

Mesenchymatous collagen is synthesized in fibroblasts. Hydroxylation of proline to hydroxyproline maintains the hydrophilic nature of the chain.

Hydroxyproline serves as metabolic marker for collagen.

Hydroxylysine is also a characteristic amino acid but it occurs in collagen even less frequently and cannot be determined as easily as hydroxyproline.

The average excretion of total hydroxyproline in urine is about 30 mg/24 hours.

The major part (65% - 75%) is found in the dipeptide prolyl-hydroxyproline chain or in the tripeptide Gly-Pro-Hypro, as

LeRoy (9) has pointed out. Only about 3% is present in the free form and about 5% - 10% appears in peptides of molecular weight 1000-6500 (Hanson and Wiederanders (7)) or even in glycopeptides (Bourrilon and Vernay (2)).

The excretion of hydroxyproline is somewhat sensitive to exogenous collagen-derived components from, for example, ice cream and jellies, which cannot be avoided completely in the diet.

It can be generally stated, however, that in the gastrointestinal tract, all hydroxyproline is liberated by prolidase and then reabsorbed. In the body, it is oxidized to carbon dioxide ($CO_2$). Degradation and excretion of proline proceeds in the following manner:

| Source | | Liberated in gut | | In blood | | Excretion |
|---|---|---|---|---|---|---|
| Ingested collagen | → | Free Hypro (reabsorbed) | → | Free Hypro (oxidized) | → | $CO_2$ |

Weiss and Klein (23) have administered $^{14}$C-gelatin orally and found only 2% - 3% of the activity in urine, in contrast to 11% - 17% after parenteral administration.

Prolyl-hydroxyproline (Pro-Hypro) is a remarkably resistant product of endogenous degradation remaining in tissues and excreted in urine. On the other hand, other peptides of hydroxyproline are cleaved, and hydroxyproline oxidized and excreted through the lungs as follows:

| | | In tissues | | | | |
|---|---|---|---|---|---|---|
| Collagen tissue | → | X-Hypro | → | Free Hypro (oxidized) | → | $CO_2$ |
| | | Pro-Hypro | → | Pro-Hypro (resistant) | → | Pro-Hypro (urine) |

It has been estimated that about 70% of the excretion of collagen degradation products is through the lungs and only 30% is through the kidneys.

An uncertain factor in the evaluation of the urinary excretion of hydroxyproline is the proportion of hydroxyproline undergoing oxidation.

Prockop and Kivirikko (15) have proposed that urinary excretion of hydroxyproline is a reliable indicator of the turnover of collagen.

But we must remember that hydroxyproline can originate from collagen in its various physiological states and reflects either the formation or degradation of connective tissue. Lindstedt and Prockop (14) showed that collagen in its various physiological states can serve as a source of hydroxyproline as follows:

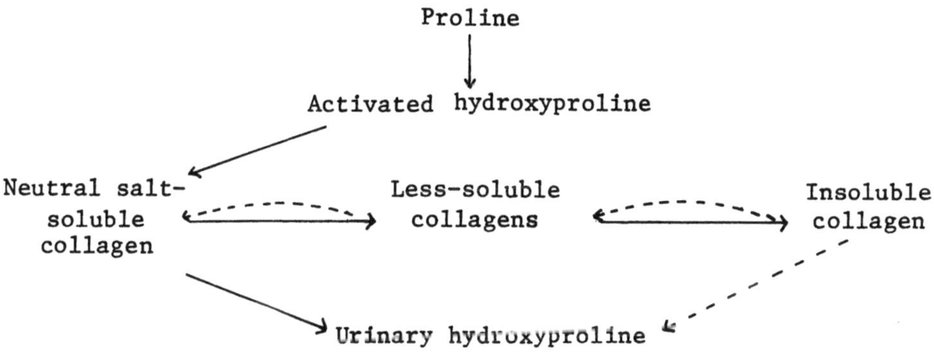


In hormonal disturbances, urinary hydroxyproline excretion is directly related to the metabolism of proteins in general.

It is customary to correlate the excretion of hydroxyproline to the body surface area or urinary creatinine, but a simultaneous estimation of the urea excretion would help to differentiate between changes in general turnover of proteins and in the metabolism of connective tissue in particular.

In children, the urinary excretion of hydroxyproline is high, indicating rapid synthesis and turnover of collagen.

Plasma contains:

1.5 µg/ml of free hydroxyproline

0.6 µg/ml of peptide-bound hydroxyproline

8.0 µg/ml of protein-bound hydroxyproline

Values for free hydroxyproline in plasma exceeding 2.5 µg/ml are due to reabsorption from the intestine.

For the synthesis of collagen both glucose and oxygen are necessary. Glucose, however, cannot be replaced by its metabolites and lactic acid is produced maximally during collagen synthesis.

The redox balance is important in many phases of collagen synthesis, as in the chain alpha-ketoglutaric acid → glutamic acid → proline → hydroxylation of protocollagen proline, and also in the formation of galactosamine and iduronic acid. On the other hand, oxygen is necessary in the hydroxylation of protocollagen proline. Increased oxygen availability favors the formation of cellular RNA in vivo as well as in subcellular particles.

The receptor of serotonin is a neuraminidase-sensitive ganglioside. It is of interest, therefore, that the neuraminic acid moiety is also important in the regulation of collagen synthesis.

## Materials and Methods

This study involved 12 cases of lymphedema of the lower limbs:

| | |
|---|---|
| Yellow fingernails syndrome | 1 case |
| Milroy's disease | 2 cases |
| Primary precox lymphedema | 1 case |
| Primary tarda lymphedema | 1 case |
| Post-infection lymphedema | 4 cases |
| Post-phlebitic lymphedema | 3 cases |

Measurements were made of proline levels in blood and in urine, hydroxyproline in blood and in urine, and urinary creatinine using the following techniques:

(1) Proline, technique of Troll and Cannan (22)
(2) Hydroxyproline, technique of Stegeman (21)
(3) Urinary creatinine, technique of Henry (8)

In addition determinations were also made of the following:

(a) $\frac{\text{millimoles of proline}}{\text{millimoles of creatinine}}$ in urine

(b) $\frac{\text{millimoles of hydroxyproline (Prol OH)}}{\text{millimoles of creatinine}}$ in urine

(c) $\frac{\text{proline}}{\text{hydroxyproline (Prol OH)}}$ in urine

(d) $\frac{\text{hydroxyproline (Prol OH)}}{\text{proline}}$ in urine

(e) estimates were made with the Sharp electronic calculator model 811.

(4) N-acetyl hydroxyproline, which served as the basis of study of urinary hydroxyproline and therapeutically with controls before and after its administration

## Discussion of Results

Oxygen and glucose are both necessary for the synthesis of collagen. Glucose cannot be replaced by its metabolites. On the other hand, all cellular functions are controlled by the genes, the expression of which is controlled by feedback signals from the cells mediated at times by substrates in enzymatic reactions.

RNA determined by a gene controls the formation of an enzyme that controls a chemical reaction. In vivo, increase in oxygen level favors the formation of cellular RNA. In children during active growth synthesis and turnover of collagen is rapid, with high urinary excretion of hydroxyproline.

An important type of feedback is the so-called enzymatic inhibition. The feedback inhibits the function of the gene and of RNA by chemicals synthesized by the cell.

Thus, there is excessive glucose in the cells, which is broken down into its degradation products. A few of these act on specific genes or on the corresponding RNA to diminish its activity. The genes then diminish the rate of formation of ribonucleic acid, thereby limiting the formation of enzymes for chemical reactions in the cell.

Such chemical reactions include reduction balance, which is involved in many steps in the synthesis of galactosamine and iduronic acid. As the receptor of serotonin is a neuraminidase-sensitive ganglioside, the neuraminic acid moiety is important in regulation of collagen synthesis.

On the other hand, the "biochemical factor" described by Földi (6) in edema and lymphatic stasis which alters cellular metabolism and leads to fibrosis is probably an alteration of normal metabolism of collagen. De Bruz (4) and Duran-Reynolds (5) discuss the enzymatic alterations in which the mucinases such as hyaluronidase, chondroitinase, and mucoidinase can alter the biological state of connective tissue, modifying the viscosity of the interstitial space and thereby influencing the hydrodynamic exchanges between the interstitium and capillaries.

High urinary hydroxyproline levels, about 5-10 times the levels of normal individuals, have been observed during rapid growth, for example, in adolescence (11-20) and in some diseases (5-11). On the other hand, the plasma levels of hypoproteins are not normally affected.

RESULTS

| | Before N-acetyl hydroxyproline | | | | After N-acetyl hydroxyproline | | | |
|---|---|---|---|---|---|---|---|---|
| Case | Plasma proline, mg % | Urinary proline, mg % | Hydroxy-proline, mg % | Creatinine, mg % | Plasma proline, mg % | Urinary proline, mg % | Hydroxy-proline, mg % | Creatinine, mg % |
| 1 | 6.5 | 11.5 | 1.76 | 45.0 | 8.5 | 9.0 | 1.94 | 56.4 |
| 2 | - | 9.0 | 3.70 | 68.5 | 6.1 | 11.1 | 2.46 | 40.0 |
| 3 | 8.5 | 9.0 | 1.94 | 56.4 | 8.0 | 2.0 | 0.79 | 4.0 |
| 4 | 7.0 | 9.0 | 1.41 | 27.4 | 4.7 | 10.6 | 2.46 | 62.4 |
| 5 | 4.7 | 12.8 | 2.56 | 84.0 | 6.1 | 15.0 | 6.80 | 111.0 |
| 6 | 6.1 | 11.1 | 2.46 | 40.0 | 6.1 | 15.0 | 6.80 | 111.0 |
| 7 | 7.5 | 11.6 | 8.10 | 68.4 | 6.5 | 2.9 | 0.61 | 9.0 |
| 8 | 8.0 | 2.0 | 0.79 | 4.0 | 6.1 | 11.1 | 2.46 | 40.0 |
| 9 | 6.5 | 2.9 | 0.61 | 9.0 | 8.0 | 2.0 | 0.79 | 4.0 |
| 10 | 4.7 | 10.6 | 2.46 | 62.4 | 8.5 | 9.0 | 1.94 | 56.4 |
| 11 | 6.1 | 5.6 | 2.38 | 25.4 | 4.8 | 5.0 | 3.44 | 127.0 |
| 12 | 5.6 | 33.4 | 6.30 | 84.0 | 4.7 | 10.6 | 2.46 | 62.4 |

$$(A) = \frac{\text{millimoles Proline}}{\text{millimoles Creatinine}} \quad \text{in urine}$$

$$(B) = \frac{\text{millimoles Hydroxyproline}}{\text{millimoles Creatinine}} \quad \text{in urine}$$

$$(C) = \frac{\text{Proline}}{\text{Hydroxyproline}} \quad \text{in urine}$$

$$(D) = \frac{\text{Hydroxyproline}}{\text{Proline}} \quad \text{in urine}$$

| | Before N-acetyl hydroxyproline | | | | After N-acetyl hydroxyproline | | | |
|---|---|---|---|---|---|---|---|---|
| Case | (A) | (B) | (C) | (D) | (A) | (B) | (C) | (D) |
| 1 | 0.25 | 0.050 | 6.5 | 0.15 | 0.16 | 0.040 | 4.6 | 0.22 |
| 2 | 0.13 | 0.060 | 2.4 | 0.40 | 0.27 | 0.070 | 4.5 | 0.22 |
| 3 | 0.16 | 0.040 | 4.6 | 0.22 | 0.50 | 0.225 | 2.5 | 0.40 |
| 4 | 0.32 | 0.060 | 6.4 | 0.16 | 0.17 | 0.045 | 4.3 | 0.23 |
| 5 | 0.15 | 0.035 | 4.9 | 0.20 | 0.13 | 0.070 | 2.2 | 0.45 |
| 6 | 0.27 | 0.070 | 4.5 | 0.22 | 0.13 | 0.070 | 2.2 | 0.45 |
| 7 | 0.17 | 0.135 | 1.4 | 0.71 | 0.32 | 0.080 | 4.8 | 0.22 |
| 8 | 0.50 | 0.225 | 2.5 | 0.40 | 0.27 | 0.070 | 4.5 | 0.22 |
| 9 | 0.32 | 0.080 | 4.8 | 0.22 | 0.50 | 0.225 | 2.5 | 0.40 |
| 10 | 0.17 | 0.045 | 4.3 | 0.23 | 0.16 | 0.040 | 4.6 | 0.22 |
| 11 | 0.20 | 0.080 | 2.3 | 0.43 | 0.04 | 0.027 | 1.4 | 0.69 |
| 12 | 0.40 | 0.085 | 5.3 | 0.19 | 0.17 | 0.045 | 4.3 | 0.23 |

In our study, we observed a constant level of plasma hypoproteins with marked abnormalities in urinary hydroxyproline.

## Conclusions

If hypoprotein levels are a function of the pool of collagen, this pool is probably distinct from the pool from which hydroxyproline peptides are derived.

If the relations between hydroxyproline and collagen are normal, plasma hypoproteins represent a parameter reflecting collagen metabolism. Because of its high molecular weight this protein is more closely related to collagen fibril than collagen metabolites.

The abnormalities which we observed suggest that envelopment of collagen is more common than indicated in histopathological studies. Under specific circumstances plasma hypoproteins can be a more sensitive index of collagen metabolism.

Thus, the study of proline and hydroxyproline in blood and in urine and a comparison with urinary studies of creatinine, while nonspecific and sometimes not sensitive enough, can be helpful in the evaluation of collagen metabolism in lymphedema. Therapeutic approaches, such as the use of a diet or various drugs, can be designed to correct these abnormalities in collagen metabolism.

## References

1. M. Battezzati and I. Donini, Il sistema linfático nella pratica clinica, Piccin Editores, Padova, 1967.

2. R. Bourrilon and J. L. Vernay, Biochem. Biophys. Acta, 117:319, 1966.

3. A. K. Cordeiro, F. F. Baracat, E. Bolanho, and A. J. Brandi, Linfedema: estudo do metabolismo do colageno (to be published).

4. De Bruz, cited by Battezzati (1), p. 180.

5. F. Duran-Reynold, La substance fondamentale du mesenchyme et les facteurs de diffusion dans l'afection, Sem. Hôp. Paris, 28:1047, 1952.

6. M. Földi, Diseases of Lymphatics and Lymph Circulation, Akademiai Kiado, Budapest, 1969.

7. H. Hanson and B. Wiederanders, Clin. Chim. Acta, 25:255, 1969.

8. M. R. Henry, Clinical Chemistry, Harper & Row, New York, 1964.

9. H. E. Jasin, W. Find, W. Wise, and M. Ziff, Relationship between urinary hydroxyproline and growth, J. Clin. Invest., 41:1928, 1962.

10. H. Keiser, E. C. LeRoy, S. Udenfriend, and A. Sjoerdsma, Collagen-like protein in human plasma, Science, 142:1678, 1963.

11. E. C. LeRoy and A. Sjoerdsma, Clinical significance of a hydroxyproline-containing protein in human plasma, J. Clin. Invest., 44:914, 1965.

12. E. C. LeRoy, Adv. Clin. Chem., 10:213, 1967.

13. E. C. LeRoy, A. Kaplan, S. Udenfriend, and A. Sjoerdsma, A hydroxyproline-containing collagen-like protein in plasma and a procedure for its assay, J. Biol. Chem., 239:3350, 1964.

14. S. Lindstedt and D. J. Prockop, J. Biol. Chem., 236:1399, 1961.

15. D. J. Prockop and K. I. Kivirikko, Ann. Intern. Med., 66:1243, 1967.

16. D. J. Prockop and S. Udenfriend, A specific method for the analysis of hydroxyproline in tissues and urine, Analyt. Biochem., 1:228, 1960.

17. D. J. Prockop, H. R. Keiser, and A. Sjoerdsma, Gastrointestinal absorption and renal excretion of hydroxyproline peptides, Lancet, 2:257, 1962.

18. D. J. Prockop and A. Sjoerdsma, Significance of urinary hydroxyproline in man, J. Clin. Invest., 40:843, 1961.

19. D. J. Prockop, Isotopic studies on collagen degradation and urinary excretion of hydroxyproline, J. Clin. Invest., 43:453, 1964.

20. J. D. Smiley and M. Ziff, Urinary hydroxyproline excretion and growth, Physiol. Rev., 44:30, 1964.

21. H. Z. Stegeman, Z. Physiol. Chem., 31:41, 1958.

22. W. Troll and R. K. Cannan, J. Biol. Chem., 200:803, 1953.

23. P. H. Weiss and L. Klein, J. Clin. Invest., 48:1, 1969.

# LYMPHATIC MALFORMATIONS AND CONGENITAL ARTERIOVENULAR ABNORMALITIES OF THE LIMBS. HYPEROSTOMY SYNDROMES IN CONGENITAL LYMPHEDEMAS

R.C. Mayall, A.C.D.G. Mayall, J.C. Mayall, U.R. Ferretti, E.T. Mehri, A. Rojas, J. Carvalho Nobre, and V. Villani

Hospital da Gamboa
Rio de Janeiro, Brasil

In the book of Malan about Vascular Malformations (Angiodysplasias, 1974) it was written on pg. 127 "Not much is to be found in the literature about lymphatic malformations associated with venous or arteriovenous malformations. It's very difficult in such cases, to ascertain whether the lymphatic lesion is a cause or a consequence of the venous or arteriovenous malformations".

It is well accepted that these vascular malformations have a common mesenchymal origin. For this reason we are studying all our patients with angiodysplasias of the limbs by a complete angiography - including routine arteriography, lymphography, and phlebography.

The angiodysplasias of the three vessels are very common and we agree with Tavero, Biglioli and Bonfati that "lymphography carried out systematically in cases of vascular malformation, has revealed the frequent participation of the lymphatic system not only in patients with visible or monstrous elephantiasis of the limbs, but also in clinically less severe cases, often disclosing the presence of lymphovenous communications".

In this paper, I will present and discuss the radiologically typical findings of hyperostomy syndrome on the legs of the patients with early congenital lymphedema, confirmed by operation, and the advantages of their treatment to improve the final esthetic result of the leg, after Charles-Josias Operation and to prevent the reciditivity of the swelling of the extremities.

Material and Method

Ten patients with congenital praecox lymphedema were selected. The angiographic examinations in these patients were made by the following methods:

1) Superficial lymphography by the Kinmonth's Technique.

2) Deep lymphography of the posterior tibial lymphatics by the technique of Romero Marques.

3) Arteriography of the posterior and anterior tibial arteries, fibular artery, by direct puncture of the popliteal artery, or by the retrograde method through the posterior tibial artery.

4) Ascending phlebography on standing position under fluoroscopy control.

5) Super selective phlebography of the posterior tibial vein by direct puncture on the retromalleolar inner region.

It was considered as typical finding of hyperostomy the following radiological findings, during a serial and fast angiography using the A.O.T.-Schonander system or a radiopaque chronometer:

1) Simultaneous filling with dye, during arteriography, of arteries and veins during the arterial phase, due to the premature venous back flow.

2) A "Bottled appearance" of the muscle mass around arteriolar branches during the second-or-arteriolo capillar phase, in the places corresponding to the abnormal thermometric and oscillographic findings of the skin.

3) Abnormal size, number, extension and direction of arteriolar branches appear occasionally with "flamesh" spots.

4) Incomplete or delayed filling of distal arteries of the leg, due to the derivation of blood through the short circuits of the calf.

These findings were more relevant on posterior tibial artery branches followed by fibular branches and seldom on anterior tibial artery.

The serial changer was the AOT-Schonander with one plate/second, during 8-10 seconds, starting the plates after a 20 ml. injection of 40 ml. volume of dye under hand pressure, and without anesthesia.

When there was a good deep lymphatic circulation the patients were submitted to the Charles-Josias Operation.

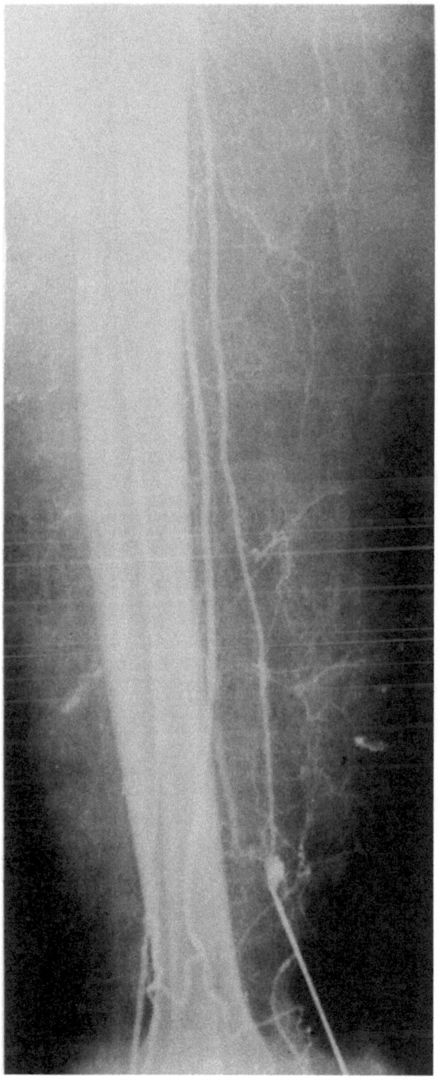

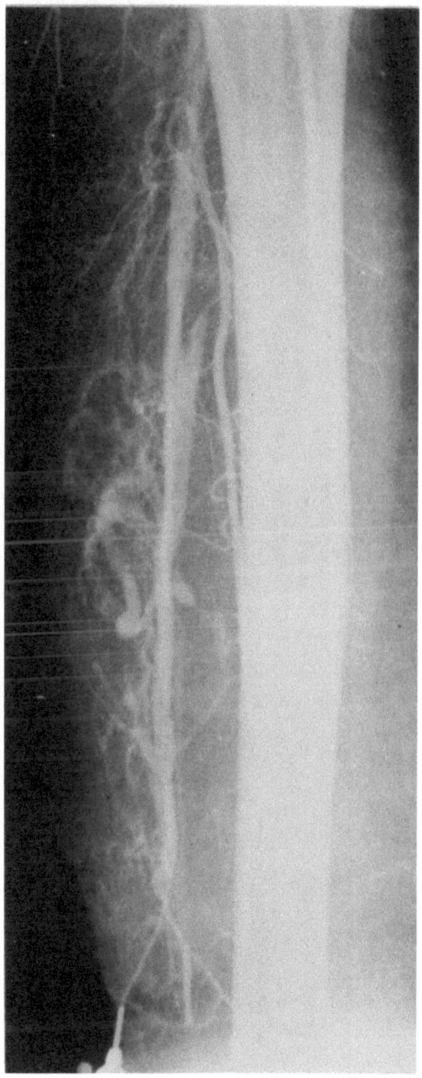

Fig. 1 - Abnormal branches of posterior tibial artery.
Fig. 2 - Bottled appearance with premature venous back flow.

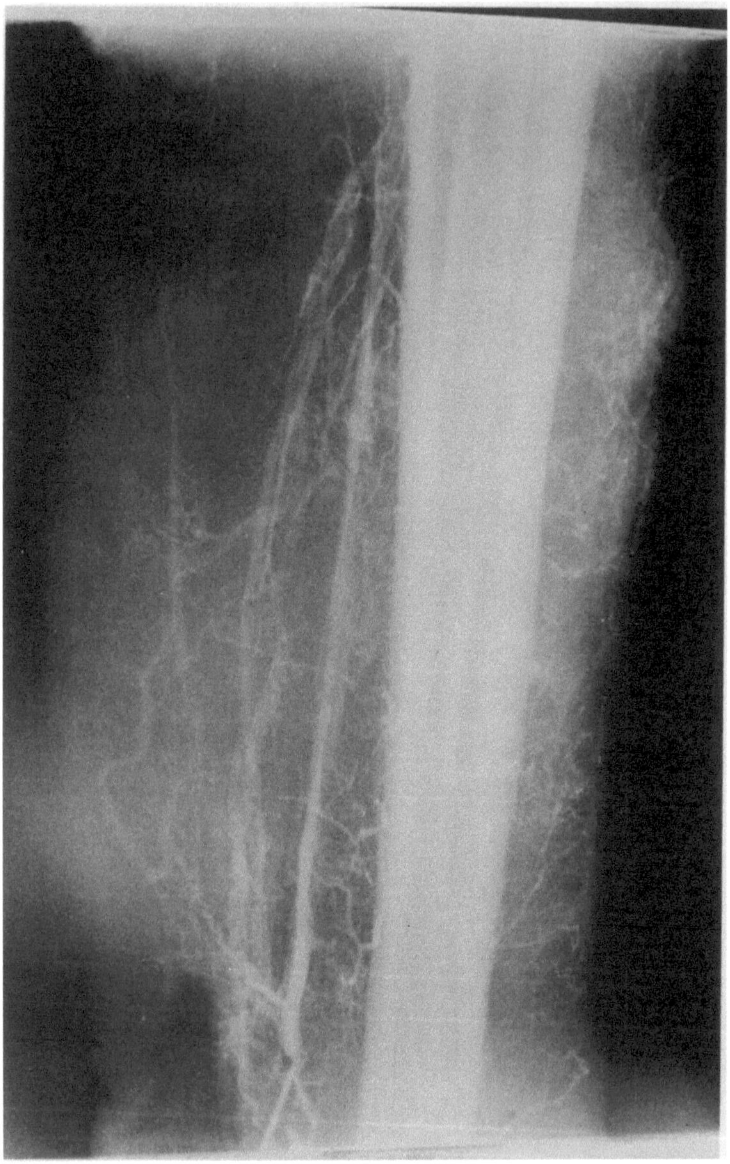

Fig. 3 - Abnormal size and direction of posterior tibial artery branch with premature venous back flow

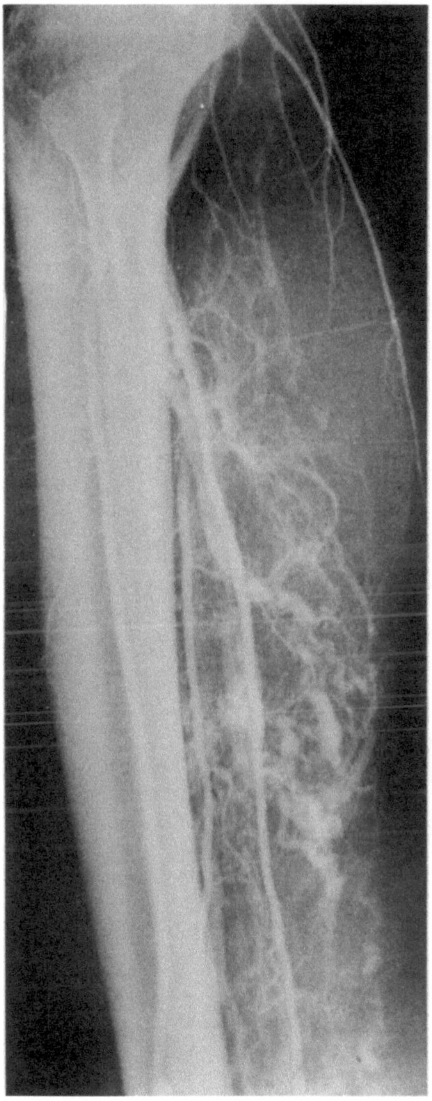

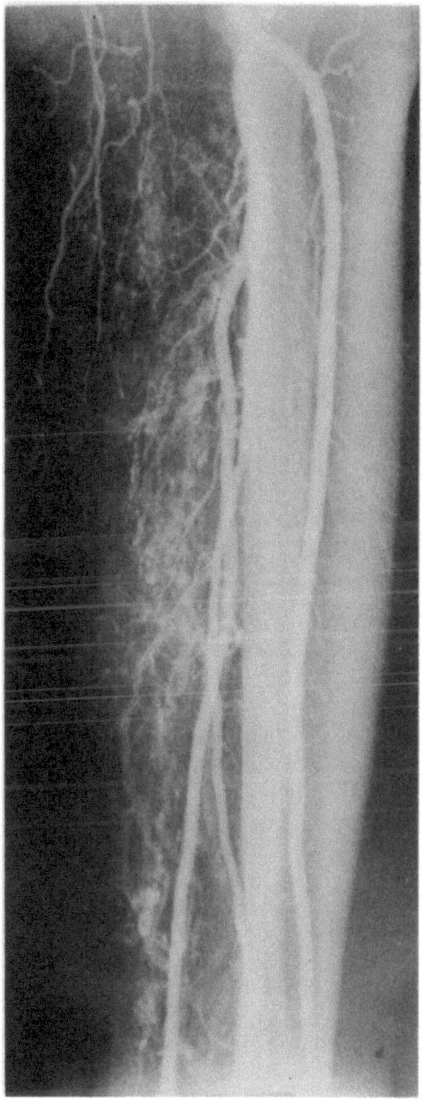

Fig. 4 - Simultaneous filling of arteries and veins during arterial phase with deep muscle veins on the leg.
Fig. 5 - Bottled appearance and flamesh spots with premature venous back flow.

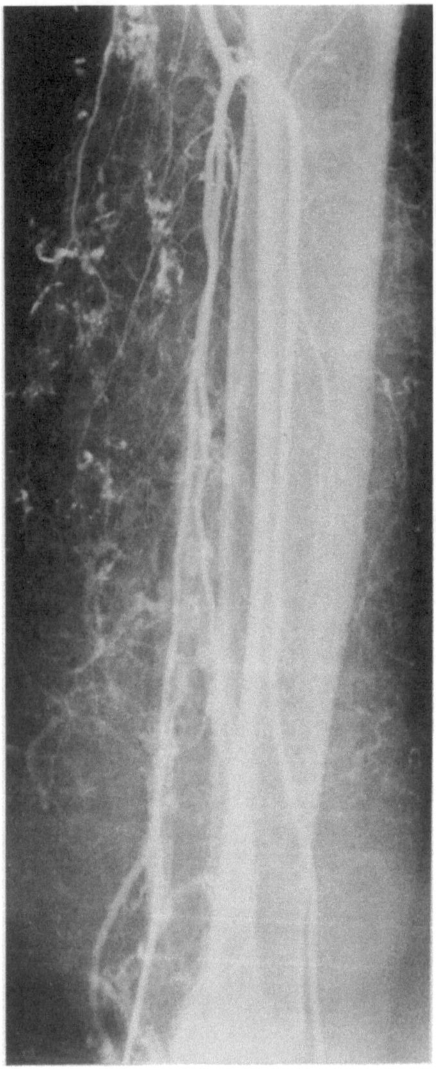

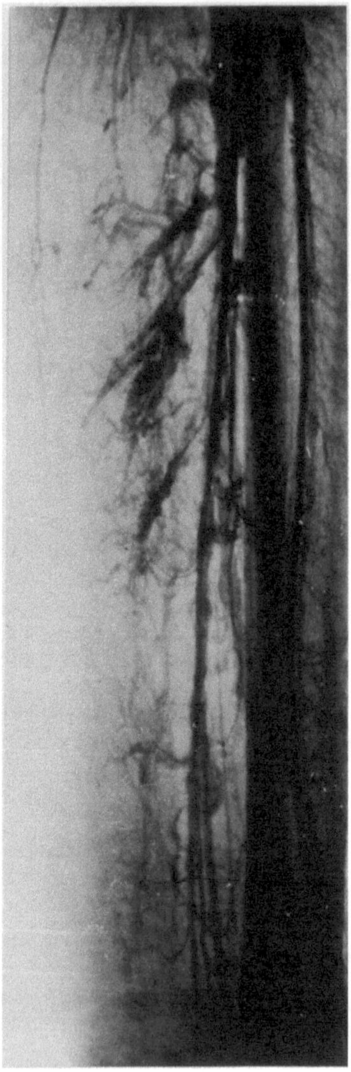

Fig. 6 - Simultaneous filling of posterior tibial and fibular arteries with bottled appearance.

Fig. 7 - Simultaneous filling of posterior tibial and fibular arteries with bottled appearance.

If these same patients presented hyperostomy syndrome we tied all the abnormal branches of the arteries of the leg. In the patients with aplasia or occlusion of the deep lymphatics of the leg, the Charles-Josias Operation was contraindicated. Only the abnormal hyperostomy branches were tied.

## Results and Discussion

The findings of the abnormal arteriovenular branching in congenital praecox lymphedemas were very common in our series.

The presence of the hyperostomy explains the associated venous stasis and chronic venous insufficiency responsible for the reciditivity of the oedema after the operation for lymphedema extremities when there is a good deep venous and lymphatic backflow. This venous stasis is also partly responsible for the lymphostasis. Based on these physiopathological explication it was recommended the surgical division of all these abnormal branches. The clinical results were very satisfying. The hardening of the lymphedema was reduced when only the division of the abnormal branches was made. The functional and final esthetic appearance was much better after a long follow up, when it was necessary to make the Charles-Josias Operation, together with the division of all abnormal branches. These patients are able to wear normal shoes, unlike the majority of patients operated on by the conventional Charles or Thompson methods.

It is difficult to prove, if these findings are primary or secondary to the lymphedema. Due to its common mesenchymal origin it is more possible to accept the simultaneous development and its physiologic worsening during the vasodilator troubles during the puberty.

It is important to make the differential diagnosis with some arteriovenous malformations whose radiological findings are different.

1) The fading of the arterial contrast is more intense distally to the fistula. In the hyperostomy the distal filling of the arteries is delayed but normal.

2) The spotty appearance on the fistula area is much more intense than the bottled appearance of hyperostomy branches.

3) The dilatation of the satellites veins is absent around the hyperostomy brances. There is only a precocious venous backflow, but the veins show a normal shape or small phlebectasis in the more advanced cases.

4) Arteriovenous fistulas commonly are diffuse on the limbs. Hyperostomy branches are more localized.

## Conclusions

The evidence of the radiological hyperostomy abnormal branches and the improvement of our patients treated according to these physio-pathological principles, justifies a warning against the routine methods of treatment of lymphedema, which are presenting very bad esthetic results everywhere, and justifies the serial and complete angiography of the arteries, veins and lymphatics on the study of all the congenital lymphedemas.

# SURGICAL CLASSIFICATION OF LYMPHEDEMAS

A. K. Cordeiro and F. F. Baracat

Instituto Arnaldo Vieira de Carvalho

São Paulo, Brazil

The classification of lymphedema is a difficult and confusing problem largely because of the lack of knowledge of the lymphatic system compared to the blood vascular system.

Winsor (11) has proposed one of the simplest classifications:

- Primary
- Secondary

The primary lymphedemas include simplex lymphedema, praecox lymphedema, congenital lymphedema, and Milroy's disease.

The secondary lymphedemas include those caused by infections, infestation, inflammation, neoplasia, and irradiation.

Allen (1,2) adds a third group to Winsor's classification, namely, inflammatory lymphedema:

- Primary
- Secondary
- Inflammatory

Martorell (9) adds essential lymphedema (primary or idiopathic) and separates the lymphedemas from lymphostatic verrucosis, chylous reflux-chyloedema, and tumorigenic lymphedema:

1. Congenital lymphedema
2. Essential lymphedema, primary or idiopathic
3. Secondary lymphedema
4. Other types of lymphedema

Martorell's further classification is as follows:

1. Congenital lymphedema

   a - simplex congenital lymphedema
   b - familial congenital lymphedema
   c - congenital lymphedema by amniotic tap

2. Essential lymphedema, primary or idiopathic

3. Secondary lymphedema

   a - tuberculous lymphedema
   b - post-lymphangitic lymphedema
   c - post-phlebitic lymphedema
   d - neoplastic lymphedema
   e - post-roentgentherapy lymphedema
   f - filarial lymphedema
   g - post-mastectomy lymphedema

4. Other types of lymphedemas

   a - lymphostatic verrucosis
   b - chylous reflux-chyloedema
   c - tumorigenic lymphedema

Földi (5,6) classifies the lymphedemas still more extensively:

<u>Classification of Lymphedema - Földi, 1969</u>

A - Malformation of lymph vessels

1. Congenital

   a - familial (Milroy's disease)
   b - nonfamilial

2. Lymphedema praecox (appears before age 35)

   a - familial
   b - nonfamilial

3. Lymphedema tarda (appears after age 35)

B - Occlusion or removal of lymphatic pathways

1. Neoplastic invasion
2. Obstructive lymphangitis (pyogenic infections, filariasis, trichophytosis, tuberculosis, syphilis)
3. Degenerative lymphangiopathy
4. Primary lymph node disease

5. Post-traumatic lymphangiopathy
6. Surgical resection (block dissection)
7. Irradiation (X-ray, radium)

C - Akinetic insufficiency of lymph circulation

1. Causalgia
2. Paralysis

Classification of Lymphedema - Földi, 1971

I. Primary forms

A - Malformation of lymph vessels

1. Congenital

a - familial (Milroy's disease)
b - nonfamilial

2. Lymphedema praecox (appears before age 35)

a - familial
b - nonfamilial

3. Lymphedema tarda (appears after age 35)

II. Secondary forms

1. Neoplastic lymphangitis
2. Obstructive lymphangitis (infections, filariasis, tricophytosis, tuberculosis)
3. Degenerative lymphangiopathy
4. Lymph node disease
5. Post-traumatic lymphangiopathy
6. Surgical resection (block dissection)
7. Roentgen or radium therapy
8. Causalgia
9. Paralysis

Battezzati (3,4) bases his classification on studies with radioactive isotopes (radio-iodinated human albumin marked $^{131}$RIHSA), lymphography, histology, and lymphodynamics:

1 - Lymphedema by disturbance of collecting function: limited to morphologic and functional modification of collectors or lymph nodes;

2 - Lymphedema by disturbance of lymphogenesis and absorption: limited to alterations of lymph production, its physico-chemical composition, and its absorption;

3 - Mixed lymphedema: limited to disturbances of collecting function of lymphogenesis and of absorption.

Other authors subdivide lymphedema by disturbances in collecting function:

A - Lymphedema from hypoplasia or agenesis of collectors
B - Lymphedema from functional insufficiency
C - Lymphedema from parietal modifications
C - Lymphedema from obstruction

Kinmonth's (8) classification is based on clinical, lymphangiographic, and histopathological studies:

A - Primary lymphedemas

1 - Unilateral hyperplasia or "megalymphatics"
2 - Bilateral hyperplasia
3 - With dysgenesis of gonads
4 - With familial pés cavus
5 - Milroy's disease (congenital familia lymphedema)
6 - Primary hypoplastic lymphedema

B - Secondary lymphedemas

a - Trauma and wounds (including surgical excision) of lymph pathways
b - Malignant disease
c - Filariasis
d - Infections and inflammations
e - Radiation

In the present paper, we present a classification of lymphedema based upon clinical, genetic, laboratory, histopathologic, and lymphangiographic studies and medical and surgical treatment.

Material and Method

453 cases of lymphedema of the upper and lower limbs, genitalia, breast, and head and neck were studied from 1960 to 1968 in the First Surgical Clinic of Santa Casa of São Paulo (head, Prof. Dr. Hermeto Jr.) and since 1969 in Instituto Arnaldo Vieira de Carvalho.

Methods of study:

1 - General and specialized physical examinations

2 - Genetic studies: secual chromatin and cariogram of patients, parents, and brothers

3 - Laboratory: blood count; hematocrit; sedimentation rate; total and fractionated proteins; blood glucose; blood urea nitrogen; lipid electrophoresis; protein electrophoresis; antistreptolysin; Na, K, and Cl blood levels; prolinemia and prolinuria; hydroxyprolinemia; and hydroxyprolinuria

4 - Histopathology: staining with HE, PAS, Masson's trichrome, Gomori's trichrome, and Alcian blue

5 - Lymphangiography: Kinmonth's technique for superficial lymphatic system; Tosati's technique for deep lymphatic system, and Romero Marques' technique for deep lymphatic system; radioisotopic lymphography with $^{198}Au$

6 - Clincal treatment

7 - Surgical treatment

8 - Follow-up

9 - Statistics

Classification and Distribution of Our Patients

| | Cases |
|---|---|
| Primary lymphedema | |
| congenital | |
| by amniotic tap | 1 |
| familial - Milroy | 9 |
| gonadal dysgenesis (Turner, Bonnevie-Ulrich) | 1 |
| + pés cavus familial | 1 |
| paecox (between birth and puberty) | 11 |
| tarda (after puberty) | 91 |
| Secondary lymphedema | |
| filarial | 5 |
| tuberculosis | 1 |
| post-lymphangitic | 50 |
| post-phlebitic | 68 |
| neoplastic | 4 |
| post-traumatic | |
| post-surgery | |
| mastectomy | 52 |
| block resection | 3 |
| plastic surgery | 1 |
| saphenectomy | 35 |

Secondary lymphedema (continued)

| | |
|---|---|
| post-radiotherapy | 75 |
| post-accident | |
| fractures | 1 |
| traffic accident | 3 |
| burning | 1 |
| animal bite | 1 |
| chylous reflux - chyloedema | 1 |
| protein-losing enteropathy | 1 |
| post-tumorigenic - lymphangiosarcoma | 1 |
| associated | |
| lympho-fibroedema | 35 |
| lymphostatic verrucosis | 1 |

## References

1. E. V. Allen, Lymphedema of the extremities. Classification, etiology and differential diagnosis. A study of 300 cases. Arch. Intern. Med., 54:606, 1934.

2. E. V. Allen, N. W. Barker, and E. A. Hines, Jr., Peripheral vascular diseases, W. B. Saunders Co., Philadelphia and London, 1965.

3. M. Battezzati and I. Donini, The morphologic and physiologic basis for a new classification of lymphoedema, J. Cardiovasc. Surg. 8:40-45, 1967.

4. M. Battezzati and I. Donini, Il sistema linfatico nella practica clinica, Piccin Editores, Padova, 1967.

5. M. Földi, Diseases of lymphatics and lymph circulation, Akademiai Kiadó, Budapest, 1969.

6. M. Földi, Erkrankungen des Lymphsystems: Grundlagen, Diagnostik, Therapie, Gerhard Witzstrock, Baden-Baden, 1971.

7. J. B. Kinmonth, G. W. Taylor, and R. K. Harper, Lymphangiography, Brit. Med. J., 1:940, 1955.

8. J. B. Kinmonth, The lymphatics: diseases, lymphography, and surgery, Edward Arnold, London, 1972.

9. F. Martorell, Angiologia. Enfermedades vasculares, Salvat Editores, Barcelona, 1967.

10. R. C. Mayall, Edemas linfaticos e venosos dos membros inferiores. Contribuição ao seu diagnostico e orientação terapeutica. Tese de Livre Docencia à Faculdade de Medicina e Cirurgia do Rio de Janeiro, Gunabara, 1970.

11. T. Winsor and C. Hyman, Enfermedades vasculares periféricas, Editoral Interamericana, Mexico, 1967.

# NEW ASPECTS IN THE THERAPY OF LYMPHOEDEMA

M. Földi

3324 Salzgitter-Ringelheim
Postfach 1, West Germany

I assume we all know the modern formulation of the classical Starling hypothesis concerning the dynamics of trans-capillary fluid exchange, based on a physiological equilibrium between the effective blood pressure in the capillary (difference between blood capillary pressure and interstitial pressure) and the effective colloid-osmotic pressure (difference between colloid-osmotic pressure in the capillaries and in the interstitium).

However, I must explain two terms introduced by me, which are already used fairly often in the literature. These are "lymphatic load" and "lymphatic transport capacity".

By "lymphatic load" I mean the amount of plasma protein plus the volume of capillary filtrate which reach the interstitium in unit time and from there cannot be transported via the venous blood capillary loops, i.e. is transported exclusively via the lymph vessels. The "lymphatic transport capacity" is the product of the total cross-section of this vessel system and of the lymph kinetics , i.e. the work which the forces active in the transport of lymph can perform in unit time. The important factors will here be mentioned only briefly: "force pumps" of the lymph initial lymphatics; rhythmic concentrations and relaxations of the lymph-vessel smooth muscles controlled by neural influences and by the work to be performed; the function of the lymph-vessel valves and lymph-vessel-wall permeability not exceeding the physiological level; contractions of the striated muscles; respiratory movements; and arterial pulsation.

Actually, any oedema must be regarded as a disequilibrium between "lymphatic load" and the "lymphatic transport capacity".

According to this definition, a lymphoedema appears when lymphatic transport capacity is insufficient to cope with the normal lymphatic load.

I would like to add at this point that to the interaction of the two forces "lymphatic load" and "lymphatic transport capacity" a third force must be added, the newly discovered process of "extralymphatic mastering of cellular plasma proteins".

We have developed a surgical method which makes it possible to produce a volumetrically standardized lymphoedema. In cooperation with Casley-Smith, histological checks have also been carried out. It was demonstrated that treatment of animals with benzopyrones - we worked with Venalot (R) - had a statistically significant and histologically clearly protective effect. In the compilation of these findings we wrote the following in the discussion of the possible action mechanism of this therapy:

1. "The formation of lymphatico-lymphatic and/or lymphatico-venous anastomoses could be promoted. This would partly eliminate the action of the lymphostasis. This possibility, however, was excluded by lymphoscopic investigations using dyes.

2. The permeability of the blood capillaries to proteins could be reduced ... It seems very improbable that vitamins would reduce the capillary permeability to a subnormal level.

3. By elimination, only one explanation remains...".

Here we put forward the hypothesis that the action of benzopyrone treatment could consist in increasing the function of histiocytes: these might be made to take up and/or digest increasing amounts of proteins. If this were the case, part of the oedema-provoking colloid-osmotic attraction force of these molecules would be made to disappear by the incorporation of plasma proteins. The result of proteolysis would be the same: amino acids are no longer "lymph-obligatory" - they are transported as crystalloid molecules via the venous blood capillaries. This working hypothesis was supported by an experiment carried out together with Kovách in 1965: by administration of benzopyrone we were able to increase the Halpern clearance, i.e. the phagocytosing activity of the RES. In further investigations we showed that a state of vitamin B deficiency leads to an increase in volume of the lymphoedema.

It is well known in immunology that vitamins influence the function of the macrophages. Before exerting their function, these cells increase their metabolism, an optimal vitamin balance being of course inevitable. Axelrod has demonstrated that vitamin deficiencies lead to a slackening of various immunological processes.

Vitale pointed out in 1974, during the opening of a symposium on nutrition and immunology, that vitamins can influence a number of immunological defence processes adversely as well as favourably.

Of course, the mechanisms discusses do not only play a part in lymphoedema, but - mutatis mutandis - in all forms of protein-rich oedemas in which any form of lymph drainage insufficiency is necessarily decisive.

In 1973 we wrote as follows:

"If it is not possible for lymph drainage to transport protein molecules escaped into the interstitium without any residue then the further fate of the tissue under consideration is largely determined by the function of the local connective tissue cells, which are to a certain extent able to take up the proteins and inactivate them colloid-osmotically. By the administration of certain vitamins the function of the connective tissue cells can be enhanced, and in the presence of vitamin deficiency it is reduced".

This theory has largely been confirmed by Casley-Smith and by Földi-Börcsök. Casley-Smith provoked lymphoedema in rats by a surgical method. Two radioactively labelled lymph-obligatory colloids were injected simultaneously into the oedematous subcutaneous connective tissue: $Cr^{51}$-albumin and $J^{151}$-polyvinyl-pyrrolidone (with a molecular weight corresponding to the albumin). The principal difference between the two substances is that the body has no mechanism that could decompose PVP, break it down into fragments of lower molecular weight, and thus inactivate them colloidosmotically. Continuous measurement of the activities corresponding to the two tracer substances showed that the injection of a benzopyrone preparation strongly accelerated the clearance of labelled albumin, but not that of PVP.

In another experimental series Casley-Smith incubated peritoneal macrophages in vitro with plasma. The proteolysis was measured as a function of time (expressed in terms of liberated glycine) and was increased by 250% with statistical significance after the addition of benzopyrone.

Földi-Börcsök investigated the cell population of lymphoedema fluid in stained smear preparations 48 h after the onset of lymphostasis in rats. One group was treated with a benzopyrone preparation, another with physiological saline. It was shown that after benzopyrone the number of phagocytosing macrophages was significantly increased.

As is known, it is possible to remove macrophages selectively from the body in animal experiments by intraperitoneal injection of very fine quartz powder: the macrophages are destroyed in their efforts to phagocytose the quartz crystals. I asked Casley-Smith to provoke oedema in rats "demacrophagocytosed" in this way and to treat these animals with benzopyrones. He found that in such animals the therapeutic effect of benzopyrones disappeared almost completely.

In the experimental lymphoedema, by the way, Casley-Smith detected after the administration of benzopyrones an increase in the serum concentration of neutral proteases: this is again a sign of the part played by the macrophages. In thermal oedema, however, he found after the application of benzopyrone a rise of the acid phosphatases; this speaks in favour of the fact that microphages are also influenced by benzopyrones (above all in inflammatory processes).

For the maintenance of a constant internal environment of the connective tissue, the body is thus equipped with two devices, one involving the canalicular drainage system of the lymph vessels and one the macrophages. They assist the lymph system by the uptake, storage, and digestion of extravascular proteins.

MEDICAL TREATMENT OF LYMPHEDEMA

H. R. van der Molen

Policlinic for Phlebology
Terwolde, Netherlands

Before turning to the medical treatment of lymphedema, several physical principles will be reviewed.

When you "bandage" a cylinder, the compression force is proportional to the tension and is equal all over the surface of the cylinder (Fig. 1). When you "bandage" a cube, on the other hand, the compression of the surface is zero, however great the tension. But at the edges, especially when they are sharp, there will be a very high pressure, and when you pull hard you risk cutting the tissue (Fig. 2). This is equivalent to the statement that for a plane surface, i.e., one with a very large radius of curvature ($R_1$),

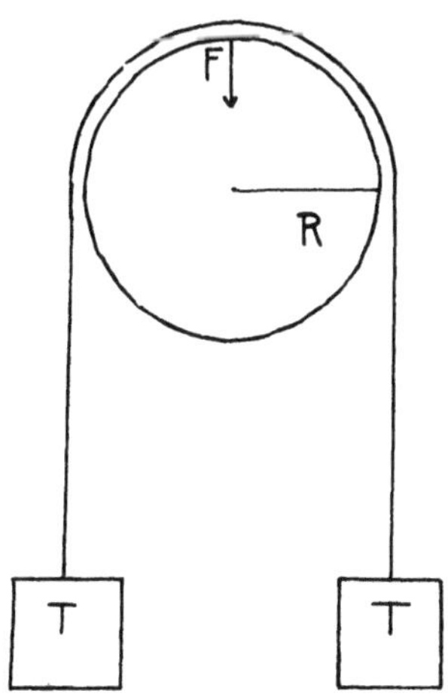


Fig. 1

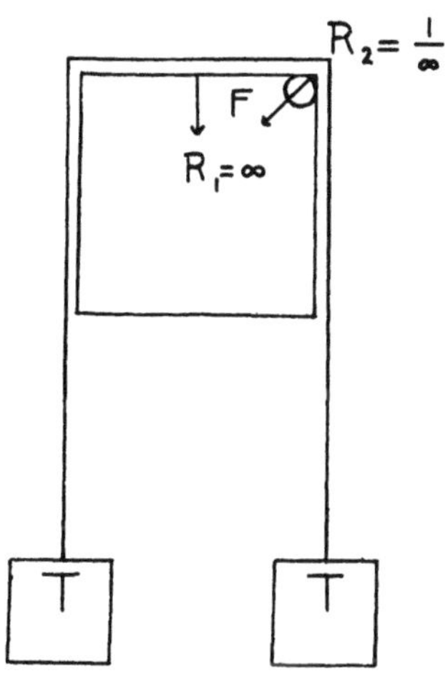


Fig. 2

$$F = \frac{T}{R}$$

Fig. 3

the pressure is small or zero, but for a very small radius of curvature ($R_2$), as is the case at an edge, the pressure on the surface is very high.

Thus, Laplace's formula can be applied: the pressure (force F) is proportional to the tension, but inversely proportional to the radius of curvature of the surface: P = T/R (Fig. 3). This principle has very important implications when applying high pressure, for instance, to the inner face of the tibia, the dorsum of the foot, and especially the retromalleolar spaces, where the radius of curvature is "negative." In those locations, you have to correct the surface in order to get a proper pressure: making the radius smaller (Figs. 4, 5) or greater (Figs. 6, 7), or changing its sign (Figs. 6, 7, 8). A different situation exists in locations where the radius is too small, e.g., the malleolus, the Achilles tendon, the lateral side of the foot, or the popliteal tendons. There the surface must be equalized with rolls (Fig. 6) or rings (Fig. 7) of carded cotton wool. A swollen foot can be compressed with the help of little balls (Fig. 5).

Considering the leg as a whole, it may be compared to a cone. Coming from the bottom up and applying ever the same traction force will nevertheless result in diminished pressure as you approach the groin and the radius becomes greater.

Now let us first consider a post-thrombotic leg with induration on the inner tibia surface. Where the lymphatics and the blood capillaries are distended, the permeability of their wall is increased. Slight trauma may reverse osmotic conditions so that reabsorption is locally impossible, and fluid accumulates in the intercellular

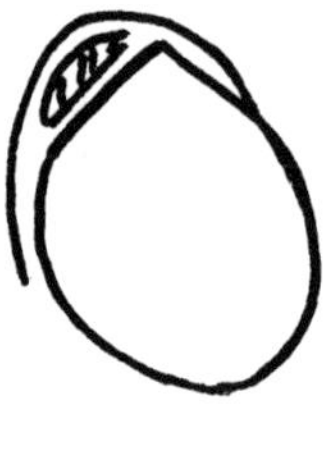

Fig. 4

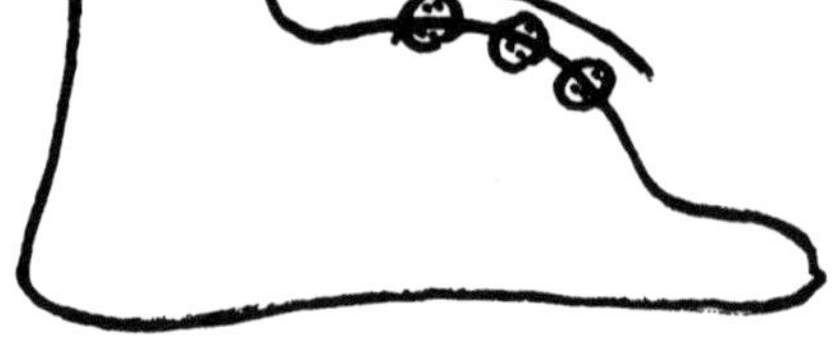

Fig. 5

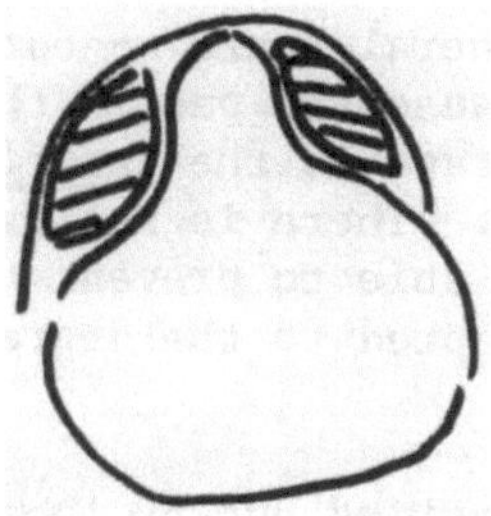

Fig. 6

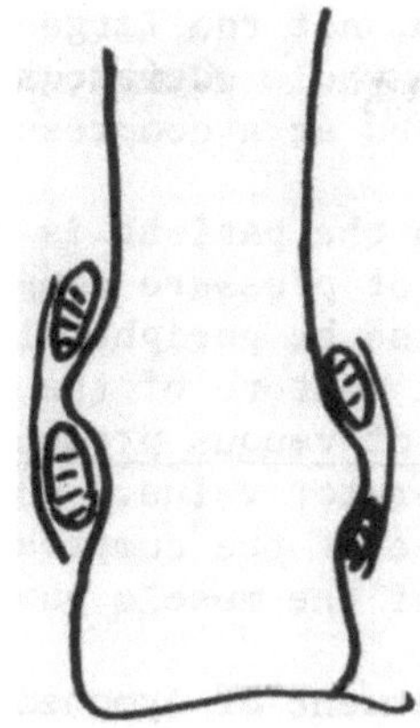

Fig. 7

spaces. Protein disintegrates, liberating vasodilator products, and there is red and painful swelling.

This condition will respond nicely to moderate compression with restoration of the circulation by removal of edema and interstitial proteins and prevention of capillary thrombosis and its consequences, especially white atrophy and pigmentation, thereby preventing ulceration.

Most induration can be cured by proper compression, which can be carried out in the following manner: The swollen area is covered with a layer of carded cotton wool over a rubber pad of 1 cm

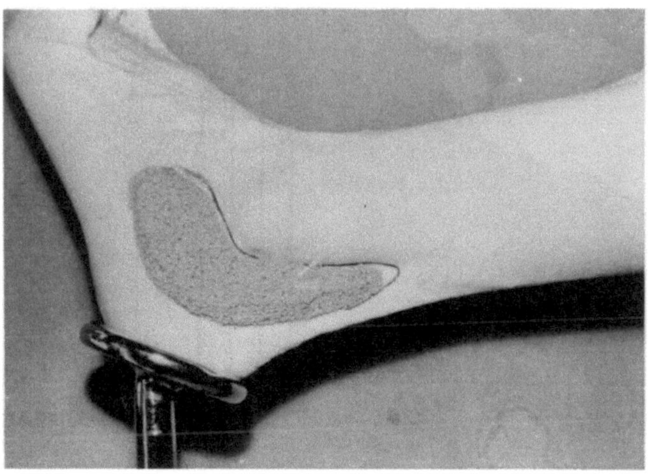

Fig. 8. Retro- and inframalleolar rubber pad.

thickness, not too large so as to avoid dead space, long enough to cover the whole edematous area. Then flannel (nonelastic) bandages are wrapped at a compression of 80 - 100 mm Hg.

When the patient is walking there will be a peripheral rhythmic increase of pressure comparable to a peripheral heart -- but there should also be peripheral hypertension because the pad is thin. The essential feature of the post-thrombotic state is the insufficient lowering of venous pressure during walking. There is reflux through the perforator veins. Only compression is able to prevent this, and the degree of the compression should be adapted to the degree of leakage of the muscle pump.

Treatment of lymphedema can also be carried out by local compression, but it should be stronger than in post-thrombotic cases. The Doppler apparatus can be used to ascertain whether there are major leaks in the venous system. In "pure" lymphedema, treatment by very strong compression is painless and can be carried out without general anesthesia, which in fact is contraindicated and leads to the rare complications associated with this procedure.

General Management

Obesity is not uncommon in lymphedema patients (Fig. 9), particularly after the age of 40, and this associated condition should be treated. Arterial hypertension, more often systolic, should also be controlled at first with a salt-free diet (Fig. 10).

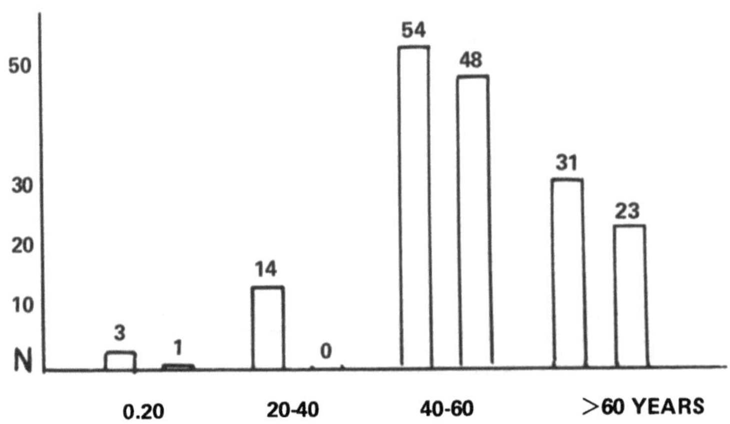


Fig. 9. Obesity in lymphedema patients. The left bar of each pair represents patients 10 kg or more overweight.

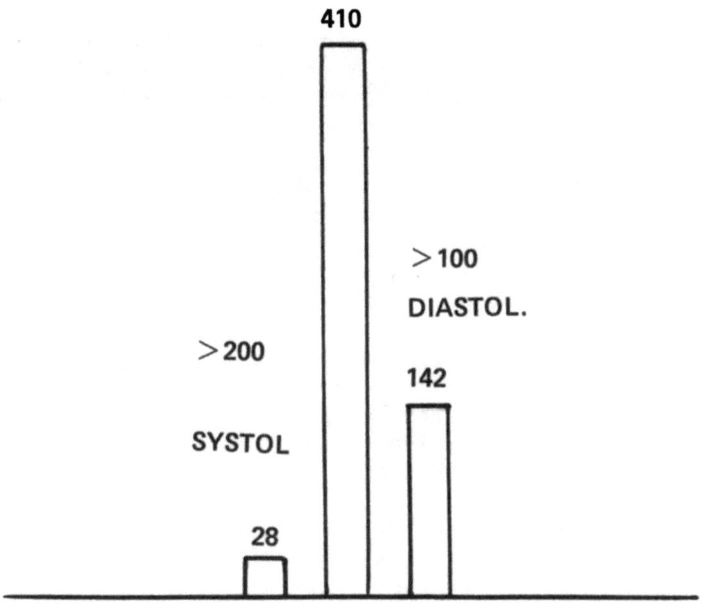


Fig. 10. Blood pressure of lymphedema patients.

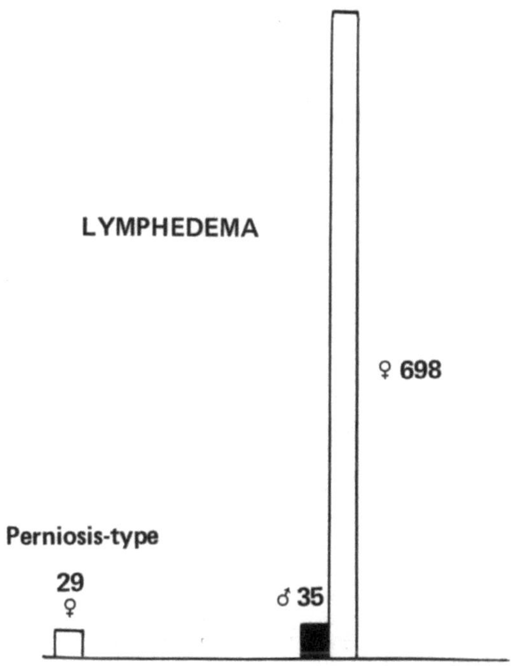


Fig. 11. Distribution of lymphedema patients by sex.

While this series is restricted to primary lymphedema, tumors in the pelvis (uterus, ovaries, prostate) can produce secondary lymphedema, and these tumors should be operated upon or otherwise treated.

The majority of patients with lymphedema are women (Fig. 11). While the reason for this is unclear, menstrual and pregnancy cycles are accompanied by great variation in vascularity, and this cyclic hyperemia may account for associated pronounced lymphatic circulatory changes in women that are not observed in men.

Lymphography and vital blue dye studies show that in most lymphedemas there is a relative lack of valved lymph vessels. The system is not truncal but rather reticular. In addition, there may be reduction in the number of lymph nodes. Total aplasia, if it exists, is very rare (Kinmonth).

Diuretics, in our opinion, are not appropriate treatment except in cases of arterial hypertension. In lymphedema, there is no renal insufficiency, so that it is not logical to make artificial kidney leaks. They may, however, be used temporarily before treatment by physical means.

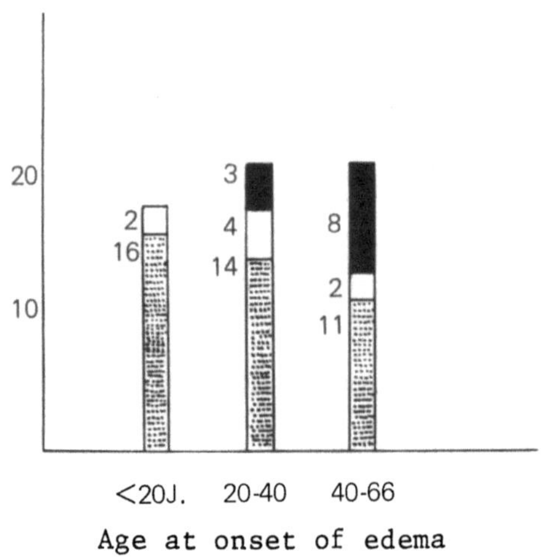


Fig. 12. Lymphedema before or after "inflammation."

edema first, "inflammation" afterwards;
edema and "inflammation" simultaneously;
"inflammation" first, edema afterwards.

Antibiotics are necessary when there are coexisting or prior recent bacterial infections whether or not they are accompanied by fever.

Lymphedematous tissue may be infected by true erysipelas or streptococcal lymphangitis. But far more often there are pseudo-erysipelas episodes: nonbacterial sterile lymphangiothrombosis. These two entities can be easily distinguished: patients suffering from lymphangiothrombosis -- just as patients with post-thrombotic induration or varico-phlebitis -- are relieved by a well applied local compression bandage. True erysipelas will not tolerate the slightest compression: it is a case of noli me tangere. The border of the lesion is also slightly elevated and progressing. In both instances, however, lymphedema will be worse after the attack. Our statistics show that such "inflammation" is rarely the cause and almost always the effect of preexisting lymphedema. In older persons, however, the reverse sequence may be seen: lymphedema caused (or revealed) by true streptococcal erysipelas (Fig. 12).

Post-filarial lymphedema is only seen in individuals who have lived in the tropics. As filariasis is no longer active when lymph-

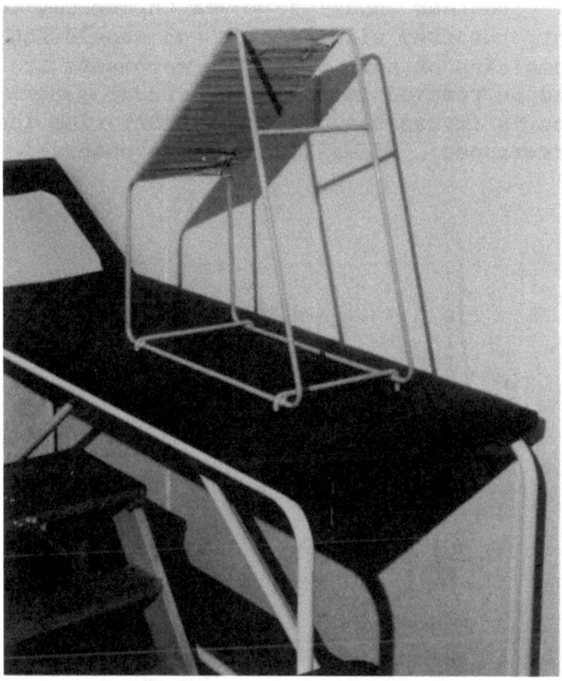

Fig. 13. Elevation at $45^{o}$.

edema is present, treatment does not differ from other forms of lymphedema. If microfilaria are found in the "midnight blood," the infestation must be treated appropriately.

Local compression treatment of lymphedema should be carried out without general anesthesia, which is not only unnecessary but may be harmful as it can lead to necrosis and paralysis. Compression treatment is performed in three stages:

1. First, elevation of the leg at a slope of 45$^{o}$ on an appropriate support for about 15 minutes (Fig. 13).

2. Next, bandaging with the very strong biflex bandages of Thuasne (Paris). When there is malleolar edema, the shape of a "culotte de zouave" with the retro- and inframalloelar spaces supercompressed with special rubber pads (2 cm rubber thickness) may be helpful (Figs. 8, 14). This shape will disappear rapidly even after the first compression treatment. When the dorsum of the foot is very edematous, one to five small hard rubber balls may be inserted under the bandage (Fig. 5), in order to produce holes in the edema. Bandaging alone will not be sufficient as the radius of the surface is too great.

The well-bandaged leg will stay in the elevated position for about 10 minutes. The toes should be moved throughout the compression treatment, but they will be blue and should not be white. If the patient complains of pain or if toe movements are impossible, the bandage should be removed immediately. Under general anesthesia proper cooperation is impossible. After a short time the biflex 18 bandages may be rewrapped. Edema fluid can be observed to come

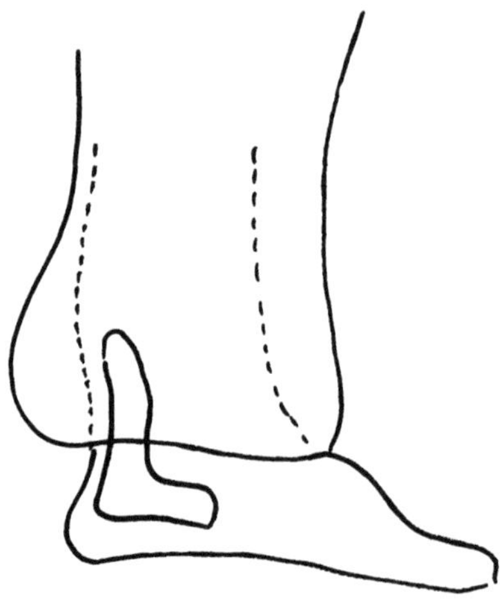

Fig. 14

upwards under the knee. Then carded cotton wool is placed in the fossa poplitea in order to protect the vessels, and a lighter elastic bandage is applied over the knee.

When this phase of the treatment does not produce a sufficient reduction in size (3-4 cm), phase 3 must be instituted.

3. Tube treatment. A soft rubber tube is used ("feuille anglaise"), 6-10 m long, 3/4 inch in diameter. First, wrap the foot including the rubber pads for the retromalleolar space and the ankles very tightly with biflex 18. Next, wind the tube around the leg until it forms a double rubber layer. When it is pulled during the winding a very strong compression is produced, measured by us at 1/2 - 2/3 of an atmosphere (5-7½ m water). After each turn a bulging protuberant circular rim, 1-1½ cm thick, will be seen progressing slowly (Fig. 15). It is best not to wind the whole leg, but to proceed in stages, i.e., one-third of the leg first. When the edema is extubated over this length, the portion is wrapped tightly with biflex 18.

In three or four repeated applications to the remaining edematous portions, the knee will be reached. This procedure is painless or almost painless in all lymphedemas having an intact venous system. The tibia periost is painful only in venous disease, but in such cases tube treatment is not necessary. The tube is left in place for 3-10 minutes and like the Thuasne bandages is taken off promptly if the patient complains of pain.

In one treatment circumference can be reduced 3-7 cm or even more on occasion. The quantity of water eliminated by the kidneys

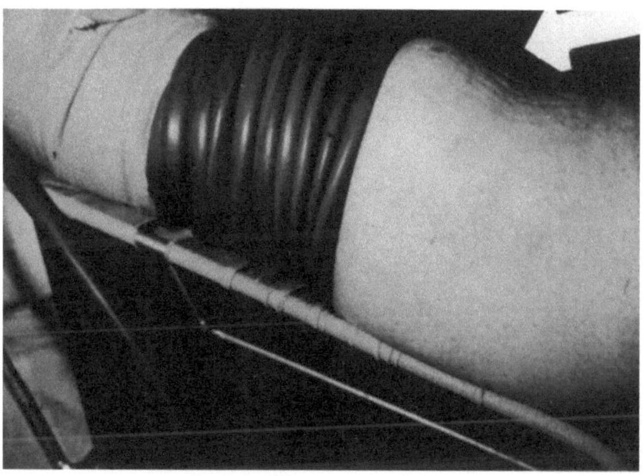

Fig. 15. Progressing edema ridge seen in "extubation."

in a few hours, even without diuretics, can be 1-2 liters, and up to 10 to 12 liters at the end of the treatment. Therefore, it is advisable to weigh the patient before an extubation. The skin becomes too loose for the extremity and it hangs like an empty sack around the leg. In a few days or weeks, however, the appearance will improve spontaneously.

The movement of lymph can be seen when vital blue is injected before the treatment (as allergic phenomena are possible with the dye, antishock measures should be at hand). The dye disperses in a cranial direction, but part of it may be taken up by deep lymphatic collectors.

Elephantiastic papillomas and keloid scars (consequences of lymph stasis) will flatten completely or partly.

Occasionally, we have to remove lymph from the thigh. Tubes should be avoided in this area so as not to disturb arterial flow. If the biflex 18 does not give sufficient compression, it can be replaced with a 5-cm-wide thick rubber-impregnated cotton bandage (tissue reference 91 E Thuasne Paris) as is used in making beds, chairs, etc. These may also be applied in cases where the tube cannot be used, e.g., where there are painful scars or old inflammation. The reduction treatment generally will last 1-2 hours at a time. It can be restarted after 1-7 days. In the meantime, the leg is wrapped with nonelastic bandages and the retromalleolar spaces filled and compressed with rubber pads, 1 cm thick. Flannel is the best material as it remains in place.

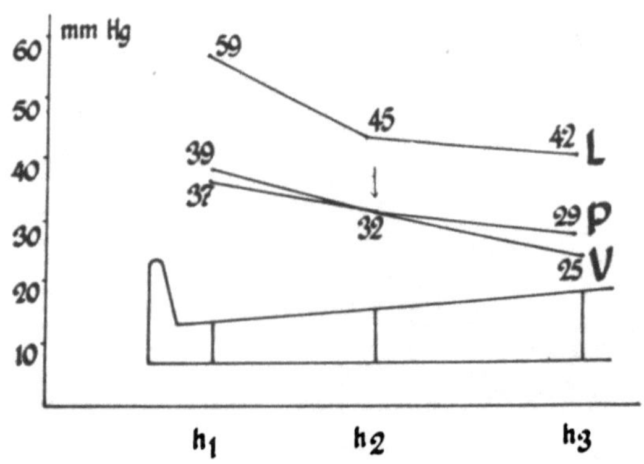


Fig. 16. Permanent compression with elastic stockings, showing the compression force required for the prevention of edema.
(L) 17 cases of lymphedema;
(P) 28 cases of post-thrombotic edema;
(V) 43 cases of varicose edema.

Why is it necessary to have a nonelastic bandage in the interval between treatments? The reason is that compression variations during walking are very great with the nonelastic bandage. This can easily be shown when you put a blood pressure tensiometer around the lower third of the leg and pump to 80 mm Hg. If you then move the toes upward you will see the pressure rising to 130–160 mm Hg: in fact the diameter will increase as the extensor tendons protrude. As the bandage cannot distend, the pressure becomes high (almost double the initial pressure).

Elastic bandages have two disadvantages. In the first place, the person who puts the bandage on cannot easily judge the degree of compression; only the patient notices when the turn is too tight. Secondly, as there is a high resting pressure, variations with walking are less: due to its elasticity, the bandage will distend.

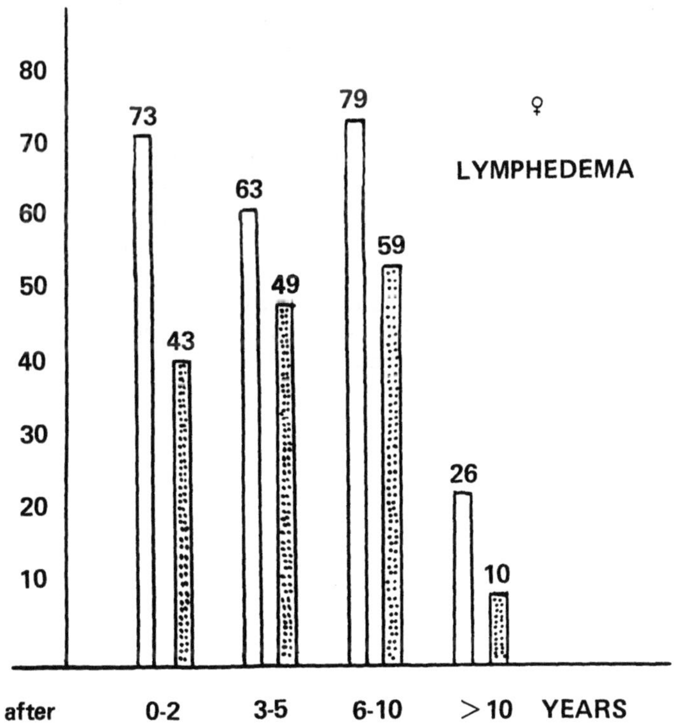


Fig. 17. Results of treatment.

□ circumference of calf diminished or increased not more than 3 cm;

⊡ increase more than 3 cm.

So a nonelastic bandage is better for a walking bandage: it is well tolerated at rest, very active in driving out edema during walking.

On the other hand, in a patient lying on a table with the leg elevated, compression is best with elastic material but for a short time only. So after treatment by elastic reduction, the patient walking with nonelastic flannel bandage will exhibit a further diminution in circumference of 1 or 2 cm by the next visit.

Treatments are repeated 2-6 times, until no further reduction is obtained. The edema will have disappeared with only fat and fibrous tissue left. Next, measurements for an elastic stocking should be taken for permanent support during working hours. When compression force is high enough, the return of edema will be prevented. For taking measurements, the circumference of the foot, ankle, and leg should be recorded with a device having centimeter gradations at an angle of 90°. Every 5-15 cm, the circumference from toes to knee or even to groin is taken.

The permanent compression force required is about 40 mm Hg in post-thrombotic cases and about 60 mm Hg in lymphedema (Fig. 16). Women naturally will prefer very thin stockings, but these are inadequate in most cases. Only very mild cases devoting considerable time to gymnastics, taking diuretics or other drugs for their dehydrating action, or using some pneumatic device might be controlled in this fashion. Most patients come to learn that only strong support will give them permanent relief, and this is why the statistics show that the best results are noted after the longest observation period (over 10 years) (Figs. 17, 18).

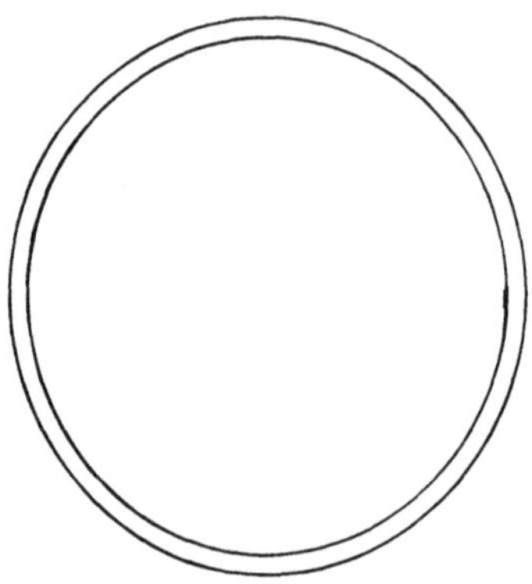

Fig. 18. Increase of calf circumference by 3 cm:
$2\pi(R_o + \frac{1}{2}) = 2\pi R_o + 3.$

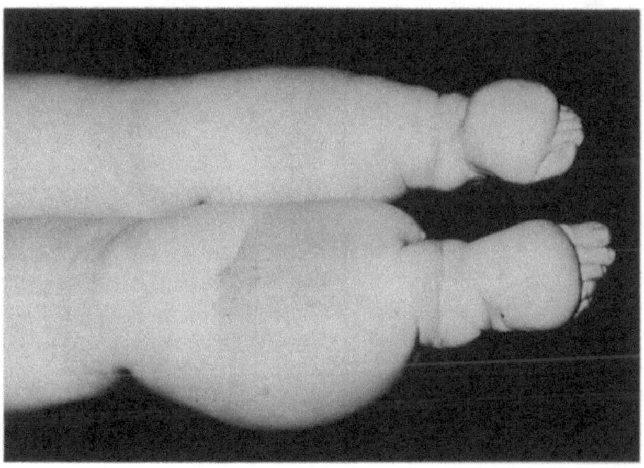

Fig. 19A. Old woman (invalid) before treatment.

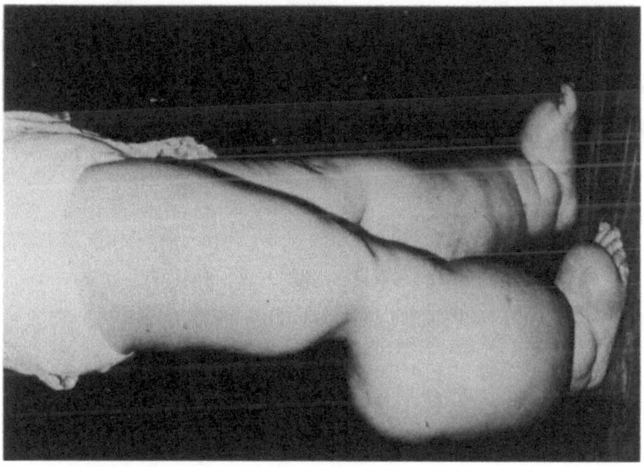

Fig. 19B. Old woman (invalid) before treatment.

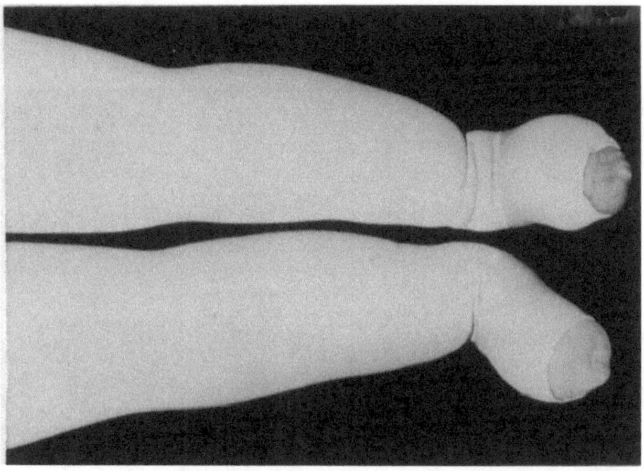

Fig. 19C. Old woman (invalid) after treatment.

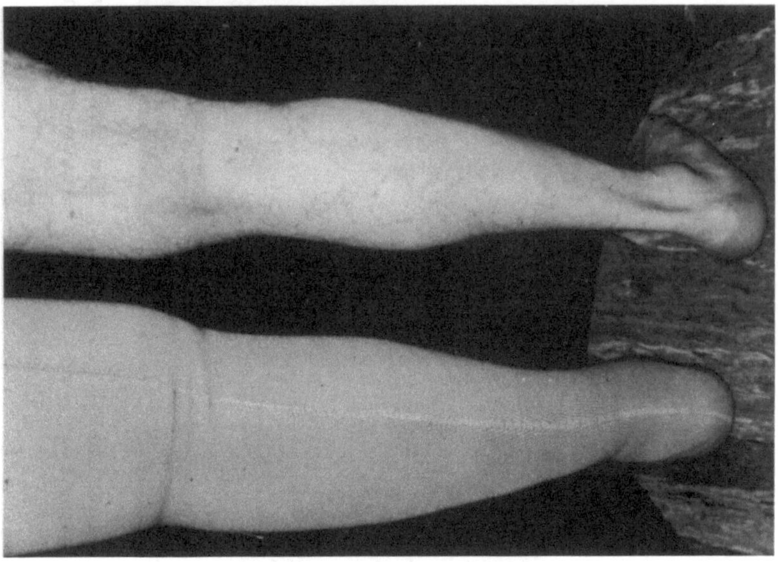

Fig. 20B. Old man after treatment.

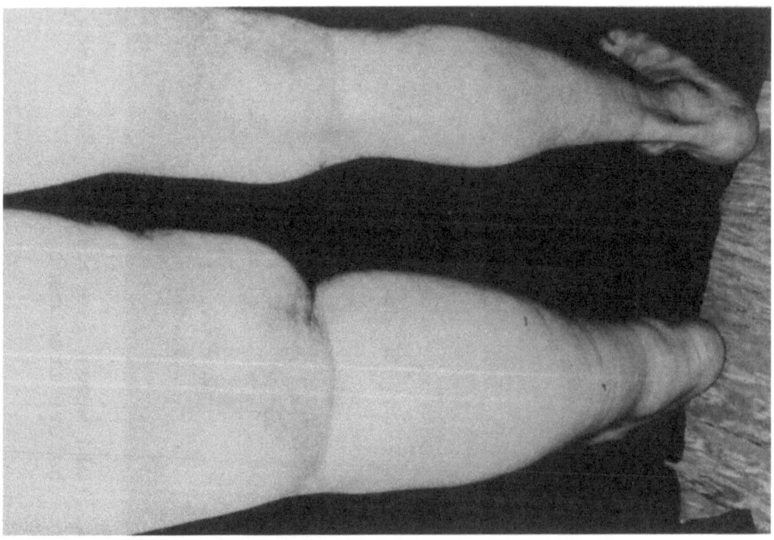

Fig. 20A. Old man before treatment.

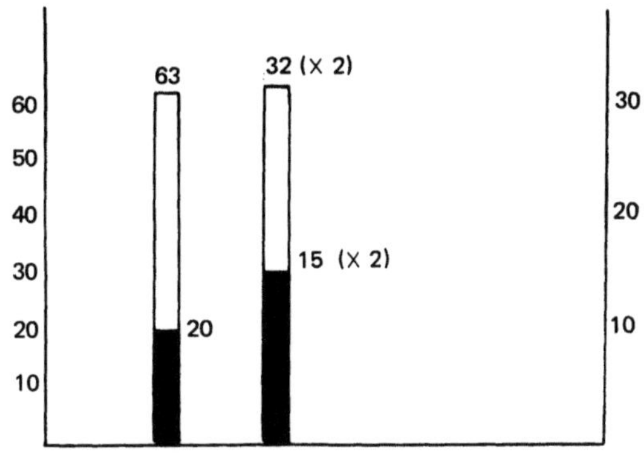


Fig. 21. 95 cases of lymphedema accompanied by "inflammation" before and after ■ treatment, with (left) and without (right) permanent elastic compression.

In a smaller number of cases, however, patients can do without stockings in subsequent years. The possibility of neovascularization with lymphatics in tissues free from edema cannot be excluded.

The strong quality of the superneodurelna varitex stockings can be utilized with success even in severe elephantiasis with lower leg circumferences of 50 cm or more (Figs. 19A,B,C, Figs. 20A,B).

Pseudo-erysipelas (lymphangiothrombosis) frequency is reduced but not abolished (Fig. 21).

Is lymphedema always "praecox?" No, the congenital scarcity of valved lymphatic vessels is often well compensated for until conditions arise overwhelming their capacity, specifically, trauma, hot climate, infections, and professions requiring standing upright for long hours.

# NEW TECHNIQUE OF LYMPHATIC-VENOUS ANASTOMOSIS FOR THE TREATMENT OF LYMPHEDEMA

Mario Degni

R. D. Viridiana 661

01238 São Paulo, Brazil

## Method

80 x 12, 80 x 15, or more rarely 80 x 18 special needles (Fig. A) are used in which one-third of the circumference has been removed to a length of 2.5 cm from the end of the needle. This superficial groove permits free passage of a curved arterial needle with 6-0 or 7-0 nylon. The lymphatics are stained with patent blue violet (PBV) according to Kinmonth's technique.

Blockage at the level of the groin lymph nodes (Fig. B) is used to exemplify this technique. Figure C shows the cutaneous incision, exposure of one lymphatic and the saphena magna vein, and one or two of its collateral branches. The lymphatic vessel is then cut and the distal stump tied or ligated (Fig. D).

Subsequently a 80 x 15 mm needle (or a needle of some other caliber) is introduced into the lumen of the vein (Fig. E) and then the lymphatic trunk is pierced (Figs. F and G) with a curved arterial needle with 6-0 nylon thread on two needles. The arterial needle either pierces the lymphatic and comes out in the opening of the lymphatic or pierces its walls on opposite sides. In this case a special maneuver, to be described later, tying the two nylon threads is applied.

In Fig. G, the curved arterial needle pierces the vein wall from the inside to the outside at a distance of 2 mm (Fig. H). We now repeat the same maneuver with the other arterial needle, keeping a distance of 1-1.5 mm between the threads. The surgeon then applies steady traction to both threads in order to introduce the

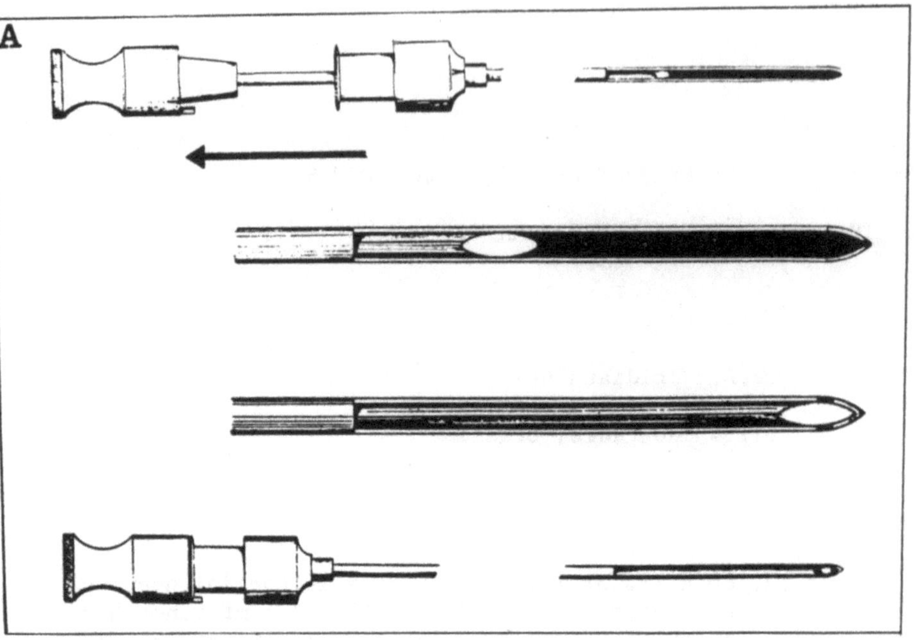
A

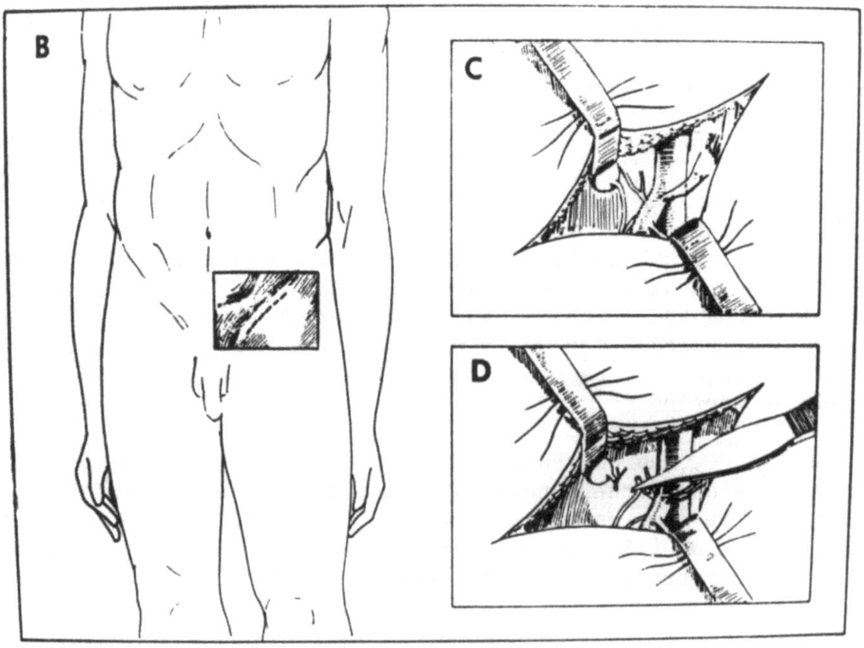
B
C
D

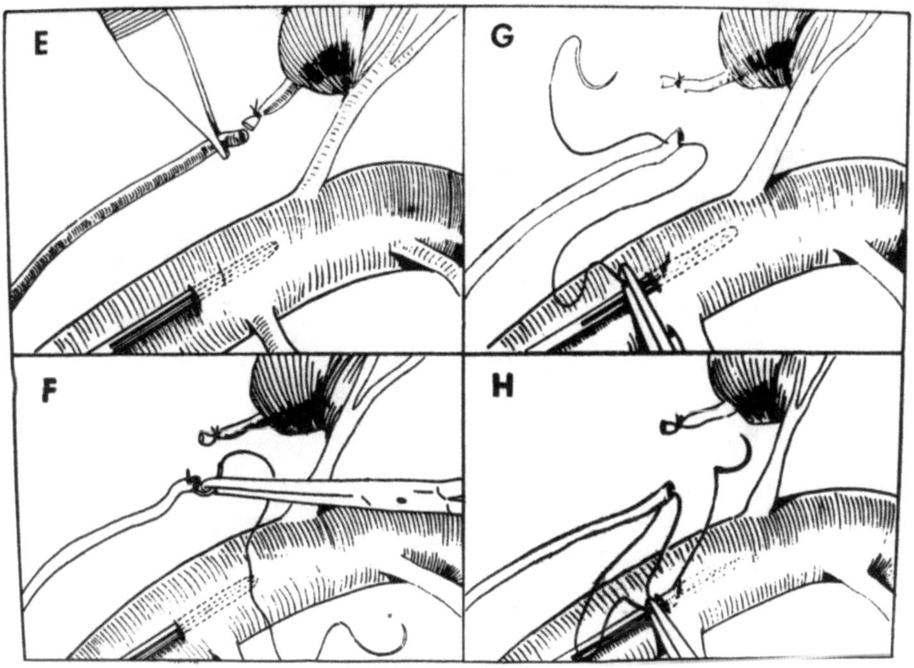
E
G
F
H

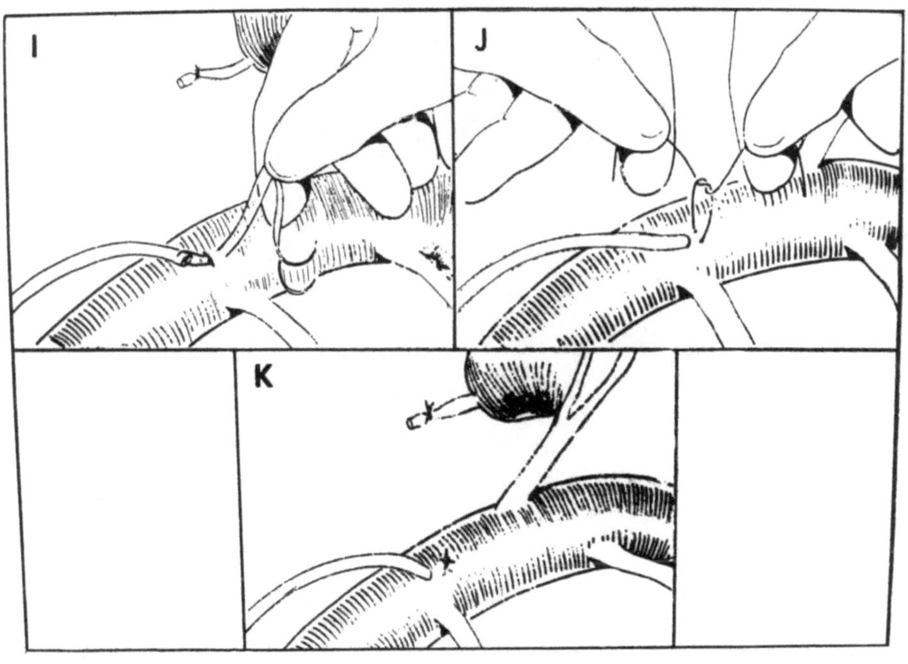
I
J
K

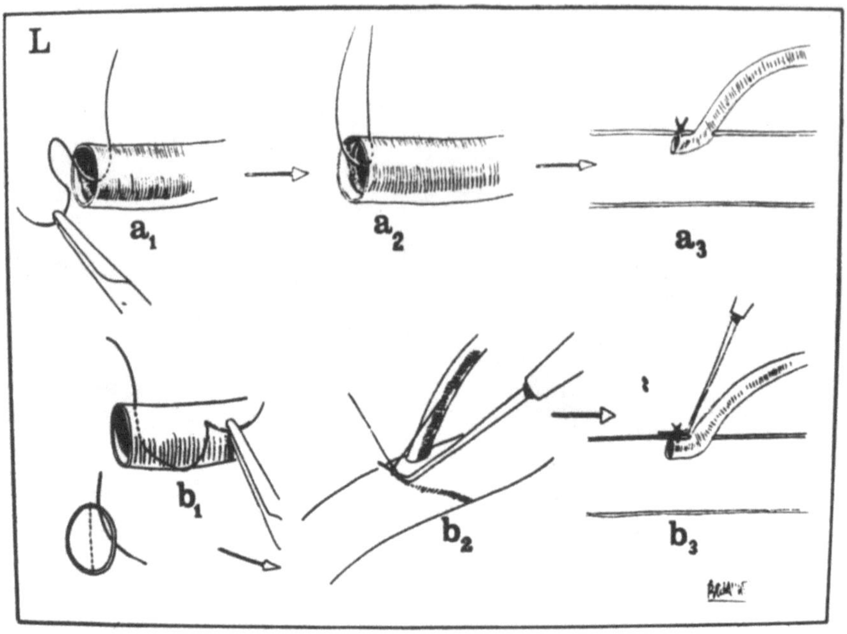


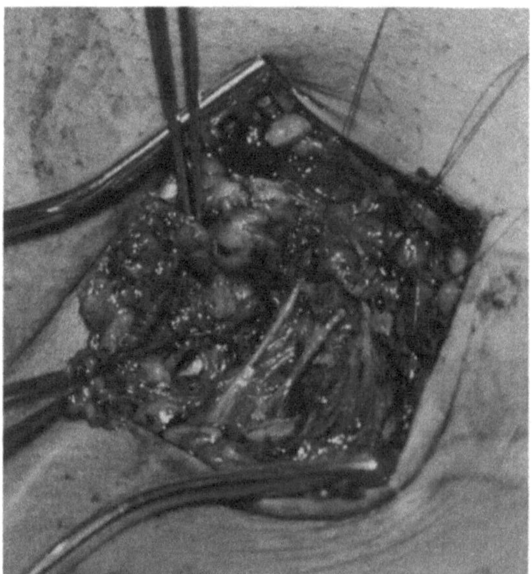

Fig. 1. Surgical dissection and exposure of three lymphatic trunks or ducts colored by PVB and a lymph node. The three lymphatics are gently pulled by a loop of cotton thread.

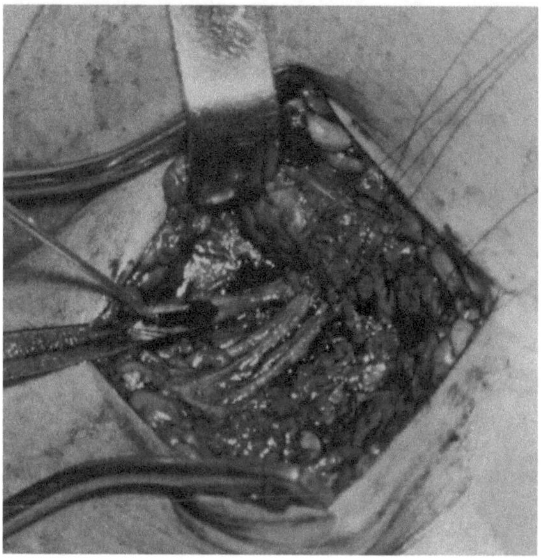

Fig. 2. The special angled needle (80 x 15) is inserted into the great saphenous vein.

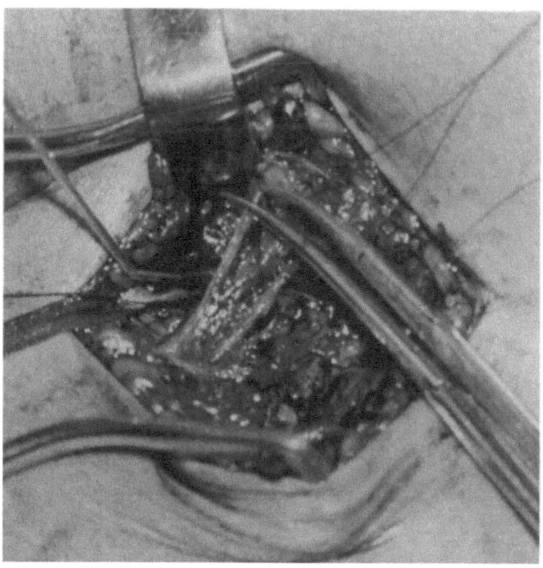

Fig. 3. The lymphatic to be anastomosed is clamped and in the process of being cut, with subsequent ligation of the end going to the lymph node.

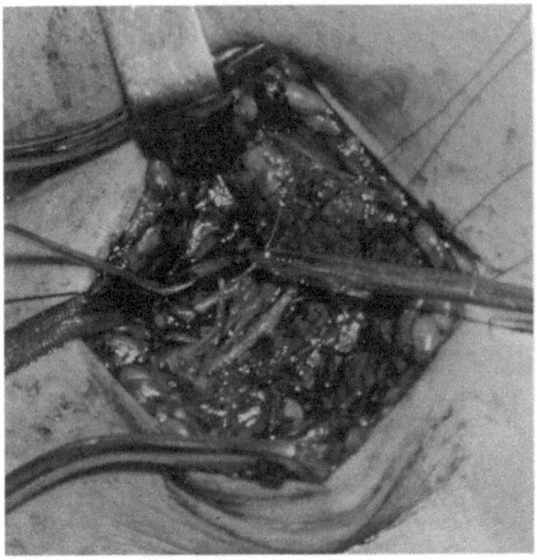

Fig. 4. One of the curved arterial needles with 6-0 nylon thread pierces the wall of the lymphatic.

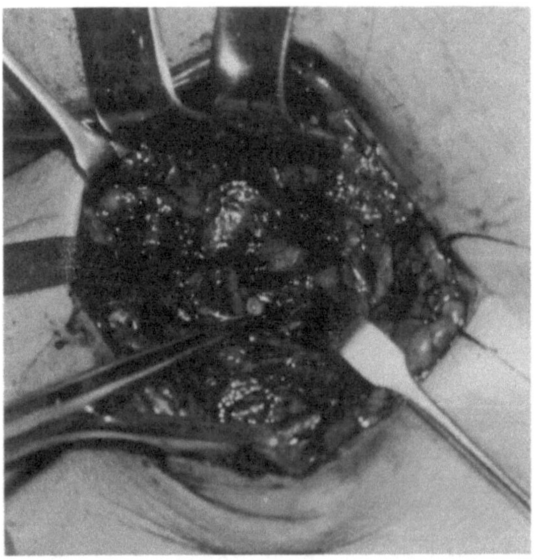

Fig. 5. The curved arterial needle emerging from the lymphatic lumen.

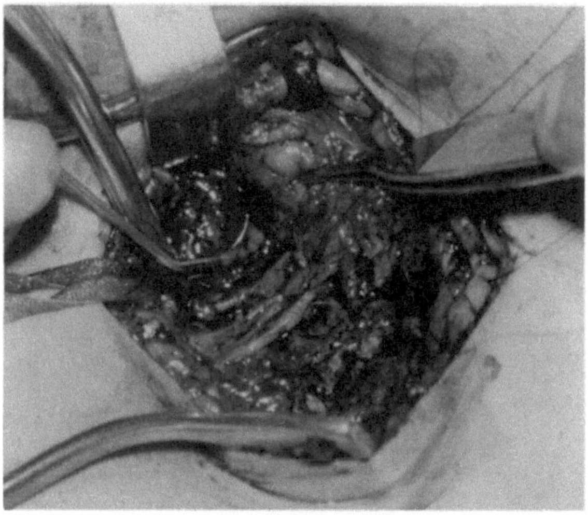

Fig. 6. In this step of the anastomosis the curved arterial needle is placed in the groove of the 80 x 15 needle and pierces the wall of the vein from the inside to the outside. The needle emerges 2 mm from the hole in the vein. The same maneuver is repeated with the other curved arterial needle, the distance between the two threads being 1-1.5 mm.

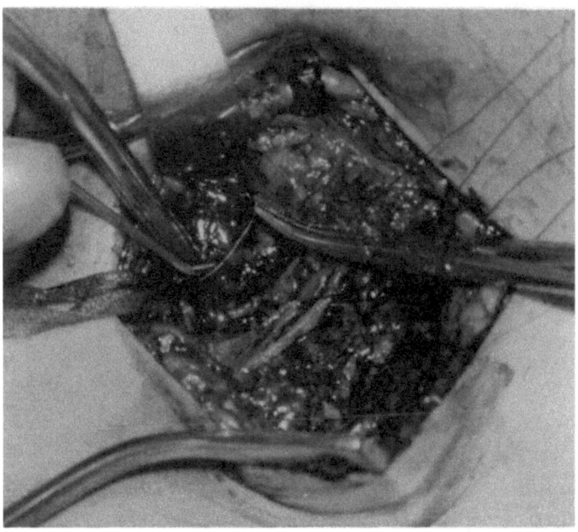

Fig. 7. The curved arterial needle emerging from the vein by means of the needle holder (in this case a curved mosquito).

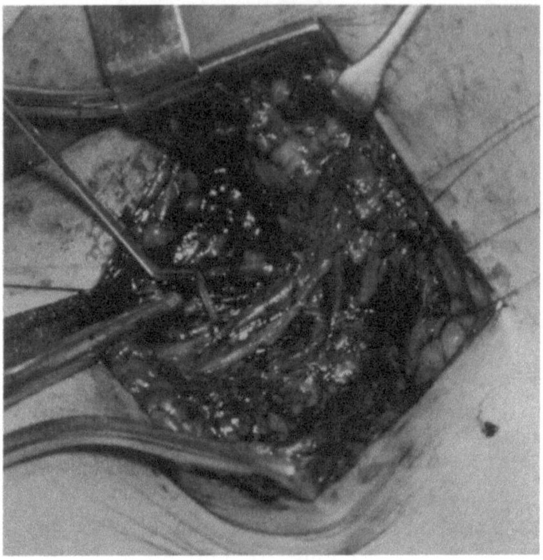

Fig. 8. The lymphatic is introduced into the vein by traction on the two threads.

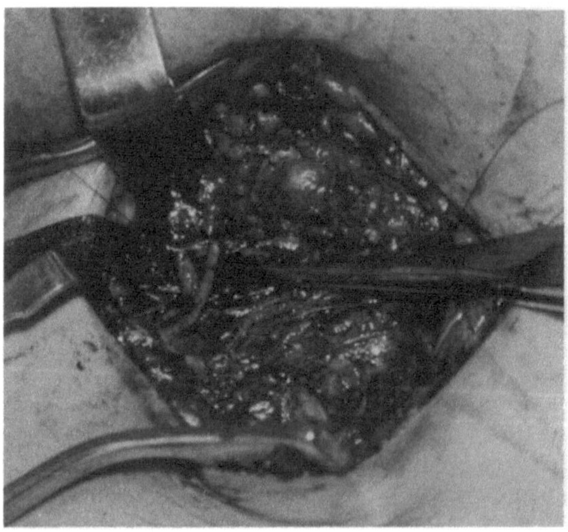

Fig. 9. Two lymphatic-venous anastomoses completed.

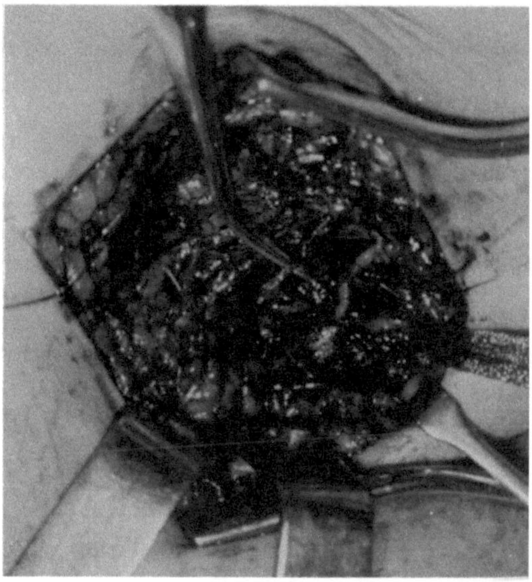

Fig. 10. Two lymphatic-venous anastomoses. By gentle squeezing of one lymphatic, PBV enters the vein demonstrating the patency of the anastomosis.

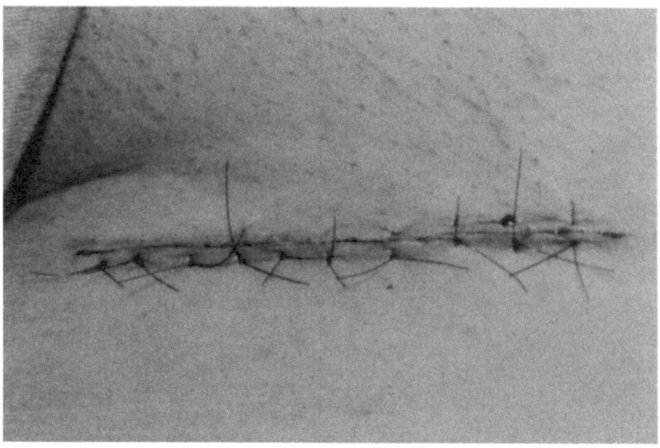

Fig. 11. Interrupted suture of the skin with 4-0 nylon thread.

lymphatic stump into the lumen of the vein (Fig. I) while the assistant removes the vein needle. To complete the anastomosis the two nylon threads are tied (Figs. J and K).

The same steps are repeated for the other anastomoses (generally 3 to 7 more).

In Fig. L ($a_1$) the best maneuver to pass the arterial needle is depicted. In Fig. L ($b_1$), when the thread pierces both walls of the lymphatic, the lumen must be maintained. The knot is tied with one stylet inside the loops, thereby avoiding stenosis of the lymphatic. Photographs of the various steps of the operation are shown in Figs. 1-11.

Reduction of edema was proportional to the number of anastomoses. In cases of megalymphatics with valvular insufficiency of superficial lymphatics, the lymphatic-venous anastomosis was constructed in the middle third of the leg. Other levels are selected according to the level of lymphatic blockage.

## Results

Fifteen patients were operated upon, with an average 63.07% reduction in edema.

# NEW TECHNIQUE OF DRAINAGE OF THE SUBCUTANEOUS TISSUE OF THE LIMBS WITH NYLON NET FOR TREATMENT OF LYMPHEDEMA

Mario Degni

R. D. Viridiana 661

01238 São Paulo, Brazil

The Handley technique of subcutaneous tissue drainage with threads, especially silk, has been extensively criticized. Our technique was conceived for a more extensive lymph drainage of the whole or part of a limb (according to the location of the edema). Multinylon thread No. 0 is utilized and triamcinolone acetonide administered postoperatively for a month or longer to avoid active fibroblast reproduction and formation of a cylinder of fibroblasts separating the thread from the interstitial fluid. The latter complication is one of the worst problems with the Handley procedure.

Special instruments were designed: three types of needles as in Figs. 1, 2, and 3, and a matching handle with a lateral groove to receive the needle and a set screw to fix it.

In Figs. 4 and 5, the concept of the net is introduced with four longitudinal threads, eight spiral threads (4 clockwise and 4 counterclockwise), and seven circular threads. All these threads are interwoven with "Paris knots," thus forming a subcutaneous net of mononylon thread No. 1.

In Fig. 6 small skin incisions are depicted arranged longitudinally along the limb up to the abdomen and buttocks. On the abdomen the thread must go above the level of the umbilicus. The incisions at the level of the malleoli are numbered No. 1 (premalleolar medial region), 2, 3, and 4 in clockwise direction, when viewed from the sole of the left foot (Fig. 6). The four longitudinal threads, numbered correspondingly, are inserted.

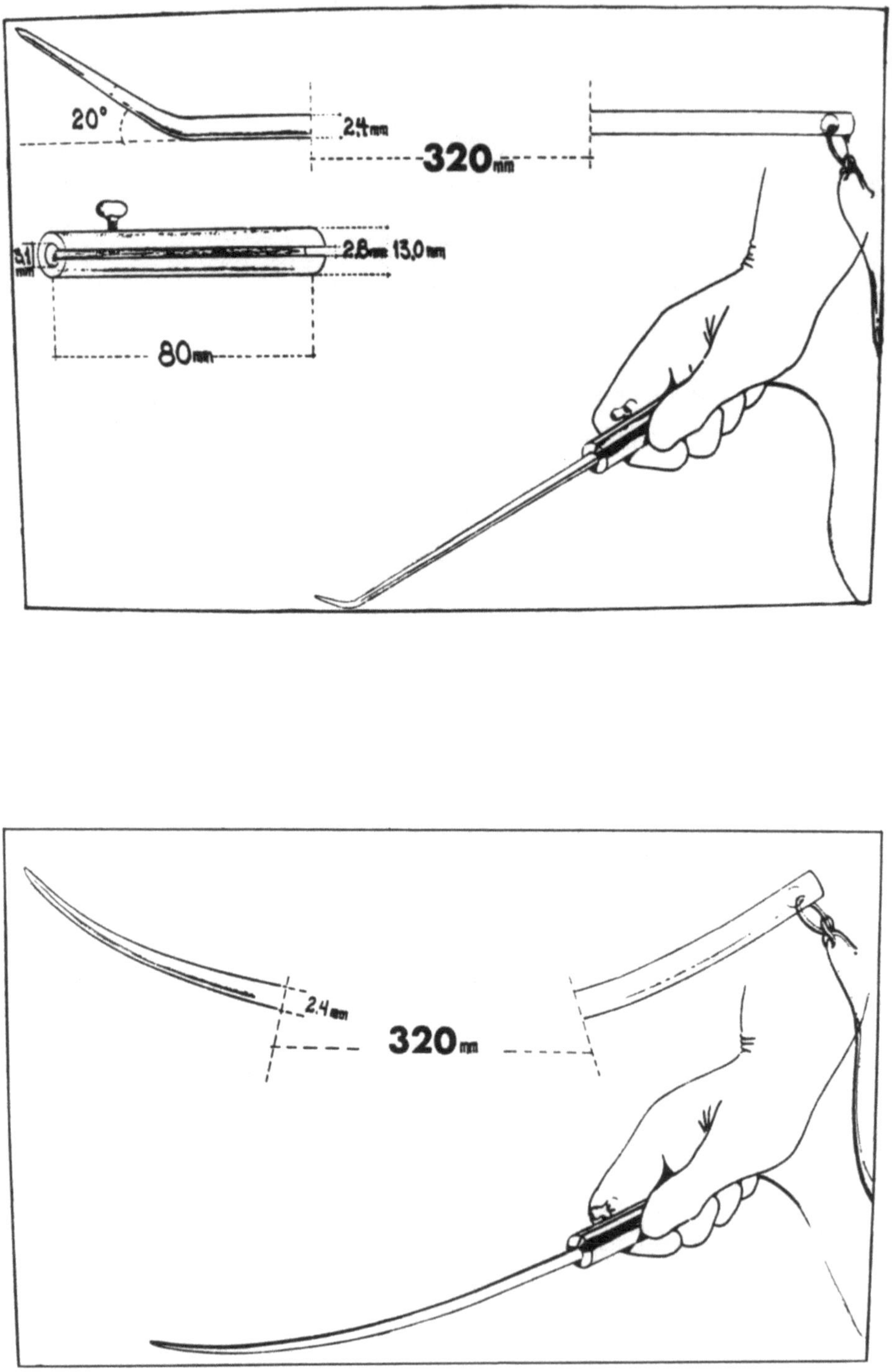


Figure 2

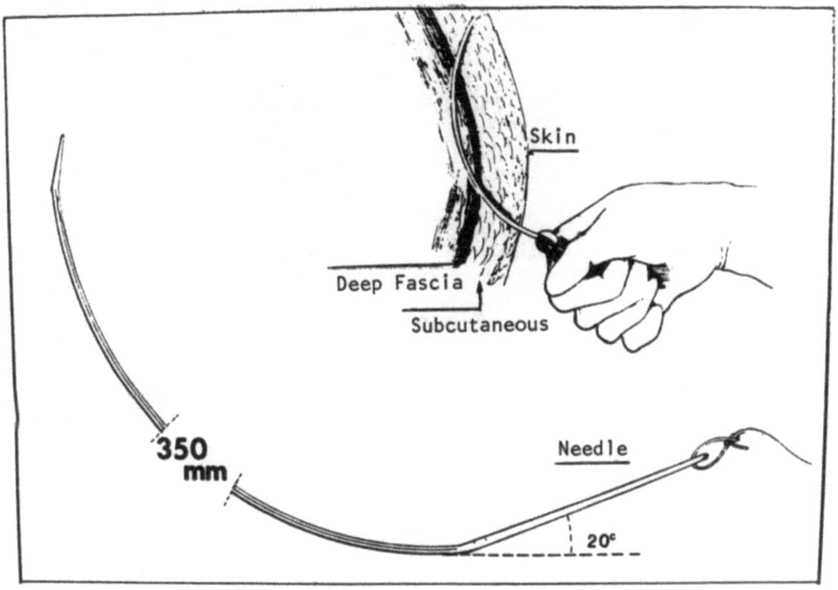


Figure 3

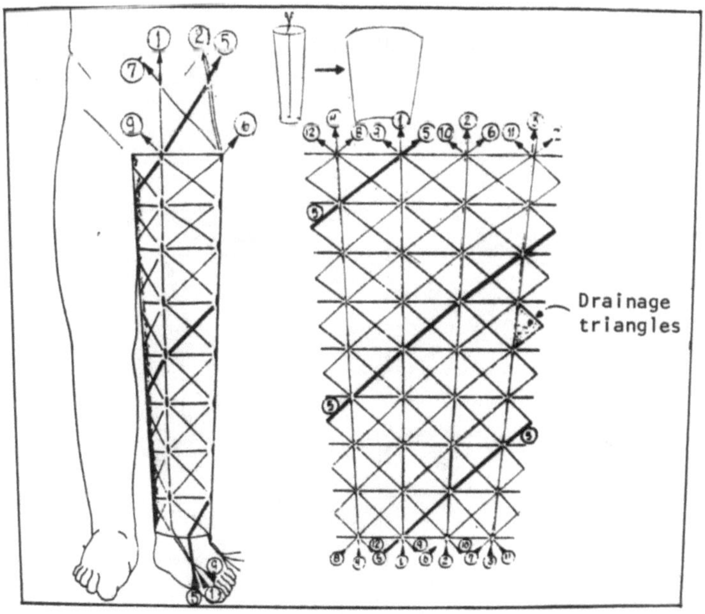


Figure 4

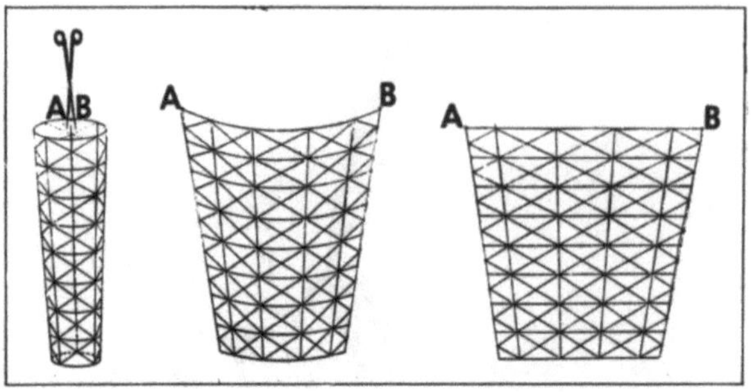


Figure 5

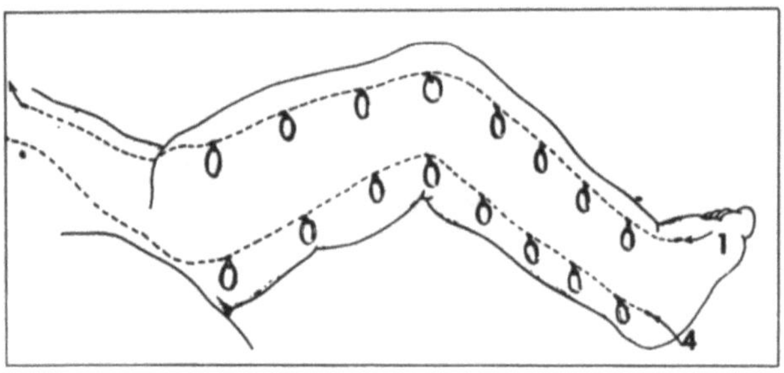


Figure 6

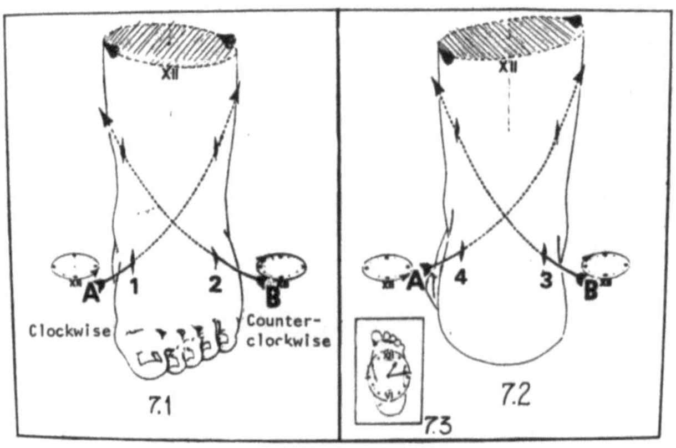


Figure 7

In Fig. 6 the loop which the longitudinal threads make at each cutaneous incision is shown maintained outside the incision by a plastic ring (diameter 2 - 2.5 cm), which facilitates the making of "Paris knots" with the spiral and circular threads. The two ends of the four longitudinal threads are fixed with mosquito forceps (Fig. 8).

Then one of the clockwise spiral threads is inserted starting at the premalleolar medial incision and ascending obliquely to the incision of the lower third of the leg corresponding to longitudinal thread No. 2 (Figs. 7 and 8).

Next the first "Paris knot" (Fig. 8a,b,c) is made, passing the needle through the same loop and ascending obliquely via the subcutaneous tissue up to the incision in the medial third of the leg (corresponding to longitudinal thread No. 3), and so on. At every loop, a "Paris knot" is made with the threads. Then all the other clockwise spiral threads are applied starting from the cutaneous incision Nos. 2, 3, and 4.

The ends of the spiral threads are fixed with the same mosquito forceps that fixes the ends of the longitudinal ones. The counterclockwise spiral threads are inserted in a similar fashion, always starting from incision No. 1 (the premalleolar medial incision).

The three ends of the threads meeting at the abdomen and buttock level and at the level of the foot are fixed with the same mosquito forceps (Fig. 8).

The net is completed with the insertion of the circular threads. These circular threads make "Paris knots" when they cross each longitudinal thread (Fig. 9). Subsequently, the opposite ends of each longitudinal thread are pulled gently in order to introduce all loops under the skin and the opposite ends of the spiral threads are also pulled. Then all plastic rings are cut and removed.

Next the upper and lower ends of all threads are cut close to the skin so that they remain buried in the subcutaneous tissue.

The rationale of this subcutaneous drainage is based on drainage triangles (Figs. 4, 10, and 11).

Supplementary longitudinal threads may be placed from the thigh to the abdomen and buttocks and to form the dorsal aspect of the foot to the lower third of the leg (Figs. 10 and 11). The drainage of the dorsal aspect of the foot is carried out with five threads (in addition to the longitudinal threads) whose positions are self-explanatory (Fig. 12).

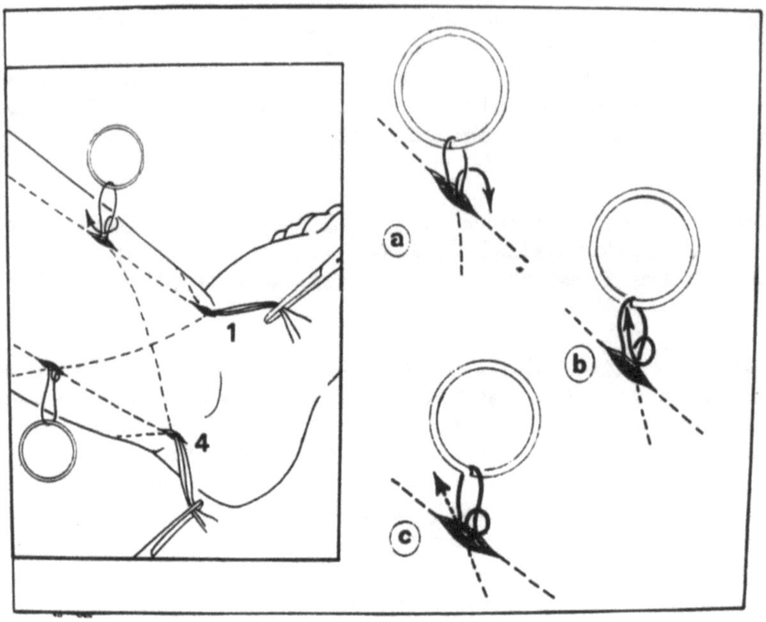


Figure 8

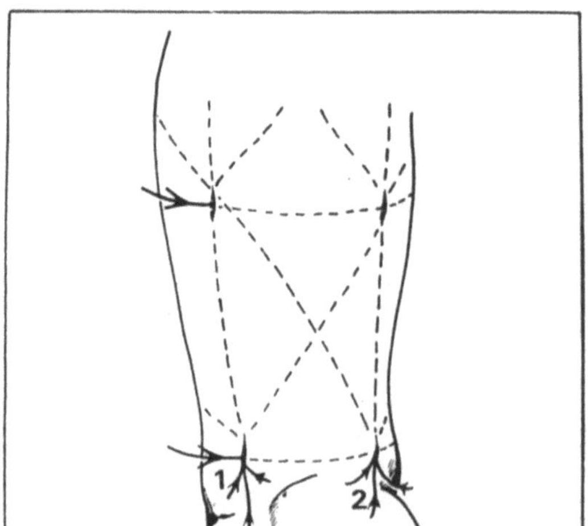


Figure 9

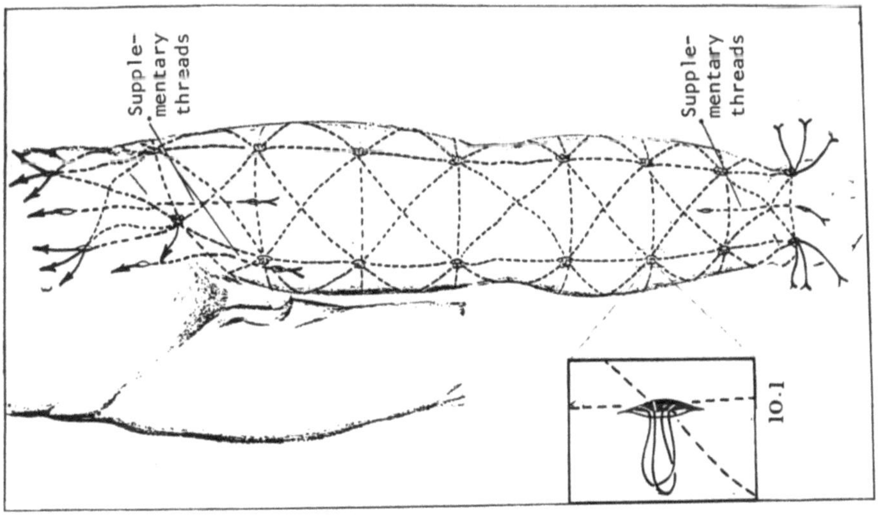


Figure 10

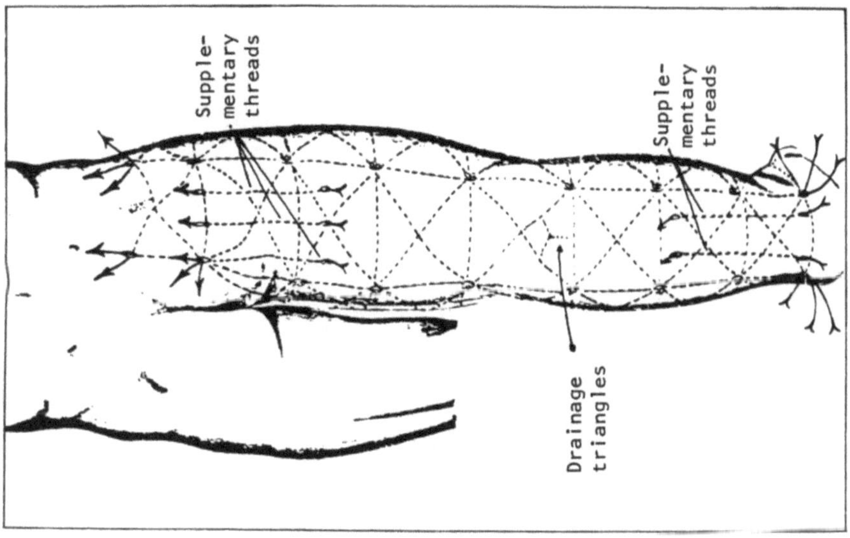


Figure 11

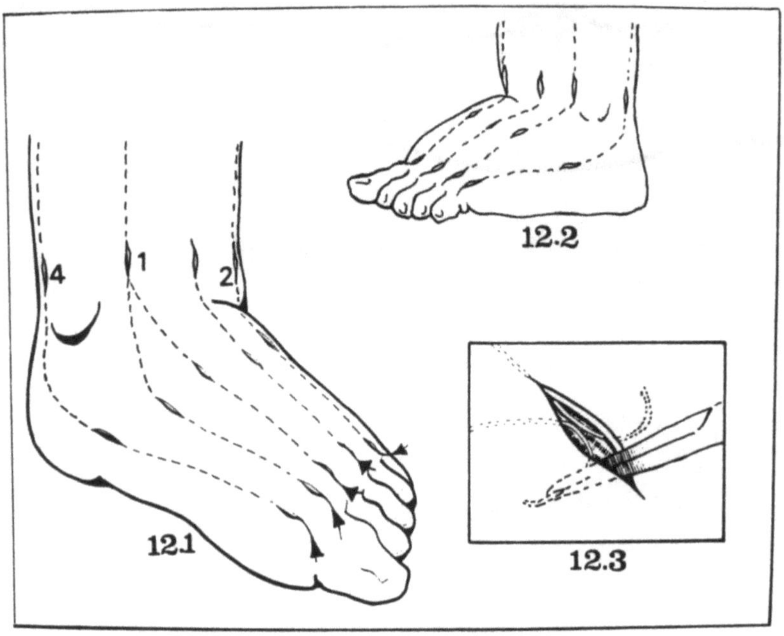


Figure 12

TABLE I

Distribution of Sex and Age of
48 Operated Patients

| Number of cases | Sex | Age |
|---|---|---|
| 13 | Males | 16 - 73 years |
| 33 | Females | 13 - 80 years |

TABLE II

Distribution of 48 Patients
by Decades

| Decade | Number of cases |
|---|---|
| 0 - 10 | 1 |
| 11 - 20 | 7 |
| 21 - 30 | 7 |
| 31 - 40 | 10 |
| 41 - 50 | 10 |
| 51 - 60 | 8 |
| 61 - 70 | 3 |
| 71 - 80 | 2 |
| Total | 80 |

TABLE III

Distribution of Unilateral Lymphedema

(37 cases)

| | Cases |
|---|---|
| Lymphedema of the foot and toes | 1 |
| Lymphedema of the foot and leg | 20 |
| Lymphedema of the foot, leg, and thigh | 16 |

Note: One case had edema of the entire limb and lower abdomen. One case had edema of the entire limb and of the penis and scrotum.

TABLE IV

Distribution of Bilateral Lymphedema

(11 cases)

| | Cases |
|---|---|
| Lymphedema of the foot and ankle | 1 |
| Lymphedema of the foot and leg | 12 |
| Lymphedema of the foot, leg, and thigh | 9 |

TABLE V

Classification of 48 Personal Cases of Lymphedema

(Based on clinical and lymphangiographic findings)

| | |
|---|---|
| A. Primary Lymphedema - 22 cases | |
| (1) Lymphedema praecox with hyperplasia | |
| a. with recurrent lymphangitis | 4 cases |
| b. without lymphangitis | |
| (2) Lymphedema praecox with hypoplasia | |
| a. with recurrent lymphangitis | 2 cases |
| b. without lymphangitis | 4 cases |
| (3) Lymphedema praecox + recurrent lymphangitis (no lymphography) | 1 case |
| (4) Lymphedema praecox with hypoplasia. Superficial and deep lymphatics not visualized by lymphography | 6 cases (1 with fibrous edema) |
| (5) Lymphedema tarda with hyperplasia | |
| a. with recurrent lymphangitis | |
| b. without lymphangitis | 1 case |
| (6) Lymphedema tarda with hypoplasia | 2 cases (1 with fibrous edema) |
| (7) Lymphedema, not classified | 2 cases |
| (8) Lymphedema congenita | |
| B. Secondary Lymphedema - 14 cases | |
| (1) Infections and inflammation | |
| a. Lymphangitis | 7 cases |
| b. Inguinal adenitis | 1 case |
| c. Erysipelas | 1 case |

(2) Latrogenic

| | | |
|---|---|---|
| a. | after stripping of varicose saphena magna vein + recurrent lymphangitis | 1 case |
| b. | after resection of lipoma of the right inguino-crural region | 1 case |
| c. | after plastic surgery of abdomen (bilateral) | 1 case |
| d. | after plastic surgery of both thighs (bilateral) | 1 case |

(3) Malignant disease

| | | |
|---|---|---|
| a. | after resection of fibrosarcoma of the left inguino-crural region invading the left inguinal fossa + radiation therapy | 1 case |

C. Lymphedema tarda, not classified - 2 cases

D. Lymphophlebedema - 12 cases

(1) Lymphedema praecox with hypoplasia

| | | |
|---|---|---|
| a. | with recurrent lymphangitis | 6 cases (1 with fibrous edema) |
| b. | with erysipelas | 2 cases (1 with fibrous edema) |
| c. | without lymphangitis | 2 cases |

(2) Lymphedema tarda

| | | |
|---|---|---|
| a. | with recurrent lymphangitis | 1 case |
| b. | hypoplastic with recurrent lymphangitis | 1 case |

TABLE VI

Lower Limb Lymphedema

| | |
|---|---|
| 48 patients | |
| 64 operations | |
| Lymphatic-venous anastomosis (see Tables VII and VIII) | 15 operations |
| Drainage with nylon net and supplementary drainage (see Table IX) | 49 operations |

TABLE VII

Lymphatic-Venous Anastomosis

| | |
|---|---|
| 13 patients | |
| 15 operations | |
| 14 lower limbs | |
| Lymphatic-venous anastomosis | 14 operations |
| Lymph node-venous anastomosis | 1 operation |

TABLE VIII

Lymphatic-Venous Anastomosis

(Total, 15 operations)

| Region of the limb | Number of operations | Lymphatic-venous anastomosis |
|---|---|---|
| Iliac fossa | 1 | 3 anastomoses with the external iliac vein |
| Inguino-crural region | 6 | Anastomosis with the saphena magna vein and/or one of its branches. 3 to 9 anastomoses performed. (1 case of lymph node anastomosis) |
| Thigh, middle third (antero-medial aspect) | 1 | Anastomosis with saphena magna vein (4 anastomoses) |
| Leg, upper third (medial aspect) | 4 | Anastomosis with saphena magna vein. 3 to 5 anastomoses performed |
| Transition of middle to lower third of leg (medial aspect) | 2 | Anastomosis with saphena magna vein (4 anastomoses in every case) |
| Popliteal region | 1 | Anastomosis with saphena parva (2 anastomoses) |

TABLE IX

Drainage of the Subcutaneous Tissue with Nylon Net

| |
|---|
| 39 patients (including 4 patients in whom the anastomosis failed - 5 operations) |
| 49 operations (nylon net + supplementary drainage) |
| 41 lower limbs |

TABLE X

Results

| | |
|---|---|
| Lymphatic-venous anastomosis, 15 operations | 5 anastomoses in 4 patients failed<br>10 anastomoses - average reduction of edema, 68% |
| Drainage with nylon net technique<br>49 operations<br>41 lower limbs | Average reduction of edema, 63.07% |
| Postoperative follow-up | Lymphatic-venous anastomosis 2-30 months<br>Drainage with nylon net 1½-36 months |

Note: All patients wearing elastic stockings.

The supplementary techniques of drainage of the subcutaneous tissue to the subfascial or subaponeurotic intermuscular tissues are not depicted.

We have carried out 64 operations on 48 patients with this technique. All the patients had few or no superficial lymphatics, and eight of them had no deep lymphatics. There was a mean reduction in edema of 67.07%. The postoperative follow-up period was 1½ to 48 months. These results are summarized in Tables I-X.

## BIBLIOGRAPHY


1 - BARROS, M.C. de: O problema etiopatogenico e terapeutico dos linfedemas progressivos. Tese para concurso de Livre Docente da Univ. Fed. Recife - Recife, 1946.

2 - BARTELS, P.: Das Lymphgefäs system. Stuttgart, Gustav Fischer Verlag, 1909.

3 - BATTEZZATI, M.; DONINI, I. e BECCHI, G.: La Linfografia Possibilitá diagnostiche e terapeutiche. Gazzetta degli Ospedali e delle Cliniche. Vol. XVI, nº 4-5, aprile-maggio, 1963, pg. 175-246.

4 - BATTEZZATI, M. e DONINI, I.: Il sistema linfático della practica clinica. Padova, Piccin Editores,1967.

5 - BATTEZZATI, M.; TAGLIAFERRO, A.; DONINI, I.; ROSSI, L.: La Linfoadenografia. Torino, Edizione Minerva e Pan Minerva Medica, janeiro 1961.

6 - FÖLDI, M.: Diseases of Lymphatics and Lymph Circulation. Budapest, Akadimiai Kiadó, 1969.

7 - FÖLDI, M.; KLÜKEN, N. and COLLARD: Praxis der Lymphgefässen und venen-erkrangunzen. Stuttgart. Gustav Fischer Verlag, 1974.

8 - HANDLEY, W.S.: Lymphangiosplasty. Lacet 1: 783, 1908. In Kinmonth, J.B. The Lymphatics, London, Edward Arnold Publishers Ltd., 1972.

9 - KAINDL, F.; MAUNHEIMER, E.; PFLEGER, L. and THURNHER, B.: Lymphangiographie und Lymphadenographier der Extremitäten. Stuttgart, G. Thieme, 1960.

10 - KINMONTH, J.B.: Studies of the lymphatics in idiopathic Lymphedema. In II Congress of the International Society of Angiology, Lisbon, 1953.

11 - KINMONTH, J.B.: Lymphography in Clinical Surgery and particularly in the treatment of Lymphedema. Ann Royal Coll. Surgery England 15: 300, 1954.

12 - KINMONTH, J.B.: Primary Lymphedema of the lower limb. Proc. Roy Soc. Med. 58: 1021-1031, 1965.

13 - KINMONTH, J.B.: The Lymphatics. London, Edward Arnold Publishers Ltd, pg.173, 1972.

14 - KINMONTH, J.B. and TAYLOR, G.W.: The Lymphatic Circulation in Lymphedema. Ann. Surg. 139: 129, 1954.

15 - KINMONTH, J.B. and TAYLOR, G.W.: Spontaneous rhythmic contractility in human lymphatics. J.Physiol., London, 133: 3, 1956.

16 - MARQUES, M.S. de B. e DEGNI, M.: Considerações sobre o Aspecto Linfoadenográfico dos membros inferiores. Rev. Bras. Cardiov. São Paulo, vol. 6, nº 2, abr-mai-jun, 1970, pg. 183.

17 - MARQUES, R.: La Lymphographie. Lyon Chirurgical, T. 56, nº 6, 801-805, 1960.

18 - MARQUES, R.: Estudo crítico da linfografia. Conferência no XIII Congresso Brasileiro de Angiologia, Recife, 1966.

19 - MARQUES, R.: Limites e alcances da Linfangiografia. Conferência no XVI Congresso Brasileiro de Angiologia. Santa Maria - RS, 1969.

20 - MARQUES, R. e CAETANO DE BARROS, M.: Linfografia. Nota prévia. Comunicação a Sociedade de Cirurgia de Pernambuco, feita em 10-7-43. Publicado na Rev. Med. Pan Americana, ano I, nº 1, vol. 3, jan-fev. 1945.

21 - MARQUES, R. e PEREIRA, L.: Análise das Técnicas de Kinmonth. Tossati, Marques e Pereira, Angiopatias, vol. 2, nº 1, jan-març. 1962.

22 - MAYALL, R.C.: Edemas linfáticos e venosos dos membros inferiores. Tese de Docência Livre da Disciplina de Angiologia da Fundação Escola de Medicina e Cirurgia do Rio de Janeiro. Editora Villani Filhos Ltda. Rio de Janeiro - Brasil, 1970.

23 - MICKELBERG, A.: Tiazidas e Edemas posflebíticas. Angiopatias, vol. 2, nº 4, out-dez., 1962.

24 - NEGREIROS, L.: Contribuição ao estudo da linfonodografia. Dissertação concurso assistente, Recife - Brasil, 1970.

25 - PEREIRA, L.: Contribuição da linfografia ao Estudo da Quilúria. Tese de Concurso. Imprensa Universitária da Univ.Fed. Pernambuco, Recife, 1968.

26 - PFLEGER, L.: Histologie und Histopathologie cutaner Lymphgefässe der unteren Extremitäten. I: Morphologie der cutanen Lymphagefässe. Arch. Exp. Derm. 221: 32, 1964.

27 - PFLEGER, L.: Histologie und Histopathologie cutaner Lymphgefässe der unteren Extremitäten. II: Pathologie der cutanen Lymphgefässe. Arch. Klin. Exp. Derm. 221: 1964.

28 - ROCHA NETO, J.M.: Da importância das anastomoses interlinfáticas e linfático-venosas. Tese de Doutoramento Univ.Fed.Santa Maria, Santa Maria-RS, Brasil, Gráfica da Univ. Fed. Santa Maria, dez. 1967.

29 - ROUVIERE, H.: Anatomie des lymphatiques de l'homme. Paris, Masson Ed., 1932.

30 - RUSZNYAK, I.; FÖLDI, M. and SZABÓ, G.: Lymphatics and Lymph. Circulation, Long Island City, Pergamon, 1960.

31 - RÜTTIMAN, A. (Editor): Progress in Lymphology. Stuttgart, G. Thieme, 1967.

32 - SERVELLE, M.: Pathologie Vasculaire, Paris, Masson, 1952.

33 - TOSATTI, E.: Lymphatiques Profounds et Lymphoedeme Chroniques de membres. Paris, Masson, 1952.

34 - VAN DER MOLEN, H.R.: Früzeitiges Lymphödemen der spontane Lymphogene Elephantiasis. Bull. Soc. Franc. Phlebol. 53: 43, 1956.

35 - VIAMONTE, M.; KOEHLER, P.R.; WITTE, M. and WITTE, C. (Editors). Progress in Lymphology II, Stuttgart, G. Thieme, 1970.

36 - ZIEMAN, S.A.: LYMPHEDEMA: Causes, Complications. Treatment of the Swollen Extremity, New York, Grune Straton.

NEW TECHNIQUES OF LYMPHOVENOUS ANASTOMOSIS FOR

SURGICAL TREATMENT OF LYPHEDEMA

A. K. Cordeiro, F. F. Baracat, F. Moreira, Jr., and R. C. Mayall

Instituto Vieira de Carvalho, São Paulo, Brazil
Faculdade de Medicina de Valença, Rio de Janeiro, Brazil

Based upon previous experiences with lymphovenous anastomosis for treatment of lymphedema, we devised numerous technical modifications that simplify the operation.

Clinical Material

These procedures were done on 86 patients including 66 with lymphedema of the legs and 20 patients with postmastectomy lymphedema of the arms. The 66 patients with lymphedema of the legs were classified as follows:

| | | |
|---|---|---|
| (1) | Primary congenital familial lymphedema (Milroy's disease) | 4 |
| (2) | Primary congenital lymphedema with gonadal dysgenesis (Turner's syndrome) | 1 |
| (3) | Primary praecox lymphedema | 1 |
| (4) | Primary tarda lymphedema | 10 |
| (5) | Primary tarda lymphedema + fibroedema | 6 |
| (6) | Secondary post-traumatic post-surgical lymphedema | |
| | (a) Post lymphadenectomy | 3 |
| | (b) Post reconstruction | 1 |
| | (c) Post varicose vein stripping | 15 |

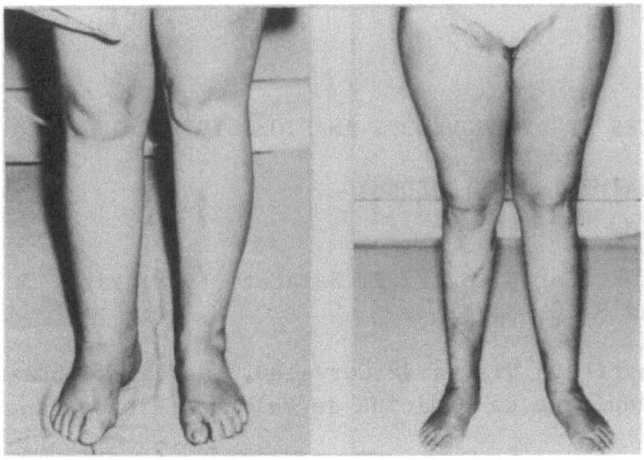

Fig. 1. Pre- and postoperative photographs of a patient with lymphedema of the legs.

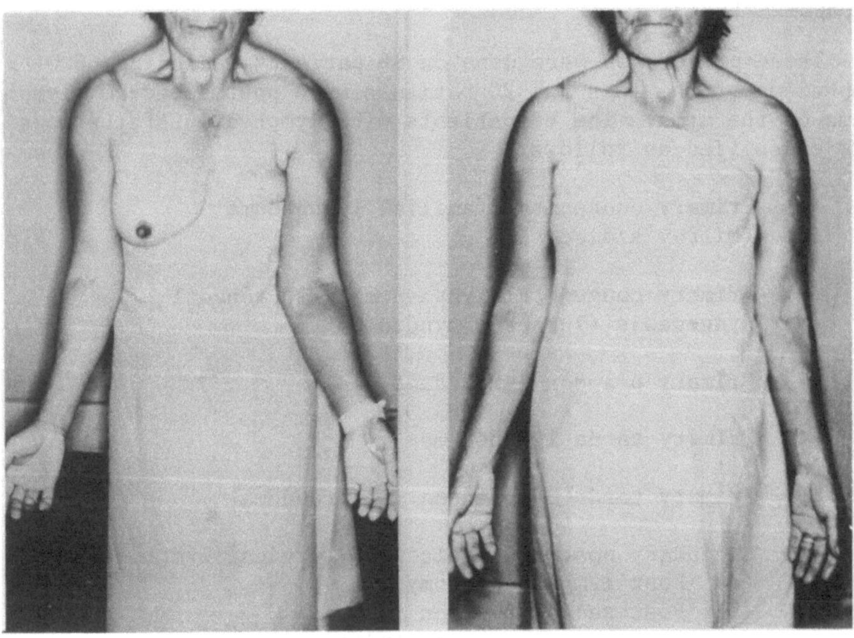

Fig. 2. Pre- and postoperative photographs of a patient with postmastectomy lymphedema of the arms.

| | | |
|---|---|---|
| (7) | Secondary post-traumatic post-accident lymphedema | |
| | (a) Traffic accident | 3 |
| | (b) Whitewash burning ($Ca(OH)_2$) | 1 |
| | (c) Animal bite | 1 |
| (8) | Secondary post-phlebitic lymphedema | 20 |

The cases of postmastectomy lymphedema of upper limbs included:

| | |
|---|---|
| Right arm | 9 |
| Left arm | 11 |

## Technique

The method used when lymphatics are too small for anastomosis as described in an earlier report (14) is a modification of Carcacia's technique.

In the previous report (14) we proposed invaginating a lymphatic trunk into the adjacent vein with the aid of specially constructed fine needles. In some instances, the lymphatic and adjacent veins were too small and anastomosis was difficult though not impossible. To overcome this shortcoming we developed a series of injection needles that can be selected and are adaptable to this technique (Fig. 3).

## Surgical Incisions

For operations on the arm an incision about 5 to 10 cm in length is made on the medial surface along the biceps muscle, and the superficial lymphatic trunks identified by previous staining by patent blue violet injected into the hand. After the lymphatic trunks are mobilized, the basilic vein is isolated. If the operation is done in the leg a similar dissection is followed using the saphenous vein or one of its major branches after pedal injection of patent blue dye for identification of lymphatic trunks. The lymphatic trunk is prepared for an anastomosis by transfixing with a double-armed 5-0 weight atraumatic needle that passes only through the adventitia. The needle and mandrel then puncture the vein, the obturator is removed, and one end of the atraumatic needle is threaded through the mandrel into the vein and transfixed to the venous wall approximately 5 mm from the puncture site. The other end of the atraumatic needle is then similarly passed into the lumen and tied gently over the vein wall (Fig. 7b). The obturator is then reinserted and the needle removed, sometimes with a slight rotation to avoid kinking of the anastomosis. These techniques are shown in Figs. 4-12.

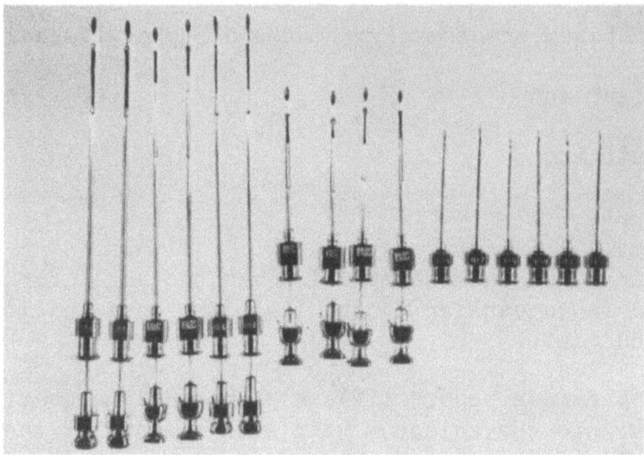

Fig. 3. Special collection of needles.

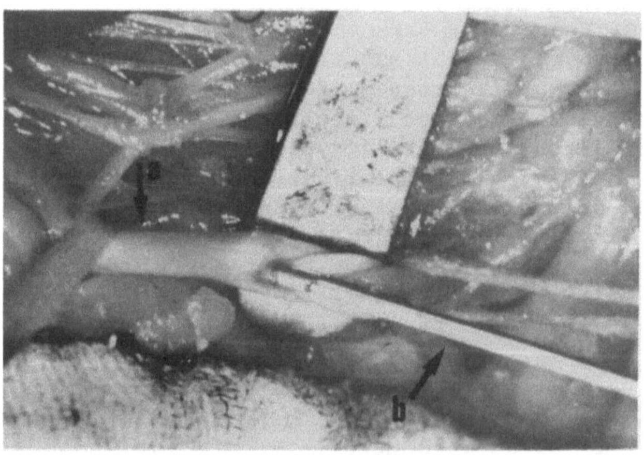


Fig. 4. (a) Dissected vein with tapes; (b) selected needle puncturing the vein.

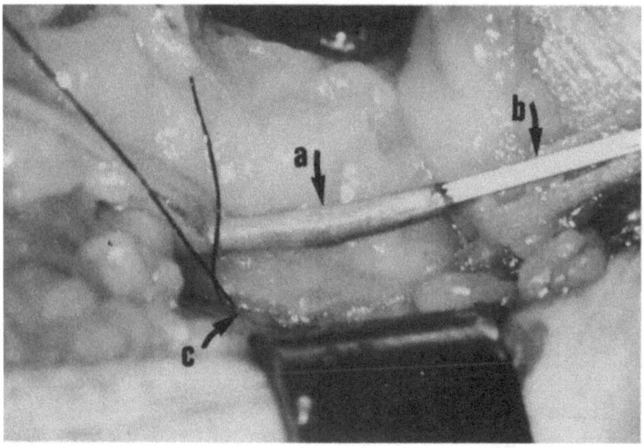


Fig. 5. (a) Dissected vein with tapes; (b) selected needle introduced into the vein; (c) dissected lymphatic trunk transfixed by 5-0 mononylon thread.

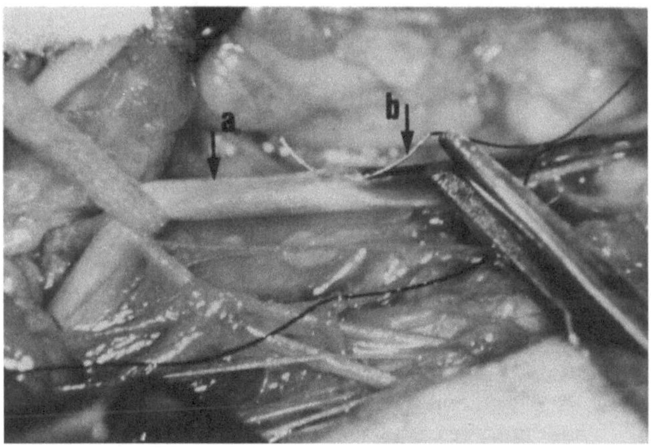


Fig. 6. (a) Dissected vein with tapes; (b) needle of 5-0 mononylon thread following the puncturing needle groove in the lumen of the vein transfixing the vein wall.

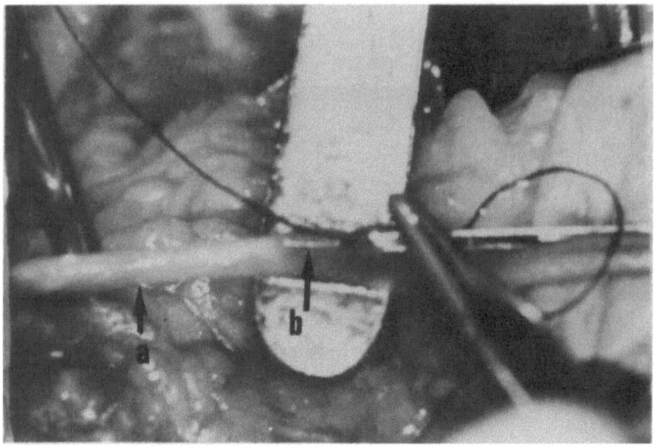


Fig. 7. (a) Dissected vein; (b) second needle used to introduce the other end of 5-0 mononylon thread following the groove guide of the puncture needle and transfixing the vein wall.

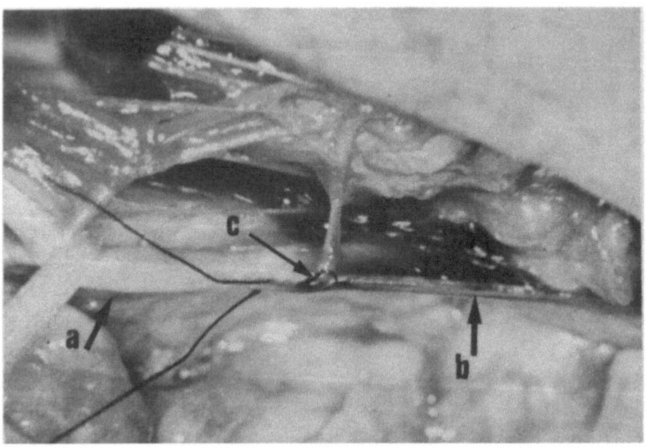


Fig. 8. (a) Dissected vein; (b) selected needle in the lumen of the vein; (c) site of passage of lymphatic trunk over the groove of the puncturing needle into the lumen of the vein.

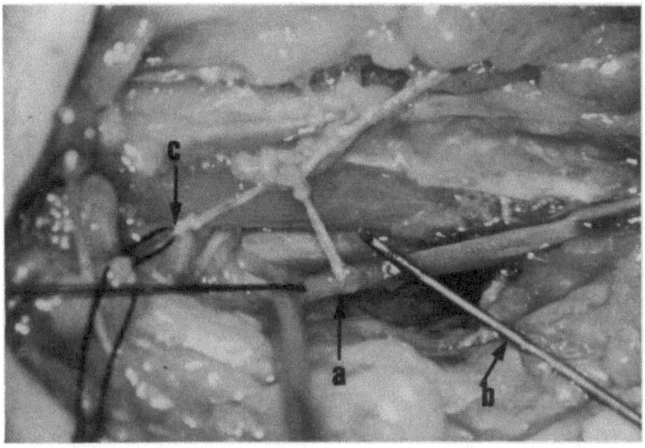


Fig. 9. (a) Lymphatic trunk in the lumen of the vein; (b) selected needle for puncture; (c) another lymphatic trunk transfixed by 5-0 mononylon thread.

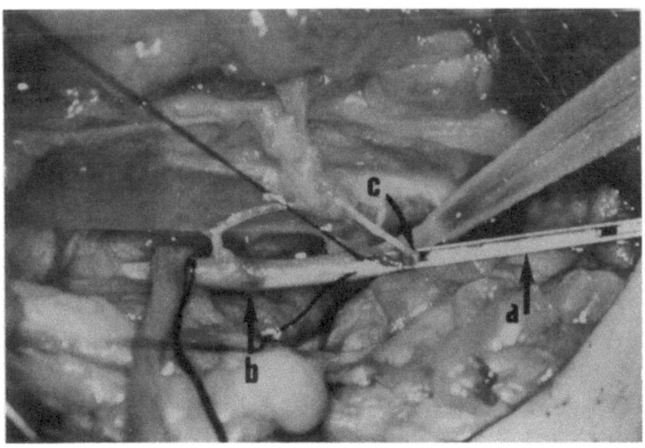


Fig. 10. (a) Selected needle puncture into the lumen of the vein; (b) lymphatic trunk tied at the vein wall; (c) another lymphatic trunk following the groove of the puncture needle and entering the lumen of the vein.

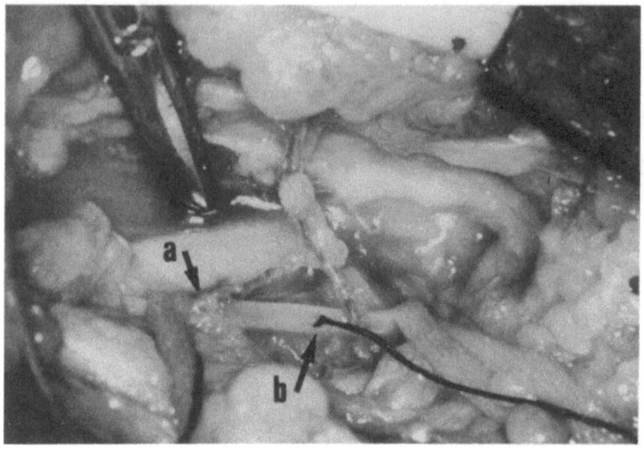


Fig. 11. (a) Lymphatic trunk fixed to the vein wall; (b) another lymphatic trunk being tied at the vein wall.

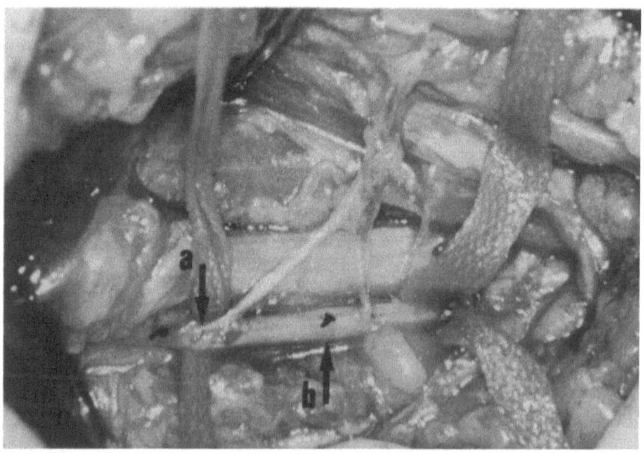


Fig. 12. (a and b) Two lymphatic trunks anastomosed to the vein. The tapes to prevent hemorrhage are open and no bleeding is seen.

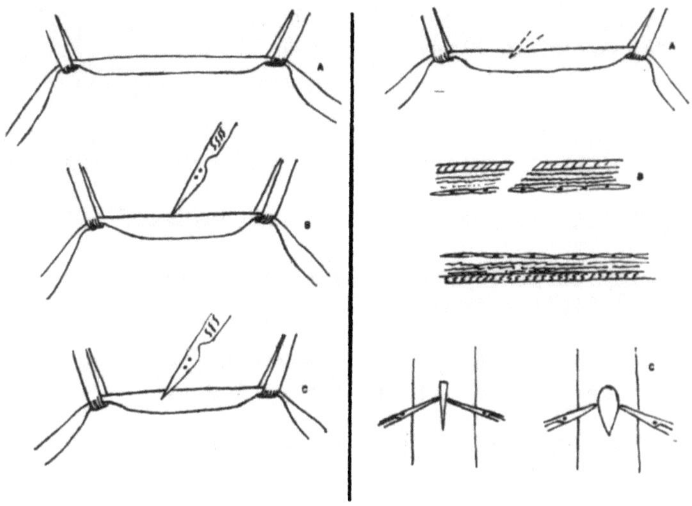

Fig. 13

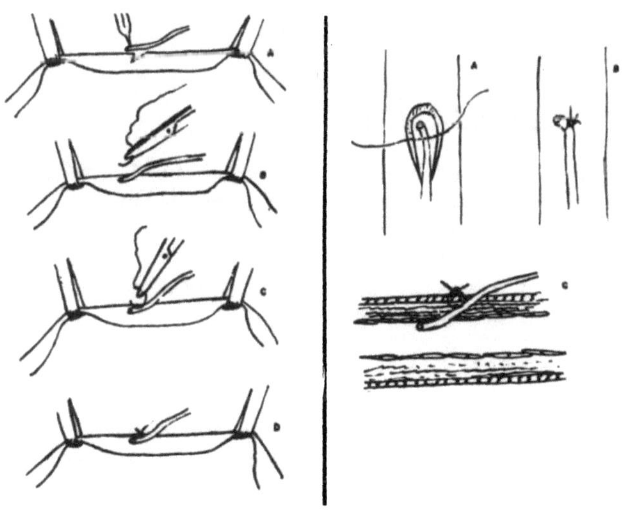

Fig. 14

An alternative technique is used when the vessels are extremely small and involves suturing in one maneuver both the adventitia of the previously open vein and the adventitia anteriorly of the lymphatic trunk as shown in Figs. 13 and 14.

## Results

These techniques, employed since 1970, have certain advantages:

(1) Simplification of lymphatic-venous anastomosis.

(2) Ability to perform the anastomosis despite the very small size of vessels.

(3) Marked reduction and sometimes disappearance of edema in a great majority of patients.

(4) Improved function and mobility of the extremities relieved of massive lymphedema.

## Complications

(1) Generalized itching that disappears spontaneously in a few days.

(2) Five patients required reoperation (4 patients in the legs and 1 in the arm). In each patient a successful LVA was carried out using the same techniques.

## Indications for this LVA Technique

Lower Limbs: In cases of lymphedema where lymphography shows patent superficial lymphatic trunks and when technical topographic difficulties preclude using our prior method.

Upper Limbs: In cases of postmastectomy lymphedema of upper limbs with or without prior radiotherapy.

## Contraindications

Lower Limbs: In cases of advanced lymphedema with severe elephantiasis; in congenital lymphedema with aplasia of lymphatics; in edematous states not primarily lymphatic in origin, e.g., cardiac, renal, allergic, etc.

Upper Limbs: With postmastectomy lymphedema with distant metastatic or local recurrence.

BIBLIOGRAPHY

1 - CARACIA,J.M. e ZUKER,M.M. - Tratamiento del linfedema. Comunicación prévia. Rev.Bras.Cardiovasc., 5:119-121, 1969.
2 - CHARLES,R.H. - A system of treatment, vol.3, A.Latham and T.C.English, Eds., Londo, Churchill, apg. 504, 1912
3 - COCKETT, A.T.K. - J. UROL. 88 (1962), 566. In 36 pag 45
4 - CORDEIRO, A.K. - Comunicações linfovenosas - Trabalho apresentado à Soc.Brasileira de Angiologia, Regional de São Paulo, jul. 1969 - São Paulo
5 - CORDEIRO, A.K. - Linfedema primario. Anastomose linfovenosa. Trabalho apresentado ao XVI Congresso Brasileiro de Angiologia, Santa Maria, R.G.S., 17-20 set. 1969.
6 - CORDEIRO, A.K. - Tratamento cirurgico do linfedema. Técnica pessoal - Trabalho apresentado ao XVII Cong. Bras. de Angiologia, São Paulo, 4-8 novembro 1970.
7 - CORDEIRO, A.K. - Tratamento cirúrgico do linfedema. Resultados. Trabalho apresentado ao XVII Cong.Bras.de Angiologia, São Paulo, 4-8 novembro 1970.
8 - CORDEIRO, A.K. - Mesa redonda sobre "Linfografia" no X Cong. Latinoamericano de Angiologia, Capitulo Latinoamericano de The International Cardiovascular Society e I Cong.Uruguayo de Angiologia, Montevideo, Uruguay, 10-14 nov. 1970.
9 - CORDEIRO, A.K. - Tratamiento quirurgico del linfedema. Tecnica personal - Trabalho apresentado ao X Cong.Latinoamericano de Angiologia, Capitulo Latinoamericano de The International Cardiovascular Society e I Cong. Uruguayo de Angiologia, Montevideo, Uruguay, 10-14 nov. 1970.
10 - CORDEIRO, A.K. - Tratamiento quirurgico del linfedema. Resultados - Trabalho apresentado ao X Cong. Latinoamericano de Angiologia, Capitulo Latinoamericano de The International Cardiovascular Society e I Cong. Uruguayo de Angiologia, Montevideo, Uruguay, 10-14 nov. 1970.
11 - CORDEIRO, A.K. - Linfedema pós mastectomia - Relator do Simpósio da Sociedade Brasileiro de Patologia Mamaria, São Paulo, 15 de outubro de 1971.
12 - CORDEIRO, A.K. - Simposio sobre: "Linfedema crônico progressivo; diagnóstico e tratamento" no XVIII Congl Bras. de Angiologia, Olinda, Pernambuco, 20-23 outubro 1971.
13 - CORDEIRO, A.K. - Surgical treatment of lymphedema including lymphovenous anastomosis - Abstracts of 4th International Congress of Lymphology - International Society of Lymphology Tucson, Arizona - March 6-10, 1973.
14 - CORDEIRO, A.K. and BARACAT, F.F. - New technique for surgical treatment of lymphedema of lower limbs and postmastectomy lymphedema of upper limbs - Trabalho apresentado ao IX Cong. Internacional de Angiologia da União Internacional de Angiologia, Florença - Italia, 3-7 abril de 1974.
15 - DEGNI, M. - New technique of lymphaticovenous anastomosis -

(buried type) for the treatment of lymphedema - Trabalho apresentado ao IX Congresso Internacional de Angiologia da União Internacional de Angiologia, Florença - Italia, 3-7 abril 1974.

16 - FOLEY, W.T. - Treatment of lymphedema - Surg.Gyn. & Obst., 101:25, 1955

17 - GILLIES,H. and MILLARD,D.R. - The principles and art of plastic surgery - Londo, Butterworth, 1957.

18 - GOLDSMITH, H.S. and de LOS SANTOS,R. - Omental transposition in primary lymphedema Surg. Gyn. & Obst., 607, 1967.

19 - HANDLEY, W.S. - Lymphangioplasty. A New method for the relief of the brawny arm of breast cancer and for similar conditions of lymphatic oedema - Preliminary note - Lancet, 1:783, 1908.

20 - HOGEMAN, K.E. - Artificial subcutaneous channels in draining lymphoedema - Acta Chir. Scandinav., 110:154, 1955

21 - KINMONTH, J.B.; ROB, C.G. and SIMEONE, F.A. - Vascular surgery - Edward Arnold (publishers) Ltda., London, 1962.

22 - KINMONTH, J.B. - The lymphatics - Diseases, Lymphography and Surgery - Edward Arnold (Publishers) Ltda., London, 1972.

23 - KOEHLER, P.R. - Lymphatico-venous anastomosis - Acta VI Intern. Angiol. Congr., 67-71, Editorial Cientifico-Medica, Barcelona, 1969.

24 - KONDOLEON, E. - Die operative behandlung der elephantiastichen oedema durch eine neue method der lymphableitung munch. Med. Wochnschr., 59:1823, 1912.

25 - LANZ, O. - Eröffnung neuer abfuhrwege bei Staum in Bauch und unteren extremitäten - Zentralbl. Chir., 38:153, 1912

26 - MACEY, H.H. - A surgical procedure for lymphedema of the extremities - J.Bone & Joint Surg., 30A:339, 1948.

27 - MALEK, P.; BELAN,A.; BABICKY,F. and KOLC,J. - Importance of lymphaticovenous communications in the regeneration of lymphatics - Progress in Lymphology II, 74-77, Georg Thieme Verlag, Stuttgart, 1970.

28 - MAYALL, R.C. - Adenolinfografias - Mesa Redonda sobre "Radiologia Vascular" do XII Cong. Bras. de Angiologia - Rev.Bras.Cardiovasc., 3 (1); 64-65, 1967.

29 - MAYALL, R.C. - Linfedemas secundarios - Acta VI Internationalis Angiol. Congr., 137-145, Editorial Cientifico-Medica, Barcelona, 1969.

30 - MAYALL, R.C.; FREITAS,J.; BARBOSA,C. e AZEVEDO,A.M.F. - Medical and surgical treatment of secondary lymphedemas - Acta VI - Internat. Angiol. Congr., 428-435, Editorial Cientifico Medica, Barcelona, 1969.

31 - MAYALL, R.C. - Edemas linfaticos e venosos dos membros inferiores. Contribuição ao seu diagnostico e orientação terapeutica. Tese de Livre Docencia à Faculdade de Medicina e Cirurgia do Rio de Janeiro, Guanabara, 1970.

32 - MOWLEN, R. - Lymphatic oedema an evaluation of surgery in its treatment, Am.J.Surg., 95:216, 1958.

33 - NIELUBOWICZ,J. and OLZEWSKY,W. - Surgical relief of lymphoedema (abst.), World Med., 1:90, 1966.
34 - PICARD, J.D.; ARVAY,N. et CHARBIT,A. - Communications lymphoveineuses - Presse Medicale (Suppl.) 74:42 - 1 - 42 -4, out. 1966.
35 - PUGNAIRE, M.R. - Linfangioplastia mesenterica en el tratamiento de las Elefantiasis de los miembros inferiores - Angiologia, 20 (3): 146-152, 1968.
36 - RÜTTIMANN, A. - Progress in Lymphology, pag. 45, Georg Thieme Verlag - Stuttgart, 1966.
37 - SISTRUNK, W.E. - Further experiences with the Kondoleon operation for Elephantiasi - J.A.M.A., 71:800, 1918.
38 - SMITH, J.W. & CONWAY,H. - Selection of appropriate Surgical procedure in lymphedema. Introduction of the hinged pedicle Plast. & Reconst. Surgery, 30:10, 1962.
39 - STANDARD, S. - Lymphedema of the arm following radical mastectomy for carcinoma of the breast. New operation for its control. Am. Surg., 116:816, 1942.
40 - THOMPSON, N. - The surgical treatment of chronic lymphoedema of the extremities - The Surg. Clin. of North America, 47:445, 503, 1967.
41 - THREEFOOT, S.A. & KOSSOVER, M.F. - Lymphatic-venous communications in man - Arch. Int. Med., 117:213, 1966.
42 - THREEFOOT, S.A. - Lymphaticovenous anastomosis - Acta VI Inter. Angiol. Congr., 53-55, Editorial Cientifico-Medica, Barcelona, 1969.
43 - THREEFOOT, S.A. - Physiology and pathophysiology of lymphaticovenous communications - Acta VI Internationalis Angiologorum Congressus, 56-61, Editorial Cientifico Medica, Barcelona, 1969.
44 - WALLACE, S. - Lymphaticovenous anastomosis. Clinical significance - Progress in Lymphology II, 87, 91, Georg Thieme Verlag. Stuttgart, 1970.
45 - WYNN, S.K. - Surgical approach to postmastectomy lymphedematous extremities - Arch. Surg., 70:418, 1953.

# Miscellanea

# TREATMENT OF FILARIAL CHYLURIA

Shoyei Yamauchi

Medical Arts Building
1010 South King Street
Honolulu, Hawaii

Chyluria remains an interesting, capricious, clinical entity, characterized by periodic voiding of milky urine containing variable amounts of blood and chyle. When the chyle content is high the urine appears milky and the term chylous urine, first applied by Prout (1816), is appropriate for its designation. Erythrocytes are always present, more commonly microscopically, but occasionally gross admixture with chyle in the urine makes such urine sanguineous and the term hematochyluria becomes the proper terminology.

## Filariasis and Chyluria

The cause and effect relationship of filariasis to chyluria is frequently difficult or even impossible to establish. The only unequivocal and acceptable criterion is the presence of microfilaremia or the adult filaria or their remains in the tissues. The possibility of exposure to filariasis is readily determined in patients' histories by their residence in an endemic area. This exposure criterion was used to designate these cases as filarial chyluria, though with one exception, filarial nematodes were not demonstrated.

Chyluria occurs as the most important late sequela of the nocturnal variety of bancroftian filariasis. In Japan it occurred in 2.5% of people living in a low density filarial endemic area (Sasa, 1970). In Polynesia, where the diurnal variety of filariasis prevails and the filarial density is high, elephantiasis is common and chyluria is rare (Manson-Bahr, 1952). No indigenous filariasis has ever been reported in Hawaii. Exposure criterion is utilized to relate filariasis as the primary cause of chyluria. Filariasis is thought to result in chylostasis and lymphatic-urinary fistulation.

Material and Method

Remissions of chyluria are induced by diminishing chylolymph stasis while permitting the lymphatico-urinary fistula to close. Between 1936 and 1970 we treated 86 personal cases of filarial hematochyluria. Microfilaremia occurred in a patient and he was treated with "Hetrazan" Lederle (diethyl carbamazine citrate). Exposure criterion related the filariasis to the chyluria in all instances - they had resided in a filaria endemic area. In 23 instances other clinical manifestations of filariasis occurred. Fifty-six patients (33 women and 23 men) received $AgNO_3$ renal pelvic lavages with a total of 122 (92/33 and 30/23) episodes of chyluria. Twenty-seven received no $AgNO_3$ lavages (these served as controls).

A chylous urine is recognized by the presence of chylomicrons, (the colloidal lipoprotein particles responsible for the milky opacity), albumin, erythrocytes, lymphocytes, and fibrin clots. Cystourethroscopy and pyelography, both excretory and retrograde, may reveal utostasis, its cause and extent, and sites and extent of pyelolymphatic backflow. Kinmonth's pedal lymphagiograms depict a comprehensive status of the chylolymph stasis in the renal, abdomino-aortic, iliac and cisterna chylithoracic duct systems related to chyluria, and reveal the relation of the chyluria to the pathology induced by filariasis. The sites of the lymphatico-urinary fistulations are determined in a progressive order by the location of egress of milky urine at cystoscopy, the beginning of pylelolymphatic backflow in pyelograms and locations of entrance of Ethiodol into the urinary stream in lymphangiograms.

Cystoscopy and pyelography (both IVP and retrograde) determine the status of the urinary tract, egress of milky urine into the urinary stream, and pyelolymphatic backflow (PLB) in pyelograms. Lymphography (pedal) follows after catheters are inserted into ureters and fixed to a Foley catheter. Fibrin clots in the renal pelvis are irrigated with water containing streptokinase and dornase. When free urine flow is established, 1 to 2% $AgNO_3$ solution, 2 cc less than the pelvic capacity as determined by water injection method (Goldstein), is instilled. Instillation is done only on one side at any one sitting. A minimum of four instillations is usually made on each side on alternating days. Larger (sized) catheters are used by choice. They drain and splint the ureter better. The tone of the ureteral musculature diminishes, spasms disappear, and the urine clears, usually after 2 to 4 instillations.

ANCILLARY SURGICAL PROCEDURES CARRIED OUT
AMONG 86 CASES OF CHYLURIA

Surgery on the Lymphatics

1) Definitive for relief of lymphostasis. Excision of retroperitoneal lymphatics from the inguinal ligament to above the renal pedicle (50% removal) in one case only (Samoan).

2) For diagnostic study. Excision of lymph nodes or trunks incidental to lymphography (feet or groin), renal pedicle (nephropexy, renal exploration for cyst or renal stones), and common iliac nodes (during hysterectomy).

Definitive Surgery for Relief of Urinary Stasis

Prostatectomy for BPH
Nephropexy for nephroptosis and U-P obstruction
Nephrotomy for intra-renal cyst
Nephrectomy for intra-renal cyst and tumor
Hysterectomy and other gynecological operations for relief of urinary stasis

Results

Follow-up results in 1970 (Fig. 1): 32/56 treated with $AgNO_3$ were well without clinical recurrence; 10 had occasional slight to moderate clouding which was controlled by restricting fat from diet; 13 were dead from intercurrent disease, 9 probably with and 4 without chyluria.

Pregnancy precipitated recurrence on 37 occasions and other conditions related to urostasis in 17 instances (Fig. 2). Pyuria occurred some time during the eposides of chyluria 35 times. Staph aureus was most frequently cultured in the younger group and enteric organisms, including pseudomonas, in the elderly debilitated women. An elderly woman who had 3 courses of therapy died of pulmonary insufficiency and a severe biochemical disturbance in 1965 with uncontrolled chyluria.

Benign prostatic hypertrophy precipitated recurrent episodes of chyluria in 11 men (Fig. 3). After definitive therapy for the conditions associated with urostasis, chyluria spontaneously remitted in some patients; others required therapy outlined. One of the patients had 3 courses of therapy from 1944 to 1959 when adequate control was no longer possible and he was still having chyluria when he died at home.

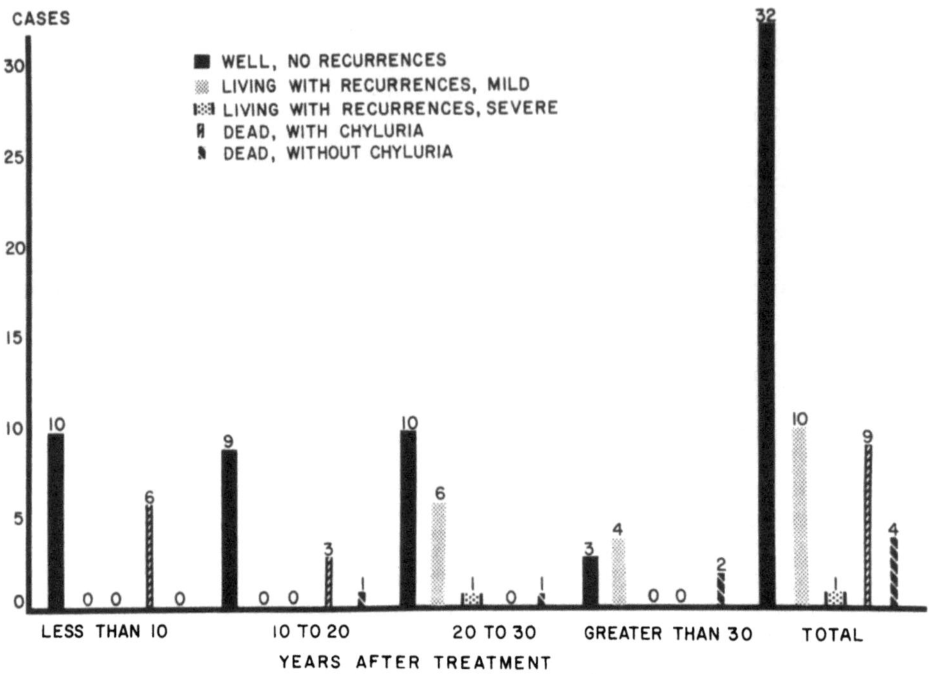


Fig. 1. Post-Treatment Follow-Up of 56 Cases.

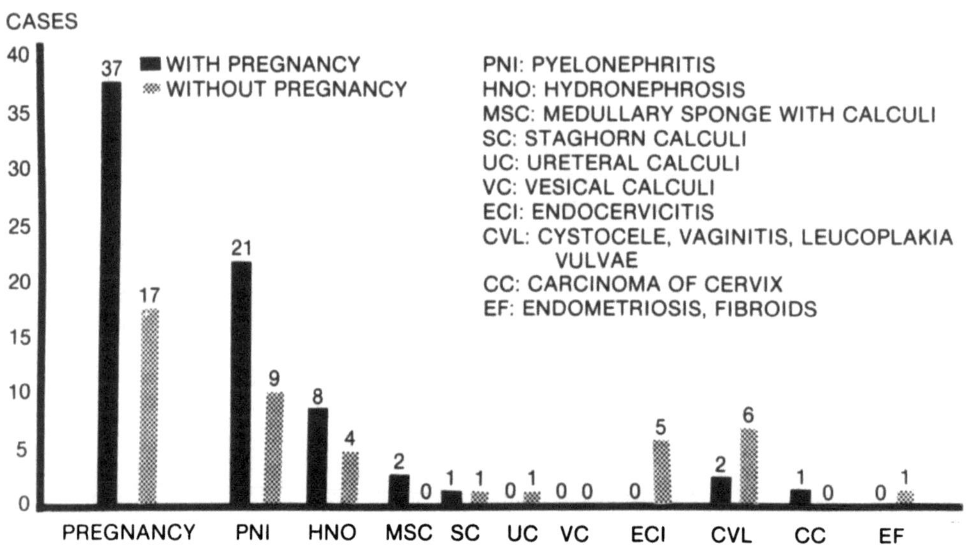


Fig. 2. Recurrent Chyluria in 33 Women after $AgNO_3$ Pelvic Lavages.

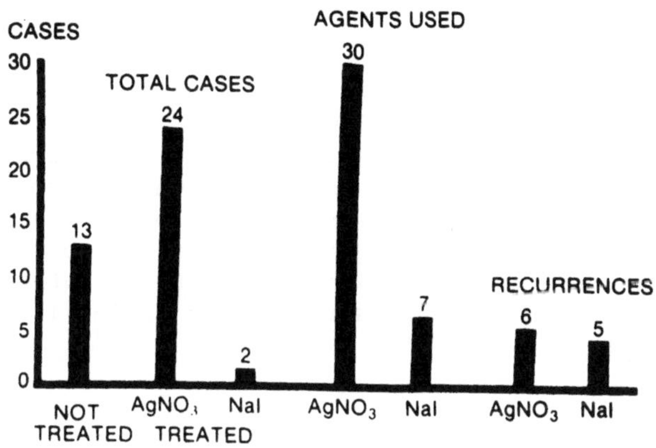


Fig. 3A. Treatment of 39 Men with Chyluria.

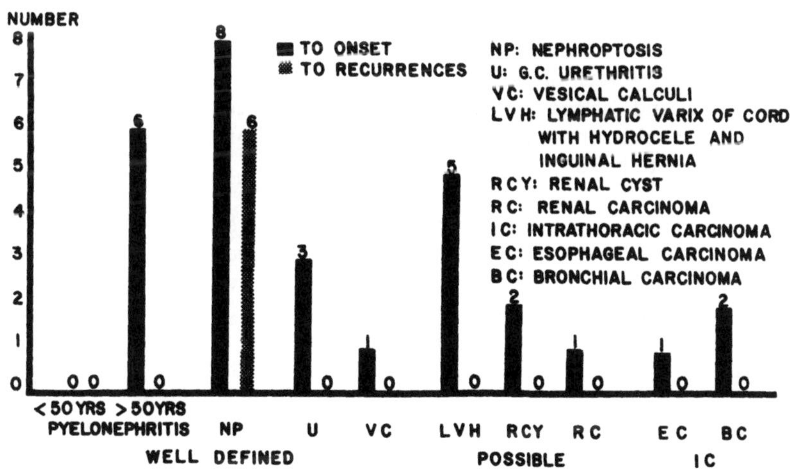


Fig. 3B. Contributory Factors to Urinary Stasis in Male Chyluric.

Short chain fatty aid, MCT oil (Portagen, Mead Johnson) substitute for ordinary fat in a diet which is restricted severely improves the nutritional status in the elderly debilitated and alleviates the intense anxiety many experience when passing bloody or opaque milky urines.

Conclusion

Combined management with low fat diet, correction of urologic conditions that cause urostasis, and renal intra-pelvic lavages with $AgNO_3$ solutions (1-2%) induces a sufficient number of long-term remissions of filarial chyluria. As shown in lymphangiograms done several years after such a remission, the persistence of renal lymphatic reflux indicated that the prechyluric anatomic state persists. Vigilance, therefore, is maintained during life for possible recurrence.

## SURGICAL THERAPY OF HEMATOCHYLURIA

Curative surgical therapy for hematochyluria should be directed at the existing chylolymph stasis in the abdomino-aortic lymphatics of which the renal lymphatics are important components. The central lymphostatic pool appears to arise from the peripheral lymphatics, both visceral and truncal, based on segmental or regional pathology resulting from filariasis. The incremental additive effects of lymph flow from the numerous collaterals in a state of stasis and tension appears to influence the chylolymph dynamics in the renal and calyceal lymphatics resulting in fistulation into the urinary stream and hematochyluria. The same mechanism is probably responsible for the unpredictable, labile, capricious remissions characteristic of this disease.

To reduce the central lymphostasis, lymphangio-adenectomy of the vessels and nodes involved in ectasia was done in a young Samoan man, aged 27 years. He was first seen with hematuria in 1963, treated with diethylcarbamazine in 1964 for active filariasis (microfilaremia), and lymphangio-adenectomy in November, 1969. Lymphatic varices and nodes along the iliacs, external and common, para-aortic, paracaval, and precaval trunks and nodes were excised from the femoral canal to above the level of the renal vessels. No attempt was made to remove the retrocaval vessels or nodes on the right side, nor the retroaortic lumbar vessels or nodes on the left side. The operation was performed through a median transperitoneal approach opening the posterior wall peritoneum over the large abdominal vessels and their branches. By retraction of the root of the small bowel mesentery cephalad, a satisfactory exposure was obtained for removal of lymphangiectasia and nodes in one stage

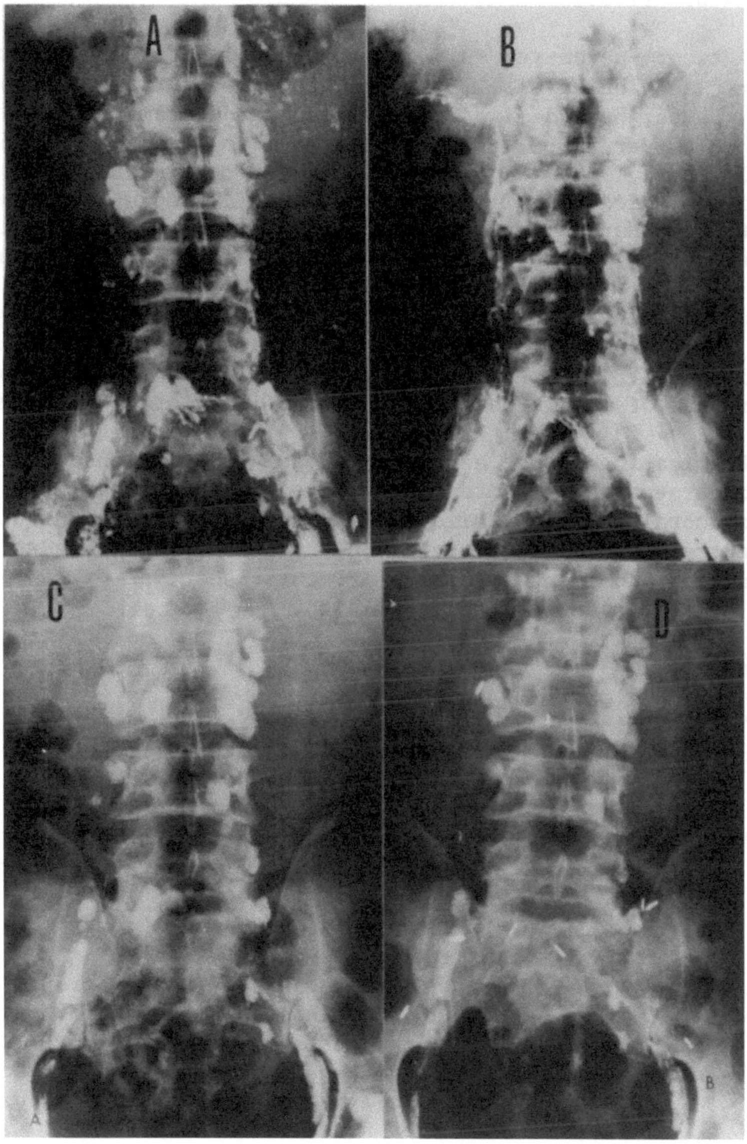


Figure 4

from the inguinal ligaments to above the renal vessels. The extent of lymphangiectasia and pre- and post-operative lymphadenograms is depicted in Fig. 4.

C 80: H.D. (T.S.)

A twenty-seven-year-old Samoan-Caucasian-Chinese electrician was first seen on May 15, 1963 with gross hematuria. Born on Niue Island, Samoa, he had lived in American Samoa from his 8th year to his 18th year (1961) when he emigrated to Hawaii. In 1955, 1956 and 1957 "hard lumps" developed in his left groin and lateral upper thigh accompanied by chills and fever. Cold compresses caused them to abate. In March, 1961 a pole fell on his right back during a hurricane storm. Since then he had suffered right back pains.

On May 1, 1963, he was seen by an internist with gross hematuria, preceded by right lumbar CVA dull aching pain for 3 months. Preadmission IVP was reported by the radiologist: "Suspicious pressure defect middle calyx, left, with inferior displacement."

Examination showed a well developed and nourished youth. Deep tenderness was elicited across the mid-epigastrium and the costovertebral angle. A mild lumbar lordosis was present with prominent erector spinae muscles due to spasm. Groin nodes were enlarged and prominent. A large irregular scar was present on the anterolateral aspect of the left thigh.

Observations 1963-1974

May 1, 1963 - Hematuria with dysuria, frequency and urgency
Staph epidermidis cultured from urine
(Dept. Health Lab.)

May 16, 1963 - 10 cc. blood samples drawn at 10 p.m., 12 midnight and 9 a.m. all contained microfilaria
$R_X$ - Hetrazan 2 mg/kg for 4 weeks

- Cystoscopy, pyelography, lymphography (50% Hypaque direct nodal injection into groin node - unsuccessful)
PLB in right pyelograms; ectatic iliac vessels in lymphograms "Stromal fibrosis" of removed nodes

February 16, 1964 - Lymphography (Kinmonth's pedal method).
Ethiodol: Rt. 10 cc.; Lt. 14 cc.
Severe lymphostasis and lymphatic ectasia of entire caudal primary channels with

RPCL (bilateral) but no fistulation. Thoracic duct ectatic, tortuous and layered below the diaphragm. Ectatic and distorted lumbar trunks. Ectatic cross-over channels and collaterals. Stasis prominent in afferent channels of abdomino-aortic nodes. Pulmontory node level to 11. Nodes remained opacified till October, 1969, when the second lymphography was done.

July 15, 1965 - Suffered deep laceration of lower thigh with electric saw. Transsected belly of the vastus medialis; wound extended into joints. Blood from wound contained microfilariae.

July 26, 1965 - Effective Hetrazan therapy.

1967 - 1969 - Progressive swelling of scrotum with continuing discomforts referred to GI and GB tracts; GB and GI studies. Urological studies. Orthopedic care.

November 2, 1969 - Second pedal lymphograms (Kinmonth's method). Dr. Uyeda.

November 18, 1969 - Excision of ectatic nodes and Varices, iliacs to L1 with repair of hydrocele and varicocele.

October 8, 1974 - Third pedal lymphogram (Dr. Sakuda). Partial block above right common-iliac with distal lymphostasis and reflux. Lymphostasis in the abdomino-aortic lymphatics reduced markedly.

## Results and Conclusion

Symptomatic improvement occurred with abatement of the pains and discomfort which had plagued him for many years. Except for occasional backaches, he was asymptomatic. Lymphography (October 8, 1974) right side only (left unsuccessful). Filling phase showed evidence of partial obstruction at the proximal level of the common iliac channels with cross-over to the left lumbar nodes. Ectatic channels with reflux occurred distally. RPCL prominent in two previous lymphangiograms were only barely visualized on the right; none on the left. Lymphostasis in the abdomino-aortic lymphatics appeared reduced.

# THE LYMPH CIRCULATION IN THE POST-THROMBOTIC SYNDROME

Nobert Klüken

Hufelandstrasse 55

Essen, Germany

At the beginning of my lecture I would like to emphasise that the object of this paper is to discuss the accompanying lymphatic components of venous diseases. I can only deal with the venous-lymphatic disturbances from this aspect and not in a general view. Well-known lymphologists like Professor Földi are more competent to do this.

If we speak of venous lymphatic interrelations, we shall first give a survey of the venous diseases we are interested in here.

In Fig. 1 the aetiopathogenetic relations of varicosis, superficial and deep thrombophlebitis vulgaris, are shown in relation to their sequelae. Varicosis leads through varicophlebitis to the varicose symptom complex. The post-thrombophlebitic syndrome, on the other hand, is more rarely a sequel to superficial thrombophlebitis vulgaris relapsing for years, but much more frequently to a deep thrombophlebitis vulgaris.

The varicose symptom complex and post-thrombophlebitic syndrome are generally grouped together nowadays as chronic venous insufficiency. This term was coined by VAN DER MOLEN. It forms a collective term for the sequelae of all the venous diseases to be discussed here.

The clinical symptoms appear as follows: oedema, pigmentation, hypostatic erythema, corona phlebectatica paraplantaris and ulcers of the lower leg. In the initial stage and in the centre of the clinical symptoms stands oedema, which first appears as a malleolar or perimalleolar (also called Bisgaard's oedema of the calcaneo-malleolar region) or a pretibial oedema.

This oedema is mainly a filtering oedema in cases in which the venous process is far from the stasis and has thus caused increased pressure in the venous area. Occasionally the type of oedema is shown by its composition, such as is found in inflammatory oedema. This occurs when phlebitic processes appear in the oedematous area. We shall discuss details later.

## The pathogenesis of venous oedema

Through hindrance of drainage, there is an increase of pressure in the blood capillaries which chiefly appears in the venous part of the capillaries. Instead of reabsorption of low-molecular substances, a transudation arises as a result of increased pressure in the venous system. This tissue lymph increases. There is a reduced absorption of lymph through the venous lymphatic anastomoses because of lymphatic hypertension with increasing volume of the lymphatics.

This in turn leads to insufficiency of the valves of the lymph vessels and the vessel walls. Fibrosis develops in the walls of the lymphatics. These last factors are the basis of the mechanical insufficiency of the lymph vessels. The same sequela may also be caused by thrombophlebitis accompanied by lymphangitis.

The central point of the process of the pathomechanism of oedema of venous origin is the lymph vascular system and the terminal flow paths.

## The exchange of liquid and material in the region of the blood and lymph capillaries.

On the arterial side of the capillaries a transudation of liquid and low-molecular substances develops. The reabsorption of liquid and low-molecular substances occurs in the venous part of the capillaries. Some of the liquid, high-molecular substances and corpuscular fractions are taken up by the lymph capillaries.

## The physiological process of absorption and reabsorption may be disturbed by the prolonged effect of hydrostatic pressure.

This happens on sitting for a long time in railway trains, in aeroplanes or in front of the television screen. Thus the hydrostatic pressure, which is normally about 110 cm $H_2O$ in the region of bone, can affect the venous part of the capillaries,

In movement, on the other hand, the hydrostatic pressure falls to about 40 cm $H_2O$ through the action of the muscular suction pressure pump.

Because of the lack of pressure gradient, the continuous effect of high hydrostatic pressure leads to transudation instead of reabsorption in the venous part. The arterial and venous parts transude liquid and low-molecular substances. The so-called "tissue pressure" reacts to the hydrostatic pressure to a certain extent. Now, the tissue pressure is, strictly speaking, a fiction, because the necessary physical conditions are lacking. Pressure can only arise in the tissues if fluid - i.e. oedema - is present. But oedema is always a pathological condition. For oedema to occur a pressure is necessary which is able to force open the normal fine structure of the connective tissue. This would therefore be the so-called tissue pressure, which, we think, is better named potential tissue pressure. In addition to this potential tissue pressure, which can be calculated to be about 75 cm $H_2O$ under physiological conditions, a colloid osmotic pressure of about 35 cm $H_2O$ is to be added. Basically, the hydrostatic pressure is to be identified with the colloidal osmotic pressure plus the potential tissue pressure, With the longer effect of the hydrostatic pressure, the lack of reabsorption in the venous part of the capillaries causes a shift of the potential tissue pressure and especially of the colloidal osmotic pressure, particularly if the lymph vessel system cannot take over the failure of function of the terminal venous capillary network. A filtering oedema then occurs which is the more marked, the longer the muscular pump is not active.

<u>The origin of oedema in chronic venous insufficiency</u>.

The hydrostatic pressure is slightly raised and cannot be compensated because of the insufficiency of the muscular suction pressure pump. The potential tissue pressure can be reduced on constitutional grounds (structure of the connective tissue). Therefore a marked filtering oedema occurs. Reabsorption can only take place through the lymph vessels, which are overburdened. This leads to greater dilatation and valvular insufficiency in the lymphatics with increased pressure and lymphatic hypostasis.

In chronic venous insufficiency, the increased pressure in the venous area is transmitted to the lymph vascular system through venous-lymphatic anastomoses. These lymphangial high pressures lead to further increases in the oedema.

In addition to the purely filtering oedema there is also an exudate, rich in proteins, arising from phlebitic and periphlebitic changes. This is also a therapeutic problem, insofar as it is not so reversible as the filtering oedema. If it remains for some time, organisation of the oedema occurs with proliferation of the tissues, and it is then no longer reversible.

In thrombotic processes of the veins which, - as we showed in the beginning - can also occur in the sequelae of chronic venous insufficiency, transitions into the lymph vessels have also been known. These thrombotic processes of the lymph vessels create additional difficulties for lymph drainage.

Not with local oedema, but rather in the extensive rapidly developing oedemata due to changes in the circulation of blood and lymph, i.e. if it is a matter of the extravasation of larger amounts of fluid from the blood capillaries and of a considerable decrease in the circulating plasma volume, a dehydration reaction can occur. This brings about a mobilisation of aldosterone, so that sodium is reabsorbed by the kidney in increased amounts. Such dehydration reactions can be produced experimentally as a disorder of systemic regulation by ligating the inferior vena cava with a considerable reduction of the effective plasma volume. However, ligation of the inferior vena cava and the increased capillary filtration caused thereby only leads to oedema when the disturbed safety-valve effect of the local lymphatic system can no longer be compensated. In spite of the manifold and complicated mechanisms, the static moments of chronic venous insufficiency stand out. This also explains why in bedridden patients oedema regresses relatively quickly, because the static pressure is considerably reduced while lying down.

# RECURRENT ACUTE TOXIC LYMPHANGITIS

Joseph Beninson, M.D., D.V.M.

Henry Ford Hospital

Detroit, Michigan, 48202 - U.S.A.

Over the past 18 years the author has seen 15 patients who have had essentially the same repetitive course of illness. After discussing these patients with my colleagues at meetings for the past decade, they have convinced me that they should be reported. Having mentioned them in related writings, I will now define the clinical picture more specifically (1,2). I believe this entity is aptly described by the title "Recurrent Acute Toxic Lymphangitis".

An ancillary problem arose in several instances when the patients were supposedly allergic to penicillin and I had to prove or disprove this diagnosis for effective therapeutic and prophylactic therapy. Today this is easily accomplished by testing for the major and minor determinants of penicillin.

As clinicians we are acquainted with the occasional patient who comes in telling of the sudden onset of chills and fever associated with malaise and headaches, as well as red streaks, diffuse cellulitis, or both. These patients respond to penicillin therapy within 2 to 3 days and may not have another episode for many years, if at all.

In this original series (see Table I) there were 6 females and 9 males ranging in age from 6 years to 51 years. Twelve lower and three upper extremities were involved. Of the upper extremities, two were post-mastectomy with attendant lymphatic obstructive disease and one had hand involvement. Two of the twelve lower extremities followed post-surgical ablative maneuvers - not associated with primary genetic lymphatic dysplasia. (3,4)

TABLE I

| RECURRENT ACUTE TOXIC LYMPHANGITIS | |
|---|---|
| SEX | 6 female, 9 male |
| AGE | 6-51 years |
| RACE | 13 white, 2 colored |
| LOWER EXTREMITY | 12 |
| UPPER EXTREMITY | 3 |

TABLE II

| RECURRENT ACUTE TOXIC LYMPHANGITIS | | | |
|---|---|---|---|
| Symptom or Sign | No. of Pts. | Symptom or Sign | No. of Pts. |
| HEADACHE | 9 | DELIRIUM | 10 |
| MALAISE | 11 | COMA | 5 |
| CHILLS | 15 | PURPURA | 5 |
| FEVER | 15 | BULLAE | 3 |
| DIARRHEA | 5 | DELAYED EDEMA | 15 |
| NAUSEA | 9 | DELAYED DOLOR | 15 |
| EMESIS | 5 | DELAYED KALOR | 15 |

Patients with recurrent acute toxic lymphangitis (see Table II) classically report the sudden onset within one to two hours of alternating chills and fever to 103-105.5, usually associated with or preceded by malaise. About two-thirds report nausea, a third vomiting, and one-third have reported diarrhea. However, the ones that have had the diarrhea have not necessarily aldo had the emesis. Almost two-thirds of them go on to delirium and about one-third become comatose.

Usually all of the above symptoms precede tenderness and swelling of the involved extremity by as much as 6 to 36 hours and rarely up to 72 hours. About 20% have a prodrome of stiffness, pain or tenderness in a specific area of the extremity, i.e. the groin, a toe or the medial paramalleolar region.

After the lapse of time noted, swelling of the extremity occurs with or without any combination of rubor, localized cellulitis and bullae with or without hemorrhage but red streaks are almost never seen. Of the 15 cases cited, only one-fifth had associated bullae and one-third had purpura. The majority had neither erysipelas nor localized tenderness. All of them had the swelling after the time lapse and about one quarter had a blotchy erythema of minimal color.

The puzzling initial gastric phase, present in almost two-thirds of the cases, preceded the swelling of the lower extremity in one instance by 72 hours. This had resulted in one patient having three complete G.I. series and another having two complete G.I. series. In a third patient, where the prodrome involved the big toe, she was treated for gout by her L.M.D.

Because of the delayed onset of the swelling, usually not associated with any erythema of a nature to suggest any other diagnosis, all of these 15 patients had been treated repetitively for acute thrombophlebitis. The most severe case in this group had been treated for thrombophlebitis upwards of 40 times and despite his youth, had been arrested and jailed for being intoxicated on at least a half-dozen occasions before being transferred to the hospital and treated for thrombophlebitis. In this particular patient, phlebography showed completely normal veins.

Cases of streptococcal lymphangitis which involve the superficial collecting lymphatics of the subcutaneum are clinically recognized by the red streaks draining toward the regional lymph nodes.

The "prairie fire" type of streptococcal lymphangitis spreads rapidly and primarily through the superficial avalvular lake of the superficial lymphatic capillaries. It may also involve the valved 1st and 2nd or 3rd superficial lymphatic capillary arcades, as demonstrated in this slide, to create the picture which we recognize clinically as erysipelas.

The above 15 patients tended, in general, not to exhibit these manifestations of superficial lymphatic disease.

In recurrent acute toxic lymphangitis the primary disease appears to involve the deep lymphatic circulation and therefore simulates acute deep thrombophlebitis. As mentioned previously, red streaking is almost never seen in this group and localized erysipelas only occasionally. Where the localized erysipelas is associated it is clearly not the cause of the massive edema involved.

In reviewing these cases, it is noted that the more episodes the patient has, the closer they come to the full clinical picture.

In treating these patients, oral penicillin was employed because it was the cheapest, required no injection, and because to my knowledge no one has ever demonstrated that any streptococcal organism is resistant to penicillin. Further, there is less proclivity for patients taking oral penicillin to develop penicillin sensitivity as opposed to injections of penicillin.

Patients were asked to take 200,000 units or 400,000 units of penicillin p.o., b.i.d. or t.i.d. depending on the severity of their lymphatic disease and body weight. When they acquired an upper respiratory infection they were instructed to double toe dosage. If despite this precaution, they had any suggestive symptoms, they were to triple the dosage.

As noted earlier, because of the patients in this group who had histories of penicillin allergy, it was extremely important to determine whether this was truly the case. Actually, in the past three years, despite suggestive histories of allergy to injected forms of penicillin over the years, I have been fortunate enough to run into no untoward reactions when following the patients in the office over the course of a day and deliberately feeding them a crushed penicillin tablet. Starting with dust, and gradually upping the dosage at 15 minute intervals for the first two hours, they are then given progressively larger particles for the next five hours, until a 200,000 unit tablet has been given in its entirety. The probable answer to these negative provocative tests must be in one of several areas:

1. The patient was responding to another drug given concomitantly at the time that the supposed penicillin reaction occurred.

2. The patient may have had a toxic erythema which was confused with a penicillin reaction.

3. The patient may have been allergic to the vehicle in which the penicillin was given by injection. (Eight-two percent of patients are allergic to the beeswax or peanut oil used as the depository vehicles of the injected penicillin.)

4. The patient was not allergic to penicillin given by the p.o. route.

I might add that none of the patients so tested have become penicillin reactors despite prolonged therapy. It is highly unlikely that they may have become hyposensitized by this p.o. technique. The possibility of desensitizing a patient to any specific antigen by any modality is for all intents and purposes purely theoretical.

The patients included in this group have been on prophylactic penicillin therapy in some instances for the past 12 years and have only had recurrences when they stopped penicillin therapy, quit using pressure-gradient supports, permitted their pressure-gradient supports to get too looses, did not increase their penicillin dosage with the onset of an upper respiratory infection, or have had unusual trauma to the involved extremity.

In some patients, due to the marked edema, it was necessary to decompress the extremity prior to the use of pressure-gradient sleeves, knee-lengths or leotards. (1)

Diagnostically, the importance of suspecting this entiry arises in differentiating it from all the other causes which bring comatose patients into the emergency room. Making this diagnosis almost always precludes the use of anticoagulants. The needless G.I. studies and gout therapy cases have already been cited. The malaise lingering between frequent episodes has been interpreted as laziness and dullness by the teachers, parents, employers and physicians involved.

## SUMMARY

The author presents the clinical courses of 15 patients he has collected over the past 18 years. They have had essentially the same clinical picture and he proposes that they be considered a new entity entitled "Recurrent Acute Toxic Lymphangitis".

He points out that these patients can be effectively controlled by a specific prophylactic penicillin regimen and pressure-gradient therapy.

In those instances where the patients also had obstructive lymphangitis or symptomatic primary genetic lymphatic dysplasia, they required decompression therapy as well.

An office procedure for determining the presence of true penicillin allergy presumably acquired by injection, using a per orum technique, was detailed. Today the testing for the major and minor determinants of penicillin supercedes this procedure. A negative test series does not rule out sensitivity in 100% of the cases; however, almost never does one get any reaction if the penicillin is taken p.o.

## BIBLIOGRAPHY

1. Beninson, J.: Six Years of Pressure-Gradient Therapy. Angiology, 12:1, pp. 38-45, Jan. 1961.

2. Beninson, J.: Superficial Lymphatics and Their Clinical Significance. NEWER VIEWS OF SKIN DISEASES, Yaffee (ed.), Little, Brown and Co.(Inc.) pp.145-152, 1966.

3. Beninson, J., Jacobson, H.S., Eyler, W.R. and DuSault, Lucille A.: Preliminary report on genetic lymphedema as studied by venography, lymphangiography, and radio-isotopic tracers, $NA_{22}$ and RISA. In <u>Progress in Angiology</u>, Proceedings of the Internationalen Gespräches über Angiologie, 1962. Darmstadt, Germany, Dr. D. Steinkopff Verlag, pp. 114-122, 1963.

4. Beninson, J., Jacobson, H.S., Eyler, W.R. and DuSault,L.A.: Additional Observations on Genetic Lymphedema as Studied by Venography, Lymphangiography and Radioisotopic Tracers, $NA_{22}$ and RISA. Vas. Surg., 1:1, pp. 43-52, April 1967.

INDEX

FSC
www.fsc.org
MIX
Papier aus verantwortungsvollen Quellen
Paper from responsible sources
FSC® C105338

If you have any concerns about our products,
you can contact us on
**ProductSafety@springernature.com**

In case Publisher is established outside the EU,
the EU authorized representative is:
**Springer Nature Customer Service Center GmbH**
**Europaplatz 3, 69115 Heidelberg, Germany**

Printed by Libri Plureos GmbH
in Hamburg, Germany